Probiotics and Prebiotics in Food, Nutrition and Health

Probiotics and Prebiotics in Food, Nutrition and Health

Editor: Jaxson Gilkeson

AMERICAN
MEDICAL PUBLISHERS
www.americanmedicalpublishers.com

AMERICAN
MEDICAL PUBLISHERS
www.americanmedicalpublishers.com

Cataloging-in-Publication Data

Probiotics and prebiotics in food, nutrition and health / edited by Jaxson Gilkeson.
p. cm.
Includes bibliographical references and index.
ISBN 978-1-63927-789-6
1. Probiotics. 2. Prebiotics. 3. Probiotics--Health aspects. 4. Prebiotics--Health aspects.
5. Probiotics--Physiological effect. 6. Prebiotics--Physiological effect. 7. Probiotics--Nutritional aspects.
8. Prebiotics--Nutritional aspects. 9. Dietary supple I. Gilkeson, Jaxson.
RM666.P835 P76 2023
615.329--dc23

American Medical Publishers,
41 Flatbush Avenue,
1st Floor, New York,
NY 11217, USA

ISBN 978-1-63927-789-6 (Hardback)

Contents

Preface

Probiotics are referred to as live cultures, such as those bacteria that are naturally found in the gut. These active cultures aid in repopulating or changing intestinal bacteria to maintain the balance of gut flora. These bacteria work to improve health and immunity but specially focus on gut health. Fermented dairy foods such as certain cheeses, yogurt and kefir generally comprise live cultures like Lactobacilli and Bifidobacteria. These live cultures might work as probiotics. On the other hand, prebiotics occur naturally, and are non-digestible food components, which promote the development of helpful bacteria in the gut. Prebiotics can help in enhancing gastrointestinal health and improve calcium absorption. They consist of fructooligosaccharides including galactooligosaccharides and inulin. Including health-promoting functional foods in the diet, such as foods that comprise both prebiotics and probiotics, helps in maintaining a healthy life. This book elucidates the importance of probiotics and prebiotics in nutrition and health. A number of latest researches have been included herein to keep the readers up-to-date with the usage of probiotics and prebiotics. Those with an interest in food and nutrition would find this book helpful.

The information shared in this book is based on empirical researches made by veterans in this field of study. The elaborative information provided in this book will help the readers further their scope of knowledge leading to advancements in this field.

Finally, I would like to thank my fellow researchers who gave constructive feedback and my family members who supported me at every step of my research.

Editor

In-Vitro Growth Inhibition of Bacterial Pathogens by Probiotics and a Synbiotic: Product Composition Matters

Jacek Piatek [1,*], Hanna Krauss [1], Arleta Ciechelska-Rybarczyk [2], Malgorzata Bernatek [3], Paulina Wojtyla-Buciora [1] and Henning Sommermeyer [1]

1 Department of Medicine, The President Stanisław Wojciechowski State University of Applied Sciences in Kalisz, Nowy Świat 4, 62-800 Kalisz, Poland; hjk12@poczta.fm (H.K.); paulinawojtyla@gmail.com (P.W.-B.); h.sommermeyer@pwsz-kalisz.edu.pl (H.S.)

2 District Sanitary-Epidemiological Station in Jarocin, Waska 2, 63-200 Jarocin, Poland; mikrobiologia@psse-jarocin.pl

3 State Hospital Jarocin, Szpitalna 1, 63-200 Jarocin, Poland; drpiatek@o2.pl

* Correspondence: drpiatek@interia.eu

Abstract: A variety of activities potentially contribute to the beneficial effects of probiotic bacteria observed in humans. Among these is a direct inhibition of the growth of pathogenic bacteria in the gut. The present study characterizes head-to-head the in-vitro pathogen growth inhibition of clinically relevant infectious bacterial strains by different types of probiotics and a synbiotic. In-vitro growth inhibition of *Escherichia (E.) coli EPEC, Shigella (Sh.) sonnei, Salmonella (S.) typhimurium, Klebsiella (K.) pneumoniae* and *Clostridioides (C.) difficile* were determined. Investigated products were a yeast mono strain probiotic containing *Saccharomyces (Sac.) boulardii*, bacterial mono strain probiotics containing either *Lactobacillus (L.) rhamnosus GG* or *L. reuteri DSM 17938*, a multi strain probiotic containing three *L. rhamnosus strains (E/N, Oxy, Pen)*, and a multi strain synbiotic containing nine different probiotic bacterial strains and the prebiotic fructooligosaccharides (FOS). Inhibition of pathogens was moderate by *Sac. boulardii* and *L. rhamnosus GG*, medium by *L. reuteri DSM 17938* and the *L. rhamnosus E/N, Oxy, Pen* mixture and strong by the multi strain synbiotic. Head-to-head in-vitro pathogen growth inhibition experiments can be used to differentiate products from different categories containing probiotic microorganisms and can support the selection process of products for further clinical evaluation.

Keywords: gut microbiome; antimicrobial activity; pathogen overgrowth

1. Introduction

The invention of antibiotic therapy some 100 years ago was a major step forward in medical practice, allowing medical practitioners to manage otherwise deadly infections caused by pathogenic bacteria. However, in the recent past, the rapid increase of bacterial antibiotic resistance has become a pressing problem of global healthcare [1]. More sensible and less widespread use of antibiotics is necessary to counteract the increasing loss of their efficacy. While it is clinically challenging to implement, antibiotics should only be used where their usage is appropriate, and best only in confirmed cases of bacterial infections. In addition to a careful usage of antibiotics, probiotics or synbiotics should be considered as prophylactic measures, at least for patients at risk of certain bacterial infections (e.g., the elderly admitted to an intensive care unit), as complementary therapy during and after antibiotic therapy, or even as standalone therapy under certain specific circumstances for bacterial infections.

Every orally taken antibiotic is leading to alterations of the gut microbiota, in some patients with symptoms (e.g., diarrhea), in others without symptoms [2]. While antibiotic-associated diarrhea (AAD) is worrying, the disturbance of the gut microbiota by antibiotics can have more severe consequences. Among these severe side effects is, for example, pseudomembranous colitis [3], which is caused by a pathogen overgrowth of the gut, in this case by *C. difficile*. Pathogenic bacteria are omnipresent in the human gut. However, as long as the gut microbiota is well balanced and diverse, no pathogen overgrowth will take place [4]. Disturbance of the equilibrium of the gut microbiota can result in loss of this pathogenic overgrowth control. Such a can loss then lead to a strong proliferation of pathogens in the gut and finally result in disease manifestation. Supplementation with certain probiotics or synbiotics (mixtures of probiotic bacteria with a prebiotic component) during and after antibiotic therapy has been demonstrated to reduce occurrence of AAD [5].

Today, a huge variety of products containing probiotic microorganisms are available. These products can be categorized according to their composition: (i) yeast and bacterial products, (ii) mono strain and multi strain products or (iii) probiotic and synbiotic products. In the present study, the inhibitions of five bacterial pathogens, *E. coli EPEC, Sh. sonnei, S. typhimurium, K. pneumoniae* and *C. difficile* by representatives of different categories of products containing probiotic microorganisms are studied. The evaluated probiotics are the clinically well-established mono strain probiotics containing either *Sac. boulardii* [6], *L. rhamnosus GG* [7] or *L. reuteri DSM 17938* [8], and two newer products, one being a multi strain probiotic containing a mixture of three different *L. rhamnosus* strains *(E/N, Oxy, Pen)*, the other being a complex multi strain synbiotic containing six *lactobacilli* (*L. acidophilus, L. casei, L. paracasei, L. plantarum, L. rhamnosus GG, L. salivarius*), three *bifidobacteria* strains (*Bifidobacterium (B.) bifidum, B. longum, B. lactis*) and the prebiotic FOS.

Most published in-vitro growth inhibition studies focused on the characterization of only one pathogenic bacterium and one or a limited number of products containing probiotic microorganisms. The present study evaluated the antagonistic activity of a range of products in head-to-head in-vitro growth inhibition experiments with a number of different bacterial pathogens, which can support the selection of products for future, more in-depth investigations.

2. Materials and Methods

2.1. Probiotics and Synbiotic

The yeast *Sac. boulardii* probiotic Enterol® (Biocodex, Gentilly, France) contains in each capsule 4.5×10^9 colony forming units (CFU) of the *Sac. boulardii* strain CNCM I-745. Dicoflor® (Bayer Sp. z o.o., Warszawa, Poland) contains 6×10^9 CFU of *L. rhamnosus GG* ATCC© 53103 per capsule. BioGaia®, (InfectoPharm Arzneimittel und Consilium GmbH, Heppenheim, Germany) contains 10^8 CFU *L. reuteri DSM 17938* per 5 drops. Lakcid® (Biomed-Lublin S.A., Poland) contains a total of 2×10^9 CFUs as mixture of the *L. rhamnosus* strains *E/N* (40%), *Oxy* (20%) and *Pen* (40%), [9]. The complex multi strain synbiotic Multilac® Baby (Vivatrex GmbH, Aachen, Germany) is a freeze-dried powder. Each sachet contains a total of 10^9 CFUs as a mixture of equal CFU amounts of *L. acidophilus LA-14; L. casei R0215; L. paracasei Lpc-3; L. plantarum Lp-115; L. rhamnosus GG, L. salivarius Ls-33, B. lactis Bl-04, B. bifidum R0071, B. longum R0175* and 1.43 g of the prebiotic ingredient FOS.

2.2. In-Vitro Growth Inhibition of E. coli EPEC, Sh. sonnei, S. typhimurium and K. pneumoniae

For the in vitro pathogen inhibition experiments with *E. coli EPEC* (clinical isolate, collection number 3410/19 *E. coli* 025), *Sh. sonnei* ATCC© 9290™ (ATCC, Manassas, VA, USA), *S. enterica subsp.*

enterica serovar typhimurium ATCC© 14280™ (ATCC, Manassas, VA, USA) and *K. pneumoniae subsp. pneumoniae* ATCC© 700603™ (ATCC, Manassas, VA, USA) the respective pathogen was inoculated on Columbia agar with 5% sheep blood (CM0331, Fisher Scientific GmbH, Schwerte, Germany) and incubated at 37 °C under aerobic conditions for 24 h [10]. Suspensions (100 µL) of the five tested products (mono strain probiotics *Sac. boulardii, L. rhamnosus GG, L. reuteri DSM 17938*, the multi strain *L. rhamnosus E/N, Oxy, Pen* and the complex multi strain synbiotic) each containing 10^6 CFU were inoculated on MRS agar (CM0361, Fisher Scientific GmbH, Schwerte, Germany) and incubated for 48 h in the presence of 5% CO_2 [11]. After the incubation, 10 mm diameter bars were cut out and transferred to a Mueller–Hinton agar (CM0337, Fisher Scientific GmbH, Schwerte, Germany) previously inoculated with the respective pathogen strain with a density of 2 on the McFarland scale. The tested cultures were stored at 4 °C for 4 h, followed by incubation at 37 °C for 24 h under aerobic conditions.

2.3. In-Vitro Growth Inhibition of C. difficile

For the in-vitro pathogen inhibition studies with *C. difficile* ATCC© 9689™ (ATCC, Manassas, VA, USA), the pathogen was cultivated under anaerobic conditions at 35–37 °C for 24–48 h on Schaedler agar (CM0437, Fisher Scientific GmbH, Schwerte, Germany) [12]. Suspensions each containing 10^6 CFU of the five evaluated products were inoculated on MRS agar and incubated for 48 h in the presence of 5% CO_2. 10 mm diameter bars were transferred to a Mueller–Hinton agar with 5% horse blood and 20 mg/L NAD (PP0972, E&O Laboratories Ltd, Bonnybridge, UK) and incubated under anaerobic conditions for 24 h.

2.4. FOS Control and Measurement of Growth Inhibition

For testing a potential pathogen growth inhibitory effect of FOS, 100 µL of a solution containing 14.3 mg/mL FOS (F8052, Sigma Aldrich, St. Louis, Missouri, USA) was applied to a 10 mm filter disk that was then administered to respective pathogen testing plates. The multi strain synbiotic was tested on the same plates as a positive control.

At the end of the incubation, measurements of inhibition zones around the tested colonies were taken from the outer edge of the colonies to the outer edge of the clear zones. Each test was performed in triplicate and the arithmetic means of the radii measuring from the edges of the colonies to the edges of the clear zones were calculated as well as the standard deviations SD (Excel, Microsoft, Redmont, WA, USA). Independent T-test statistical analyses of datasets were conducted with GraphPad Prism software version 8.2 (GraphPad Software, San Diego, CA, USA), Datasets were considered as significantly different when a p-value < 0.01 was achieved.

3. Results

In-Vitro Pathogen Growth Inhibition

In-vitro growth of all five tested pathogenic bacteria were inhibited by all evaluated products. However, the extent of in-vitro growth inhibitions by the products varied significantly for all tested pathogens (Figure 1).

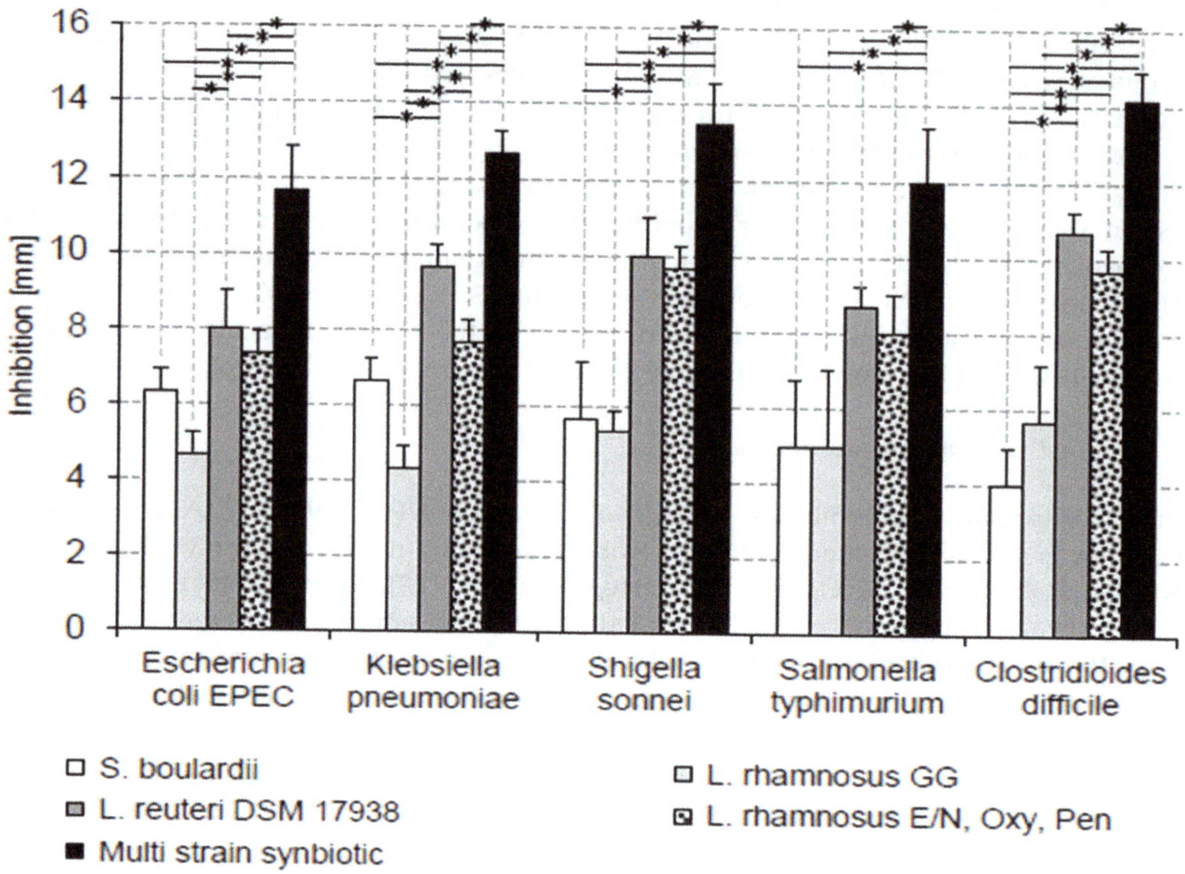

Figure 1. In-vitro growth inhibition of pathogens by different probiotics and a multi strain synbiotic. The *L. rhamnosus E/N, Oxy, Pen* mixture contains the three different probiotics in a CFU ratio of 40/20/40. The multi strain synbiotic contains a mixture of equal CFU amounts of *L. acidophilus LA-14; L. casei R0215; L. paracasei Lpc-3; L. plantarum Lp-115; L. rhamnosus GG, L. salivarius Ls-33, B. lactis Bl-04, B. bifidum R0071, B. longum R0175* and the prebiotic fructooligosaccharides (FOS). Significant differences (p-values < 0.01) between the inhibitions by different products are indicated by horizontal lines marked with an asterisk (*).

The inhibitory patterns found for *E. coli EPEC* and *K. pneumoniae* were similar. The antagonistic effects of the tested products ranked from weak to strong inhibition as follows: *L. rhamnosus GG* < *Sac. boulardii* < *L. reuteri DSM 17938* = multi strain probiotic *L. rhamnosus E/N, Oxy, Pen* < complex multi strain synbiotic.

For the inhibition of *Sh. sonnei* and *S. typhimurium* an inhibition ranking from weak to strong of *Sac. boulardii* = *L. rhamnosus GG* < *L. reuteri DSM 17938* = multi strain probiotic *L. rhamnosus E/N, Oxy, Pen* < complex multi strain synbiotic was found. While there was a significant difference (p-values < 0.01) between the inhibitions of *Sh. sonnei* by *Sac. boulardii* or *L. rhamnosus GG* and the *L. reuteri DSM 17938* probiotic or the multi strain probiotic *L. rhamnosus E/N, Oxy, Pen*, the difference of the inhibitions by these two groups of probiotics of *S. typhimurium* was not significant (p-values > 0.01).

The inhibition of the gram-positive *C. difficile* by the tested products resembled that of *Sh. sonnei* and *S. typhimurium*. The weakest inhibitions were found for *Sac. boulardii* and *L. rhamnosus GG*. Inhibitions by *L. reuteri DSM 17938* and the multi strain probiotic *L. rhamnosus E/N, Oxy, Pen* were intermediate and the best inhibitory effect was found for the complex multi strain synbiotic.

As shown in Figure 2, FOS alone had no inhibitory effect on *E. coli EPEC*. FOS also had no inhibitory effect on the growth of the other four tested pathogens (data not shown).

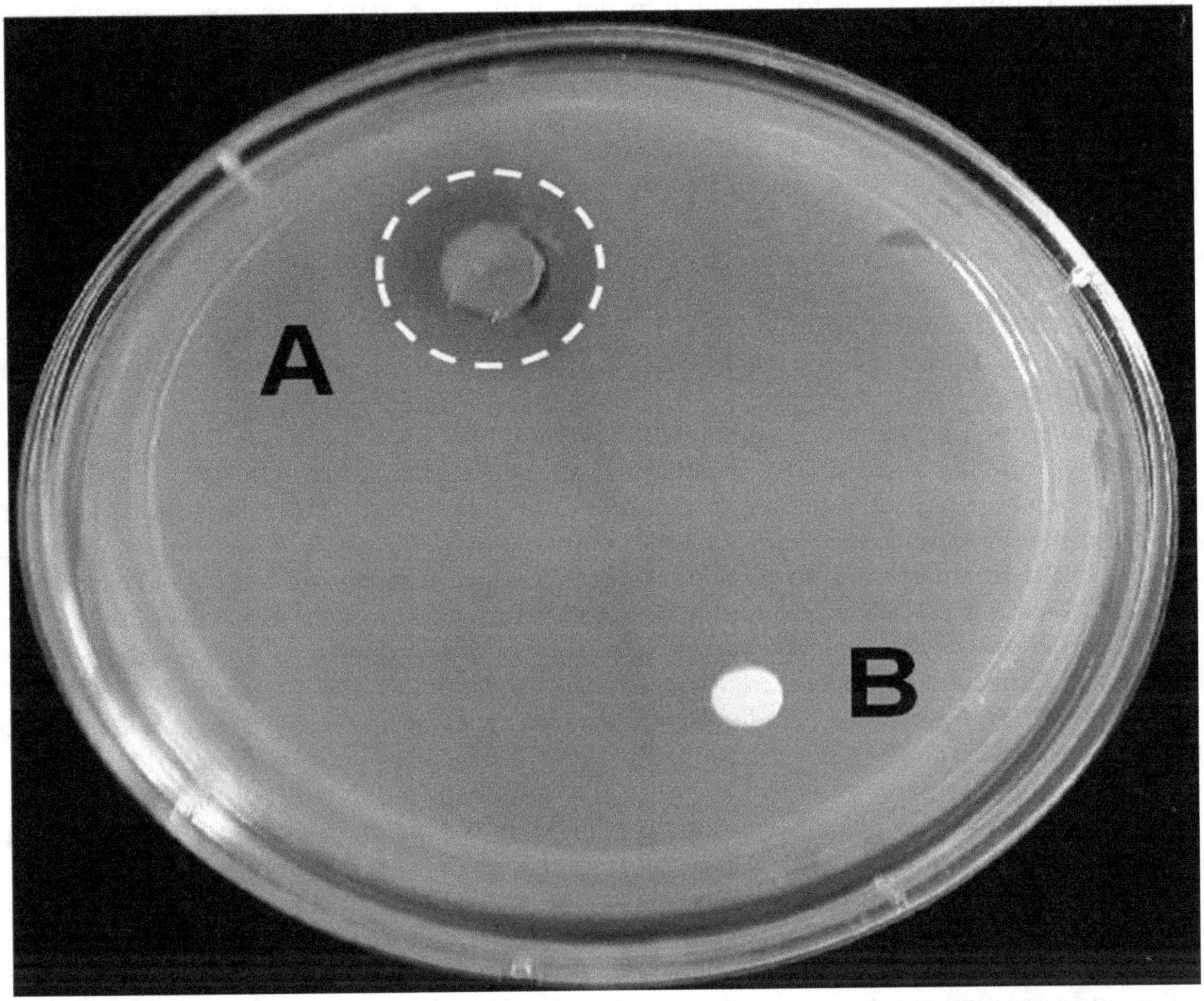

Figure 2. Example of the effects of the multi strain synbiotic (**A**) and FOS (**B**) on the in-vitro growth of *Enteropathogenic E. coli EPEC.*

4. Discussion

A large number of studies have been published which are characterizing the in-vitro pathogen growth effects of individual probiotic microorganisms. There are also studies which compare the growth inhibitory effects of individual strains in head-to-head experiments. Less data are available for the in-vitro growth inhibitory effect of individual multi-strain products. To our knowledge there is no study published which compares the in-vitro pathogen growth inhibitory effects of probiotic products from different categories (yeast, bacteria, mono-strain, multi-strain, probiotic, synbiotic) head-to-head. The present study compares the in-vitro pathogen growth inhibitory properties of products containing probiotic microorganisms commonly used by physicians in Poland. The in-vitro pathogen growth inhibition experiments of the present study are not aiming to identify the underlying mechanisms of growth inhibition or to identify the causes of potential synergistic effects of probiotic bacteria in the multi-strain products, but to focus primarily on establishing a ranking of efficacy in this one particular experimental set-up. Inhibition of pathogen growth is only one potential effect exhibited by probiotic bacteria in the gut and other activities (e.g., inhibition of the adherence of pathogens to the gut mucosa, stimulation of the host immune system) are also potential contributors to their efficacy. However, in-vitro pathogen growth inhibition testing is a helpful measure that can be used to support the selection of products for further investigation, e.g., in clinical trials.

For the in-vitro growth inhibition testing, five bacterial pathogens were selected which physicians encounter in their day-to-day practice. All five selected bacterial pathogens represent major health care concerns. As outlined in the following, infections with these pathogens are not always requiring antibiotic therapy. In addition, the increasing rate of developing antibiotic resistance in these bacteria has stimulated the interest in probiotics as prophylactic, alternative or adjuvant therapy for infections caused by them.

Enteropathogenic E. coli EPEC is a major cause of infant diarrhea [13]. As long as there is no evidence for a systemic infection, antibiotic therapy is rarely indicated and should be deferred until culture results are available. Due to this, and the emerging resistance of *E.coli* against antibiotics [14], probiotics are considered as additional options to manage *E. coli* infections [15]. In-vitro pathogen growth inhibition experiments found no clear *E. coli* growth antagonism by the yeast *Sac. boulardii* [16]. In contrast, in-vitro growth inhibitions of *E. coli* have been described for a number of mono strain bacterial probiotics, among them *L. rhamnosus GG* [17], *L. reuteri DSM 17938* [15] and multi strain probiotics [15,18,19].

Shigella infections are a major public health problem in areas of poor sanitation with especially high incidence, morbidity and mortality in children [20]. Shigellosis is spread by fecal-oral transmission and ingestion of a small number of *Shigella* bacteria can already cause clinical disease. Most patients recover from Shigellosis without antibiotic treatment within 5–7 days. Various antimicrobial agents are effective in the treatment of severe cases of Shigellosis, however, a globally emerging antibiotic resistance is observed [21]. Consequently, probiotics are considered as an alternative approach to manage Shigellosis. *Sac. boulardii* has been shown to interfere with *Shigella* pathogenesis [22], however, in-vitro growth inhibition of *Sh. sonnei* by *Sac. boulardii* has not been published. Inhibition of in-vitro growth of *Sh. sonnei* has been demonstrated for *L. rhamnosus GG* [17], for *L. reuteri* [23] and a number of other *lactobacilli* [24]. For the multi strain products investigated in this study, results from in-vitro growth inhibition of *Sh. sonnei* have not been demonstrated.

Most food-borne bacterial gastroenteritis is caused by *S. typhimurium*. Antibiotic therapy is not advised for most of the patients with *S. typhimurium* infection, as the infection is often self-limiting and antibiotic resistance of the bacterium is on the rise [25]. Therefore, especially for severe cases or patients with persistent infections [26], non-antibiotic treatment alternatives are needed [27]. There is a large amount of studies, including human clinical trials, indicating that *Sac. boulardii* has potential in the prevention and treatment of infections with *S. typhimurium* [28]. However, no study has been published comparing the in-vitro growth inhibition of *S. typhimurium* by *Sac. boulardii* with that of bacterial probiotics. In-vitro growth inhibition of *S. typhimurium* has been shown for a number of individual *lactobacilli* strains, [17,29,30]. The method has also been used for the search for new *lactobacilli* strains with growth inhibitory potential against *S. typhimurium* [19,31]. Our group has recently published that *S. typhimurium* was more strongly inhibited by a multi strain synbiotic (different from that investigated in the present study) when compared with the in-vitro growth inhibition caused by its individual bacterial strains [30].

K. pneumoniae is responsible for an alarming increase in hospital infections, especially in intensive care units. More and more antibiotics have lost their efficacy against *K. pneumoniae*, and strains of *K. pneumoniae* have emerged that are resistant against most of the presently available antibiotics [32,33]. Consequently, interest in probiotics/synbiotics as alternative options to manage infections with *K. pneumoniae* has emerged. Few studies have investigated the effect of probiotics on the in-vitro growth of *K. pneumoniae* [34–36], however, all with promising results.

For an initial *C. difficile* infection (CDI), the exposure to antibiotics is the most important risk factor [37]. In this context, it is important to note that certain antibiotics (e.g., clindamycin, quinolones, cephalosporins) are associated with a higher risk of causing CDI. The pathology of CDI is characterized by a disruption of the gut microbiota, resulting in an overgrowth by *C. difficile*, production of toxins and disease development. Characteristic symptoms are diarrhea and abdominal pain. In severe cases, the CDI can result in a life-threatening pseudomembranous colitis. Recurrence of CDI is a not uncommon observation. First step in the treatment of CDI is discontinuing the therapy with the inciting antibiotic as soon as possible. Depending on severity of the CDI, three antibiotics can be considered for therapy: metronidazole, vancomycin and fidaxomicin [38]. In addition, supporting the diversity of the gut microbiota is an important therapeutic objective in the management of CDI [39].

In-vitro growth inhibition of *C. difficile* by a number of mono strain probiotics, among them *L. rhamnosus*, and *bifidobacteria* has been described [40,41]. To our knowledge, the present study is the first which compares head-to-head the in vitro-growth inhibition of *C. difficile* by representatives from different categories of products containing probiotics.

The products evaluated in the present study can be categorized by the following criteria: (i) yeast/bacteria, (ii) mono strain/multi strain and (iii) probiotic/synbiotic (containing probiotic and prebiotic components). While the in-vitro pathogen growth inhibitory effects vary among the tested products, the inhibitory effects seem not to be pathogen-dependent. Weakest pathogen inhibition is observed for *Sac. boulardii* and *L. rhamnosus GG*, intermediate for *L. reuteri DSM 17938* and the *L. rhamnosus E/N, Oxy, Pen* mixture and strongest inhibition is found for the multi strain synbiotic. This finding is in line with the hypothesis that multi strain probiotics exhibit superior growth inhibitory effects towards pathogenic bacteria because they are combining a broader range of independent antibacterial activities, some of which might even act synergistically [42,43]. However, it has to be mentioned that in-vitro characterization of the potential synergistic effects in multi strain probiotics, especially those containing a larger number of different strains, can hardly be demonstrated due to the fact that thousands, if not millions of potential combinations would have to be investigated. Synbiotics might have an additional advantage over pure probiotics, as their prebiotic component provides a source of energy, potentially supporting the proliferation of their probiotic components. Based on our experiments, we can exclude that FOS itself has an inhibitory effect on one of the tested pathogenic bacteria.

An obvious limitation of the present study is that it is using only one experimental set-up to establish an in-vitro efficacy ranking among the evaluated products. No efforts have been undertaken to investigate the underlying mechanisms of the observed pathogen inhibitions or the underlying mechanisms of potential synergies in the multi strain products. Dedicated human clinical studies will be necessary to evaluate if these in-vitro findings will translate into clinical benefits for patients.

5. Conclusions

In-vitro growth inhibition of a variety of pathogens is helpful to differentiate products and product categories containing probiotic microorganisms. Based on the results of the present study, multi strain probiotics should be preferred in case a strong in-vitro growth inhibition of a broad range of pathogens is desired. Our study results can support the product selection for future clinical investigations.

Author Contributions: Conceptualization, H.S., J.P., H.K. and P.W.-B.; methodology, A.C.-R., and M.B.; validation, J.P. and H.K.; formal analysis, J.P., H.K.; data curation, A.C.-R. and M.B.; writing—original draft preparation, H.S. and J.P.; writing—review and editing, H.S., J.P. and H.K.; visualization, H.S.; supervision, J.P.; project administration, J.P. All authors have read and agreed to the published version of the manuscript.

Acknowledgments: The authors would like to acknowledge the work of Sabine Hanna from Cambridge Assessment English for proof-reading, English style editing, and useful suggestions.

References

1. Aslam, B.; Arshad, M.I.; Khurshid, M.; Muzammil, S.; Rasool, M.H.; Nisar, M.A.; Alvi, R.F.; Aslam, M.A.; Qamar, M.U.; Salamat, M.K.F.; et al. Antibiotic resistance: A rundown of a global crisis. *Infect. Drug Resist.* **2018**, *11*, 1645–1658. [CrossRef] [PubMed]
2. McFarland, L. Antibiotic-associated diarrhea: Epidemiology, trends and treatment. *Future Microbiol.* **2008**, *3*, 563–578. [CrossRef] [PubMed]

3. Farooq, P.D.; Urrunaga, N.H.; Tang, D.M.; von Rosenvinge, E.C. Pseudomembranous Colitis. *Dis. Mon.* **2015**, *61*, 181–206. [CrossRef] [PubMed]
4. Bäumler, A.J.; Sperandio, V. Interactions between the microbiota and pathogenic bacteria in the gut. *Nature* **2016**, *535*, 85–93. [CrossRef] [PubMed]
5. Guo, Q.; Goldenberg, J.Z.; Humphrey, C.; El Dib, R.; Johnsto, B.C. Probiotics for the prevention of pediatric antibiotic-associated diarrhea. *Cochrane Database Syst. Rev.* **2019**, *4*, CD004827. [CrossRef]
6. Szajewska, H.; Kolodziej, M. Systematic review with meta-analysis: Saccharomyces boulardii in the prevention of antibiotic-associated diarrhoea. *Aliment. Pharmacol. Ther.* **2015**, *42*, 793–801. [CrossRef]
7. Szajewska, H.; Kolodziej, M. Systematic review with meta-analysis: Lactobacillus rhamnosusGG in the prevention of antibiotic-associated diarrhoea in children and adults. *Aliment. Pharmacol. Ther.* **2015**, *42*, 1149–1157. [CrossRef]
8. Urbanska, M.; Gieruszczak-Bialek, D.; Szajewska, H. Systematic review with meta-analysis: Lactobacillus reuteri DSM 17938 for diarrhoeal diseases in children. *Aliment. Pharmacol. Ther.* **2016**, *43*, 1025–1034. [CrossRef]
9. Jarocki, P.; Podlesny, M.; Wasko, A.; Siuda, A.; Targonski, Z. Differentiation of three Lactobacillus rhamnosus strains (E/N, Oxy and Pen) by SDS-PAGE and two-dimensional electrophoresis of surface-associated proteins. *J. Microbiol. Biotechnol.* **2010**, *20*, 558–562. [CrossRef]
10. Ellner, P.D.; Stoessel, C.J.; Drakeford, E.; Vasi, F. A new culture medium for medical bacteriology. *Tech. Bull. Regist. Med. Technol.* **1966**, *36*, 58–60. [CrossRef]
11. De Man, J.C.; Rogosa, M.; Sharpe, M.E. A medium for the cultivation of Lactobacilli. *Appl. Bact.* **1960**, *23*, 130–135. [CrossRef]
12. Schaedler, R.W.; Dubos, R.; Costello, R. The development of the bacterial flora in the gastrointestinal tract of mice. *J. Exp. Med.* **1965**, *122*, 59–66. [CrossRef] [PubMed]
13. Ochoa, T.J.; Contreras, C.A. Enteropathogenic, E. coli (EPEC) infection in children. *Curr. Opin. Infect. Dis.* **2011**, *24*, 478–483. [CrossRef] [PubMed]
14. Poirel, L.; Madec, J.Y.; Lupo, A.; Schink, A.K.; Kieffer, N.; Nordmann, P.; Schwarz, S. Antimicrobial Resistance in Escherichia coli. *Microbiol. Spectr.* **2018**, *6*. [CrossRef]
15. Fijan, S.; Sulc, D.; Steyer, A. Study of the In Vitro Antagonistic Activity of Various Mono-Strain and Multi-Strain Probiotics against Escherichia coli. *Int. J. Environ. Res. Public Health* **2018**, *15*, 1539. [CrossRef]
16. Rajkowska, K.; Kunicka-Styczynska, A.; Rygala, A. Probiotic Activity of Saccharomyces cerevisiae var. boulardii Against Human Pathogens. *Food Technol. Biotechnol.* **2012**, *50*, 230–236.
17. Hütt, P.; Shchepetova, J.; Lõivukene, K.; Kullisaar, T.; Mikelsaar, M. Antagonistic activity of probiotic lactobacilli and bifidobacteria against entero- and uropathogens. *J. Appl. Microbiol.* **2006**, *100*, 1324–1332. [CrossRef]
18. Shokryazdan, P.; Sieo, C.C.; Kalavathy, R.; Liang, J.B.; Alitheen, N.B.; Jahromi, M.F.; Ho, Y.W. Probiotic Potential of Lactobacillus Strains with Antimicrobial Activity against Some Human Pathogenic Strains. *BioMed Res. Int.* **2014**, *2014*, 927268. [CrossRef]
19. Jacobsen, C.N.; Rosenfeldt Nielsen, V.; Hayford, A.E.; Møller, L.; Michaelsen, K.F.; Pærregaard, A.; Sandström, B.; Tvede, M.; Jakobsen, M. Screening of Probiotic Activities of Forty-Seven Strains of *Lactobacillus* spp. by In Vitro Techniques and Evaluation of the Colonization Ability of Five Selected Strains in Humans. *Appl. Environ. Microbiol.* **1999**, *65*, 4949–4956. [CrossRef]
20. Niyogi, S.K. Shigellosis. *J. Microbiol.* **2005**, *43*, 133–143.
21. Puzari, M.; Sharma, M.; Chetia, P. Emergence of antibiotic resistant Shigella species: A matter of concern. *J. Infect. Public Health* **2018**, *11*, 451–454. [CrossRef] [PubMed]
22. Mumy, K.L.; Chen, X.; Kelly, C.P.; McCormick, B.A. Saccharomyces boulardii interferes with Shigella pathogenesis by postinvasion signaling events. *Am. J. Physiol. Gastrointest. Liver Physiol.* **2008**, *294*, G599–G609. [CrossRef]
23. Spinler, J.K.; Taweechotipatr, M.; Rognerud, C.L.; Ou, C.N.; Tumwasorn, S.; Versalovic, J. Human-derived probiotic Lactobacillus reuteri demonstrate antimicrobial activities targeting diverse enteric bacterial pathogens. *Anaerobe* **2008**, *14*, 166–171. [CrossRef] [PubMed]
24. Zhang, Y.C.; Zhang, L.W.; Ma, W.; Yi, H.X.; Yang, X.; Du, M.; Shan, Y.J.; Han, X.; Zhang, L.L. Screening of probiotic lactobacilli for inhibition of Shigella sonnei and the macromolecules involved in inhibition. *Anaerobe* **2012**, *18*, 498–503. [CrossRef] [PubMed]

25. Eng, S.K.; Pusparajah, P.; Ab Mutalib, N.S.; Ser, H.L.; Chan, K.G.; Lee, L.H. Salmonella: A review on pathogenesis, epidemiology and antibiotic resistance. *Front. Life Sci.* **2015**, *8*, 284–293. [CrossRef]
26. Marzel, A.; Desai, P.T.; Goren, A.; Schorr, Y.I.; Nissan, I.; Porwollik, S.; Valinsky, L.; McClelland, M.; Rahav, G.; Gal-Mor, O. Persistant Infections by Nontyphoidal Salmonella in Humans: Epidemilogy and Genetics. *Clin. Infect. Dis.* **2016**, *62*, 879–886. [CrossRef]
27. Liévin-Le Moal, V.; Servin, A.L. Anti-Infective Activities of Lactobacillus Strains in the Human Intestinal Microbiota: From Probiotics to Gastrointestinal Anti-Infectious Biotherapeutic Agents. *Clin. Microbiol.* **2014**, *27*, 167–199. [CrossRef]
28. Gut, A.M.; Vasiljevic, T.; Yeager, T.; Donkor, O.N. Salmonella infection—prevention and treatment by antibiotics and probiotic yeasts: A review. *Microbiology* **2018**, *164*, 1327–1344. [CrossRef]
29. Das, J.K.; Mishra, D.; Ray, P.; Tripathy, P.; Beuria, T.K.; Singh, N.; Suar, M. In vitro evaluation of anti-infective activity of a Lactobacillus plantarum strain against Salmonella enterica serovar Enteritidis. *Gut Pathog.* **2013**, *5*, 1. [CrossRef] [PubMed]
30. Piatek, J.; Sommermeyer, H.; Bernatek, M.; Ciechelska-Rybarczyk, A.; Oleskow, B.; Sommer Mikkelsen, L.; Bundvig Barken, K. Persistent infection by Salmonella enterica servovar Typhimurium: Are synbiotics a therapeutic option?—A case report. *Benef. Microbes* **2019**, *10*, 211–217. [CrossRef]
31. Dowarah, R.; Verma, A.K.; Agarwal, N.; Singh, P.; Singh, B.R. Selection and characterization of probiotic lactic acid bacteria and its impact on growth, nutrient digestibility, health and antioxidant status in weaned piglets. *PLoS ONE* **2018**, *13*, e0192978. [CrossRef]
32. Centers for Disease Control and Prevention (CDC). Vital Signs: Carbapenem-Resistant Enterobacteriaceae. *MMWR Morb. Mortal. Wkly. Rep.* **2013**, *62*, 165–170.
33. Xu, L.; Sun, X.; Ma, X. Systematic review and meta-analysis of mortality of patients infected with carbapenem-resistant Klebsiella pneumoniae. *Ann. Clin. Microbiol. Antimicrob.* **2017**, *16*, 18. [CrossRef] [PubMed]
34. Mogna, L.; Deidda, F.; Nicola, S.; Amoruso, A.; Del Piano, M.; Mogna, G. In Vitro Inhibition of Klebsiella pneumoniae by Lactobacillus delbrueckii Subsp. delbrueckii LDD01 (DSM 22106): An Innovative Strategy to Possibly Counteract Such Infections in Humans? *J. Clin. Gastroenterol.* **2016**, *50* (Suppl. 2). [CrossRef]
35. Savino, F.; Cordisco, L.; Tarasco, V.; Locatelli, E.; Di Gioia, D.; Oggero, R.; Matteuzzi, D. Antagonistic effect of Lactobacillus strains against gas-producing coliforms isolated from colicky infants. *BMC Microbiol.* **2011**, *11*, 157. [CrossRef]
36. Piatek, J.; Bernatek, M.; Ciechelska-Rybarczyk, A.; Oleskow, B.; Sommermeyer, H. Inhibition of Carbapenem-Resistant NDM-1 Klebsiella pneumoniae isolated from a Hospital Outbreak Patient by a Synbiotic: A Non antibiotic Treatment Option. *Int. J. Med. Res. Health Sci.* **2019**, *8*, 12–20.
37. Bignardi, G.E. Risk factors for Clostridium difficile infection. *J. Hosp. Infect.* **1998**, *40*, 1–15. [CrossRef]
38. McDonald, L.C.; Gerding, D.N.; Johnson, S.; Bakken, J.S.; Carroll, K.C.; Coffin, S.E.; Dubberke, E.R.; Garey, K.W.; Gould, C.V.; Kelly, C.; et al. Clinical Practice Guidelines for Clostridium difficile Infection in Adults and Children: 2017 Update by the Infectious Diseases Society of America (IDSA) and Society for Healthcare Epidemiology of America (SHEA). *Clin. Infect. Dis.* **2018**, *66*, e1–e48. [CrossRef]
39. Chang, J.Y.; Antonopoulos, D.; Kalra, A.; Tonelli, A.; Khalife, W.T.; Schmidt, T.M.; Young, V.B. Decreased Diversity of the Fecal Microbiome in Recurrent Clostridium difficile -Associated Diarrhea. *J. Infect. Dis.* **2008**, *197*, 435–438. [CrossRef]
40. Naaber, P.; Smidt, I.; Štšepetova, J.; Brilene, T.; Annuk, H.; Mikelsaar, M. Inhibition of Clostridium difficile strains by intestinal Lactobacillus species. *J. Med. Microbiol.* **2004**, *53*, 551–553. [CrossRef] [PubMed]
41. Schoster, A.; Kokotovic, B.; Permin, A.; Pedersen, P.D.; Dal Bello, F.; Guardabassi, L. In vitro inhibition of Clostridium difficile and Clostridium perfringens by commercial probiotic strains. *Anaerobe* **2013**, *20*, 36–41. [CrossRef] [PubMed]
42. Timmerman, H.M.; Koning, C.J.; Mulder, L.; Rombouts, F.M.; Beynen, A.C. Monostrain, multistrain and multispecies probiotics-A comparison of functionality and efficacy. *Int. J. Food Microbiol.* **2004**, *96*, 219–233. [CrossRef] [PubMed]
43. Ouwehand, A.C.; Invernici, M.M.; Furlaneto, F.A.C.; Messora, M.R. Effectiveness of Multistrain versus Single-Strain Probiotics: Current Status and Recommendations for the Future. *J. Clin. Gastroenterol.* **2018**, *52* (Suppl. 1), S35–S40. [CrossRef] [PubMed]

2

Microbial Medicine: Prebiotic and Probiotic Functional Foods to Target Obesity and Metabolic Syndrome

Miranda Green [1], Karan Arora [1,2,3] and Satya Prakash [1,*]

[1] Biomedical Technology and Cell Therapy Research Laboratory, Department of Biomedical Engineering, Faculty of Medicine, McGill University, 3775 University Street, Montreal, QC H3A 2B4, Canada; miranda.green@mail.mcgill.ca (M.G.); karan.arora@mail.mcgill.ca (K.A.)

[2] Department of Bioengineering, Faculty of Engineering, McGill University, 3775 University Street, Montreal, QC H3A 2B4, Canada

[3] Biena Inc., 2955 Rue Cartier, Saint-Hyacinthe, QC J2S 1L4, Canada

* Correspondence: satya.prakash@mcgill.ca

Abstract: Obesity has become a global epidemic and a public health crisis in the Western World, experiencing a threefold increase in prevalence since 1975. High-caloric diets and sedentary lifestyles have been identified as significant contributors to this widespread issue, although the role of genetic, social, and environmental factors in obesity's pathogenesis remain incompletely understood. In recent years, much attention has been drawn to the contribution of the gut microbiota in the development of obesity. Indeed, research has shown that in contrast to their healthier counterparts the microbiomes of obese individuals are structurally and functionally distinct, strongly suggesting microbiome as a potential target for obesity therapeutics. In particular, pre and probiotics have emerged as effective and integrative means of modulating the microbiome, in order to reverse the microbial dysbiosis associated with an obese phenotype. The following review brings forth animal and human research supporting the myriad of mechanisms by which the microbiome affects obesity, as well as the strengths and limitations of probiotic or prebiotic supplementation for the prevention and treatment of obesity. Finally, we set forth a roadmap for the comprehensive development of functional food solutions in combatting obesity, to capitalize on the potential of pre/probiotic therapies in optimizing host health.

Keywords: microbiome; probiotics; prebiotics; obesity; metabolic syndrome; inflammation; bile acid (BA); short chain fatty acid (SCFA); metabolic syndrome (MetS)

---

1. Introduction

Obesity has become among the largest global health challenges that currently face our society, comprising what is currently considered an "epidemic" of non-communicable pathology. Recent estimates from the International Obesity Task Force (IOTF) suggest that 1.1 billion adults are overweight, including 312 million who are obese [1]. In some industrialized countries there has been an alarming rise in the prevalence of obesity in the previous decade alone, with rates doubling or nearly tripling among the general population [2,3]. Furthermore, due to the rapid global proliferation of the so-called "Western lifestyle", comprising high-fat, high-refined carbohydrate diets and largely sedentary daily routines, this trend is not confined to the North America but rather materializing on an international scale [3].

In parallel to growing waistlines and body mass indices across the globe, modern society is also experiencing a dangerous increase in prevalence of obesity-associated metabolic derangements. A collection of such risk factors, known as metabolic syndrome, affects an estimated one in four adults worldwide [4]. This condition is defined as a clustering of diagnostic symptoms including elevated blood triglycerides, blood sugar, blood pressure, and fasting blood glucose, in addition to abdominal adiposity and low HDL cholesterol [5]. According to the World Health Organization (WHO) definition, at least two of these criteria coupled with evidence of insulin resistance must be present in order to substantiate a diagnosis [6].

The global economic and social burden of obesity and metabolic syndrome demands sustainable, fundamental changes in nutritional and lifestyle standards that are based on a sound understanding of metabolic pathology. Much work remains to be done to understand the origins and salient factors promoting obesity and its physiological impacts, such that potential therapeutic avenues for directly targeting metabolic pathology can be developed and effectively implemented.

Among such factors the human gut microbiome has recently taken center stage, bolstered by modern research demonstrating its central role in modulating human health. Previously ignored by much of the medical literature, the trillions of microbial cells colonizing our gut are now known to be a central metabolic hub, promoting physiological homeostasis and immune function through a close symbiotic relationship to the host [7]. Furthermore, the role of the human microbiome has been found to span beyond the GI tract, mediating a variety of critical communications between the gut, enteric nervous system (ENS), and the brain [8]. In accordance with these findings, perturbations to the gut microbiome, or "dysbiosis", has been linked to a myriad of metabolic, gastrointestinal, and cognitive pathologies.

The ability of the gut microbiome to interconnect genetics, the environment, the immune system, and the brain implies it could account for previously undescribed variables underlying the development of obesity and its metabolic complications. In this regard, multiple mechanistic axes connecting the gut microbiota to obese pathophysiology are being explored. Early evidence suggests perturbations to the microbiome in obesity favor increased energy harvest from food, resulting in perturbed nutrient partitioning [9] and development of adiposity. This is consistent with the role of the microbiome in regulating fat metabolism, in which bacterial fermentation of non-digestible carbohydrates can lead excessive production of short-chain fatty acids (SCFAs) and other lipogenic precursors [10]. In addition, a dysbiotic microbiome contributes to initiation of numerous pro-inflammatory pathways that are a hallmark of obese phenotypes. These include increased absorption of bacterial lipopolysaccharide (LPS) expressed on the surface of Gram-negative strains, as well as modulation of gut barrier permeability leading to translocation of bacterial endotoxins into systemic circulation [11]. Finally, the signaling activity of bacterial SCFAs modulates the hormonal milieu of the gastrointestinal tract and viscera, making the microbiome a key mediator of gut–brain communications involving satiety and energy state of the host [12].

In light of these and other functions, modulation of the gut microbiome through dietary intervention has been proposed as a potential treatment for obesity. Similar to how development of obesity involves the interplay of numerous genetic, social, and environmental factors, an individual's microbiome composition is partially established early in life yet highly dynamic and susceptible to change. Indeed, there is considerable evidence suggesting dietary factors are a key determinant of host microbiome diversity and structure, in addition to innate characteristics such as sex and genetic background. Data suggests that up to 57% of gut microbial composition is explained by diet alone, compared to the mere 12% accounted for by genetic variation [13]. Furthermore, the effects of dietary intervention are rapid and dramatic, eliciting visible restructuring of the gut microbiota within as little as 24 h [14]. Thus, fine-tuning host macronutrient intake to improve integrity of the gut microbiome, and potentially reverse the dysbiosis associated with pathological metabolic states, may offer an effective and minimally invasive means of combatting obesity and its associated comorbidities.

The goals of this review are to, first, explore recent evidence elucidating the microbiome's role in the etiology of obesity, and second, discuss the therapeutic potential of dietary modification (specifically pre and probiotics) in prevention and management of obesity and metabolic syndrome.

2. The Microbiome in Obesity and Metabolic Syndrome

The complex ecosystem of the gut microbiota comprises over 1000 unique bacterial strains, with a prokaryotic population that outnumbers the total cells in the human body by an order of magnitude [8]. Only recently has research begun to unravel the intricate links between the microbiome and human health, especially in the context of host metabolism. Just like other organs in the body, the microbiome can dynamically respond to a variety of internal and external physiological cues, such as food intake, energy requirements, and stress, in order to maintain a state of metabolic homeostasis. Accordingly, perturbances to the microbiome that lead to an unstable or "dysbiotic" state are linked to the pathophysiology of various metabolic conditions, including obesity.

The first studies establishing a causal link between the microbiome and an obese phenotype were performed in germ free (GF) mice, which were initially found to be resistant to diet-induced obesity even under conditions of high-fat (HF) feeding [15]. Furthermore, an obese phenotype was transmissible to these animals via fecal transplant from either Western diet-fed or genetically obese mice, which induced greater weight gain than inoculation with wild-type microbes [9]. Similar results have been observed in colonization studies with microbiota from pairs of mono and dizygotic human twins discordant for obesity. Specifically, microbial inoculation leads to a progressively greater increase in fat mass and body weight in animals receiving microbes from the obese twin, despite no significant differences between animal groups in energy intake [16].

Inspired by these findings, a multitude of microbial survey studies have attempted to define what constitutes an "obese" microbiome, and pinpoint the specific strains that contribute to development of obesity and related metabolic symptoms. Based on such investigations, a lean phenotype has largely come to be associated with an increased *Bacteriodetes:Firmicutes* ratio, whereas this taxonomic proportion is inverted in obese individuals [17,18]. Further supporting this model, studies monitoring the microbiome of obese patients during weight loss have observed a "remodeling" of the gut ecosystem to contain a higher relative amount of *Bacteroidetes* subtypes [19,20]. However, further human studies and meta analyses have revealed this one-to-one association may not be as unambiguous as previously thought. Notably, a recent metanalysis by Sze et al. found a negligible association between the *Bacteriodetes:Firmicutes* ratio and obesity status across analytical studies, and that high levels of experimental "noise" in the form of interpersonal variation and small sample size likely confounded these early observations [21]. This, along with other inconsistency in the literature, suggests that salient differences in pathology-related microbiota may occur at a more precise phylogenetic level than the broad divisions described above.

Although it remains unclear the exact taxonomic composition that constitutes a "healthy" gut microbiota, it is evident that microbial diversity is an essential component to host health. Compared to their lean counterparts obese individuals have a markedly lower bacterial diversity, and decreased fecal microbial gene richness is associated with various physiological markers of obesity and metabolic syndrome [22].

Building on this notion, other studies have argued for the importance of a healthy "core" microbiome, comprising the diverse bacterial genes required for metabolic integrity, that is perturbed in the clinically obese [23]. This diversity-centered model aligns well with the plethora of metabolic niches occupied by the microbiome, supporting various homeostatic processes that are critical to host health. It thus follows that in absence of sufficient microbial diversity to sustain these functions, or presence of a dysbiotic gut microbiota with perturbed metabolic capacity, development of a pathological state may occur. Indeed, a normal healthy microbiota may be better defined at a functional rather than at a compositional level, such that certain essential bacterial species can dynamically respond to changes in host metabolism.

In the case of obesity and metabolic syndrome, it is important to understand not only the microbiome's contribution to metabolic function in healthy individuals, but how perturbations to the microbiome may promote a diseased state (see Figure 1). However, the interplay of these mechanisms and how they influence the overall metabolic status of an individual has yet to be fully understood.

Thus, a discussion of how the microbiome can be targeted in treatment of obesity first warrants examination of the unique channels mediating host–microbiome interactions, and the evidence for their involvement in metabolic pathology.

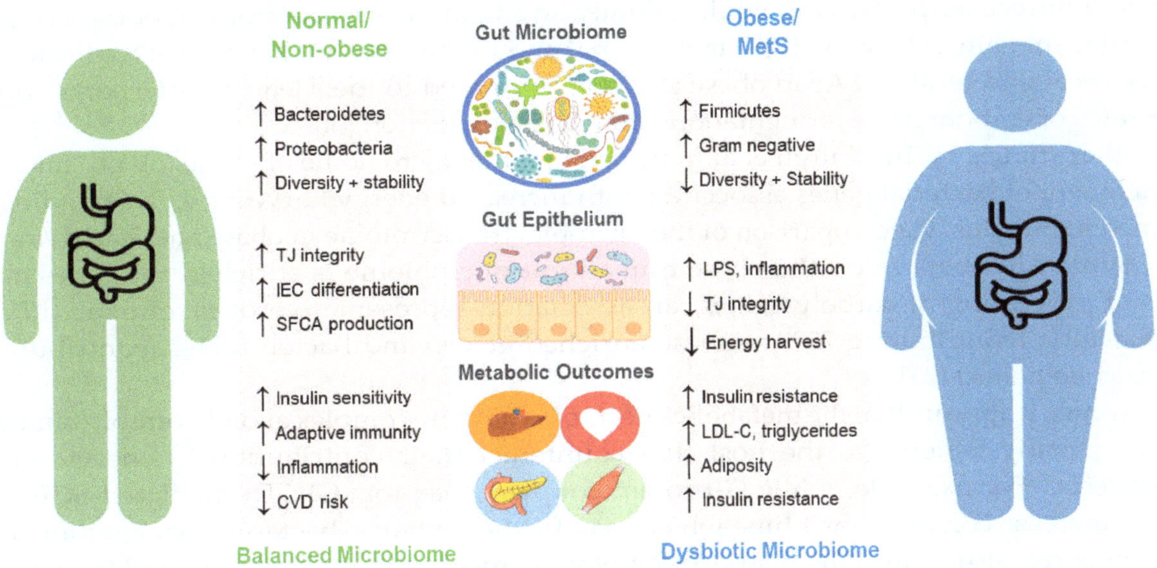

Figure 1. An overview of the microbiome's role in development of obesity and metabolic syndrome (MetS), including some of the mechanisms thought to contribute to changes in host metabolic state. Up and down arrows indicate increase and decrease, respectively. TJ = Tight Junction, IEC = Intestinal Epithelial cells, SCFA = Short Chain Fatty Acid, CVD = Cardiovascular Disease, LPS = Lipopolysaccharide and LDL-C = Low Density Lipoproteins-Cholesterol.

2.1. *The Microbiome in Energy Harvest and Expenditure*

Despite the complex genetic, social, and environmental parameters contributing to its development, the core etiology of obesity depends on a chronic positive energy balance. More precisely, dysregulation of nutrient partitioning in a state of perpetual energy surplus leads to fat storage and weight gain, with a myriad of associated disturbances to organ and tissue function [24]. The intestinal microbiota modulates energy balance by extracting calories from indigestible carbohydrates in the human diet, which are fermented into short chain fatty acids (SCFAs) and other metabolites. These by-products of microbe metabolism can subsequently serve as a form of bioavailable fuel for cellular processes in various tissues and organs. Indeed, colonocytes obtain 60–70% of their cellular energy from SCFA oxidation [25], and the fraction of substrate not consumed by the colon epithelium is transported into systemic circulation such that it can be mobilized to peripheral tissues [25]. It is estimated that through this energy extraction paradigm SCFAs provide ≈10% of daily caloric requirements in humans [26]. Different species of SCFA can also have different metabolic fates: whereas propionate is primarily a precursor for gluconeogenesis, acetate and butyrate are preferentially incorporated into fatty acids and cholesterol [27]. Furthermore, in addition to an important energy source SCFAs serve as active signaling molecules, that interact with G-protein coupled free fatty acid receptors (FFARs) in various tissues to exert a broad spectrum of effects on lipid, glucose, and protein metabolism.

An individual's intestinal SCFA profile relies on a variety of endogenous and external factors, including abundance of fermentable substrates, host–microbiome interactions, host lifestyle, and gut bacterial diversity. In turn, composition and size of the SCFA pool is an important determinant of host metabolic state [10]. The involvement of SCFAs and energy harvest in obesity was first brought to light in seminal studies performed by Bäckhed et al., in which GF mice were protected against diet induced obesity compared to their wild-type littermates [15]. In keeping with this result, GF mice also displayed reduced concentrations of intestinal SCFAs [28] and doubled their caloric excretion of undigested polysaccharides in feces and urine compared to conventional animals [29], supporting the causal role of gut bacteria in converting these substrates into a bioavailable energy source for the host. Furthermore, colonization of these mice with a healthy microbiome was sufficient to increase intestinal SCFAs and induce adiposity [15], while colonization with microbiota from an obese donor doubled this subsequent gain in fat mass [9]. Many animal and human studies have since confirmed increased levels of cecal and fecal SCFAs in obese subjects compared to their lean counterparts, indicative of higher rates of carbohydrate fermentation and energy extraction [30–33].

Further studies by Turnburgh et al. revealed that the microbiome of obese (ob/ob) mice displayed an enrichment of bacterial genes associated with increased energy harvest [9]. This finding has been confirmed in humans, via comparison of the microbial transcriptome in obese and lean di/monozygotic twins. Similar to obese mice, the obese human gut microbiome is enriched for genes involved in microbial processing of carbohydrates, an association representative of taxonomic differences in Actinobacteria (contributing 75% of obese-enriched genes) and Bacteroidetes (contributing 42% of lean-enriched genes) [23].

However, it appears that the metabolic effects of SCFAs are complex and pleiotropic, simultaneously conferring many benefits to the host that counteract their contribution to energy surplus and adipogenesis. For example, while G-protein coupled receptor (GPCR) mediated SCFA signaling serves to increase colonic transit time which may further enhance bacterial fermentation and energy extraction, it can also contribute to absorption of vital micronutrients from ingested food and promote host bowel regularity [34].

This dual role of SCFAs may in fact provide a net benefit, as multiple studies have demonstrated a function for SCFAs in protecting against diet-induced obesity. The reduction of weight gain by SCFA metabolites has been linked to a variety of mechanisms, including modulation of metabolic flux and satiety signaling. For one, SCFA signaling through FFARs 2 and 3 stimulates the secretion of glucagon-like peptide 1 (GLP-1) from intestinal cells and promotes intestinal gluconeogenesis, pathways that act twofold to enhance insulin sensitivity and reduce appetite [35,36]. Furthermore, in both mouse and human studies SCFAs have been shown to enhance intestinal production of the anorexigenic peptide YY (PYY) and the adipocyte-associated hormone leptin, both of which increase satiety levels and promote reduction of energy intake [34,37–40].

In addition to these enteroendocrine pathways, recent work has also demonstrated the neuroactive properties of SCFA metabolites, allowing direct modulation of appetite control. Particularly, acetate can cross the blood–brain barrier and enhance hypothalamic GABAergic neurotransmission, repressing appetite and reducing energy intake [41] Similarly, butyrate can suppress activity of orexigenic neurons in the hypothalamus and vagal afferents in the brainstem, an effect shown to mediate reduced food intake and protection against the effects of high-fat feeding [42,43].

Complementary to reducing food intake, many animal studies have confirmed the positive influence of SCFAs on body weight through increasing host energy expenditure. This effect is associated with upregulation of various thermogenic genes, thereby leading to enhanced mitochondrial function, browning of adipose tissue, and activation of lipid oxidation via gut–neural signaling pathways [44–47]. Specifically, den Besten et al. showed that SCFA supplementation upregulates expression mitochondrial uncoupling protein 2 and raises AMP-to-ATP ratio, thereby stimulating oxidative metabolism in liver and adipose tissue via AMPK [47]. The phenotypic outcome is dramatic increases to energy expenditure as well as reduced body weight and fat mass, despite little change in nutrient intake or high-fat feeding.

These effects have been investigated in humans, with similar overall outcomes despite providing less mechanistic insight. Canfora et al. showed that colonic administration of SCFA mixtures (comprising acetate, propionate, and butyrate) increased fasting lipid oxidation and resting energy expenditure (REE) in overweight and obese subjects [48]. Further in vivo data from human cohorts has corroborated the finding that SCFAs raise whole-body REE and lipid oxidation [49], and shown these changes to be independent of fasting glucose and insulin levels [50]. Although mechanistic studies of these SCFA-induced effects are lacking in humans, current work suggests they provide significant improvements to oxidative metabolism that may translate into long-term benefits in weight control.

2.2. Regulation of Immune Function

One of the hallmarks of obesity and metabolic syndrome is a systemic, low-grade inflammatory state. Research has shown that a wide range of inflammatory markers, including C-reactive protein and pro-inflammatory cytokines, are strongly associated with development of adiposity [51,52] and increased risk of metabolic disorders such as cardiovascular diseases, fatty liver disease, and type 2 diabetes [53]. More recently, direct mechanistic links have been suggested between obesity-associated systemic inflammation and the development of insulin resistance, the core diagnostic symptom of metabolic syndrome [54,55].

Although the causal relationships linking obesity, metabolic syndrome, and inflammation are incompletely understood, multiple lines of evidence implicate dysbiotic gut microbiota as a key modulator of immune signaling in the context of metabolic pathology. For one, lipopolysaccharide (LPS) derived from the cell wall of pathogenic Gram-negative microbes can bind toll-like receptors (TLRs) in mucosal and peripheral tissues, initiating pro-inflammatory signaling cascades [56,57]. Data from both human and rodent studies has linked an obese phenotype to elevated circulating levels of plasma LPS, a condition known as metabolic endotoxemia [58–60]. For example, in a comparative study of human subjects, baseline circulating endotoxin levels were found to be 20% higher in obesity or glucose intolerant individuals and 125% higher in type 2 diabetics compared to lean subjects [61].

Rodent studies by Cani et al. were the first to causally link metabolic endotoxemia to an obese phenotype. They found elevated plasma LPS could be induced by high fat feeding, which subsequently led to increased adiposity and metabolic dysregulation in the form of hyperglycemia and insulin resistance [62]. Interestingly, however, the same effect was achieved via artificial subcutaneous infusion of LPS into the blood plasma, even in absence of high fat feeding. Thus, not only is diet a direct factor in modulating systemic inflammation, but a pro-inflammatory state is sufficient to promote obesity and perturbed metabolic function. More recent studies have mechanistically corroborated these findings, linking microbiota-related inflammatory changes during HFD-induced obesity to Toll-like receptor 4 (TLR4) signaling and a resultant increase in plasma levels of LPS [63].

The potential contribution of the gut microbiome, especially a perturbed microbiome as seen in the context of obesity, to this phenomenon is twofold. For one, pathogenic strains that may dominate a dysbiotic gut are a rich source of LPS and other endotoxins, that may infiltrate circulation to initiate an immune response [56,57]. Second, there is strong evidence for the critical role of the gut microbiota in maintaining integrity of the gut epithelial lining, a function that if compromised would permit increased intestinal translocation of endotoxins into the blood [64].

The gut microbiome occupies the outer mucus layer of the intestinal epithelium, where it can interact with the luminal environment and metabolize dietary components. The inner mucus layer of the gut epithelium, on the other hand, is critical for limiting the exposure of epithelial cells to the microbiome and other potential pathogens entering the lumen from the external environment. However, resident bacteria also serve as a crucial line of resistance to colonisation and invasion by exogenous microbes that may harm the host [65]. Thus, the symbiotic yet complex relationship between the microbiome and gut epithelium serves to maintain a robust and tightly regulated mucosal immune defense mechanism.

Unlike pathogenic strains, many commensal species of gut microbes are known to help stabilize the mucosal membrane through promoting regular turnover of mucin glycoproteins [56,57] and stimulating intestinal endocannabinoid production that may help attenuate inflammation [66]. Furthermore, exposure to probiotic microbial species has been shown to promote upregulation of intracellular tight junction proteins [67,68] that provide an essential structural framework for maintaining mucosal barrier function.

Additional work has also pinpointed the role of bacterial SCFAs in maintenance of gut epithelial immunity. In vivo studies have demonstrated the potent trophic effects of SCFA metabolites on colonic epithelium cells. These include providing energy for cell growth, stimulating epithelial cell proliferation and differentiation, and enhancing mucus secretion, all functions that normalize intestinal permeability [69,70]. This not only further emphasizes the importance of bacterial SCFAs in promoting gut health, but provides mechanistic explanation for the observation that SCFA administration decreases systemic inflammation and immunoreactivity [71].

Thus, when considering the role of the gut microbiota in the etiology of obesity, one can attribute significant weight to the impaired intestinal barrier integrity and subsequent metabolic endotoxemia that develops in the presence of a dysbiotic microbiome structure. It follows that restoring a normal, healthy equilibrium between resident microbes and innate mucosal immunity would attenuate these systemic effects and potentially preclude development of morbid adiposity.

2.3. *Regulation of Bile Acid Metabolism*

The gut microbiota also participates in various stages of bile acid (BA) metabolism, and the bidirectional crosstalk between hepatic BA production and microbial ecology mediates a key interaction between the microbiome and the host. Postprandial primary BAs (cholic acid and chenodeoxycholic acid) released by the liver are modified and metabolized by the gut microbiota to produce bioactive secondary BAs, including deoxycholic acid (DCA) and Lithocholic acid (LCA) [72]. These microbial metabolites can bind cellular receptors including farnesoid X receptor (FXR) and Takeda G protein-coupled receptor (TGR5), thereby exerting profound downstream effects on lipid metabolism, cholesterol balance, and insulin sensitivity [73] that are particularly relevant to the discussion of metabolic pathology.

The dysbiotic microbiome structure displayed in obese phenotypes is accompanied by altered BA pool composition and metabolism, and a number of studies have associated elevated BAs and secondary BAs with chronic conditions including obesity and type 2 diabetes [72]. It has been shown that high fat feeding results in adiposity as well as an increase in total BAs across tissues (particularly deoxy- and taurodeoxycholic acid), which is associated with taxonomic microbiome restructuring to favor strains capable of BA processing [74]. Interestingly, another important property of BAs is that they exert potent anti-microbial effects, providing a feedback mechanism by which BA levels exert a strong selective pressure on the microbiota [75]. In fact, direct cholic acid supplementation has been shown to produce similar changes in microbiome composition to those seen in diet-induced obesity, including an expansion of members in the class *Firmicutes* capable of DCA production [75]. Thus, BA transformation by the gut microbiota can initiate changes in the BA pool size, while BAs can conversely initiate changes in the diversity and composition of the gut microbiota, both of which dramatically impact host physiology.

The aforementioned signaling properties of select primary and secondary BAs further complexifies this axis of microbe–host communication, especially in the context of obesity and metabolic disease. On one hand, BA-dependent TGR5 activation on the surface of enteroendocrine cells increases secretion of the incretin hormone GLP-1, which improves glycemic regulation in liver and pancreas, protects against insulin resistance, and improves satiety [76]. In addition, stimulation of TGR-5 by BAs induces browning of adipose tissue and increases skeletal muscle energy expenditure through thyroid hormone signaling, protecting against diet-induced obesity [76].

The role of FXR-mediated BA signaling in obesity is markedly more pleiotropic and complex, and is impacted by the microbiome via multiple avenues. For one, negative regulation of BA production by FXR signaling provides a mechanism by which the microbiome may directly influence the size of the BA pool and regulate lipid homeostasis [77]. This was demonstrated in elegant studies by Sayin et al. who found that in addition to regulating secondary BA metabolism the microbiome also inhibits BA synthesis in the liver by alleviating FXR inhibition in the ileum [78]. Furthermore, BA agonism of FXR can initiate the release of fibroblast growth factors (FGFs) 19 and 21, both of which contribute to insulin sensitization and hypolipedmia [79]. Finally, the bacterial enzyme bile-salt hydrolase (BSH) relieves inhibition of FXR signaling via selective cleavage of its antagonist tauro-β-muricholic acid (TβMCA). Colonization of mice with microbiota displaying enhanced BSH activity leads to reduced body weight, as well as lower serum cholesterol and hepatic triglycerides in colonized GF mice [80].

Although these findings may suggest a positive role for FXR in body weight homeostasis, other research suggests otherwise. Most notably, FXR-deficient mice are actually protected against both diet-induced obesity as well as induction of an obese phenotype via fecal transplant [81]. Furthermore, mice colonized with an obese microbiome show increased ileal BAs and FXR mRNA, suggesting a role for increased FXR signaling in microbial transmission of an obese phenotype [16]. Finally, and perhaps most interestingly, in direct contradiction to the aforementioned study Yao et al. found that knockout of *B. thetaiotaomicron* BSH in gnotobiotic mice led to reduced weight gain on a high-fat diet compared to WT-colonized mice [82]. This effect was associated with higher in-vivo levels of TβMCA, suggesting that repression of FXR signaling is key in preventing diet-induced adiposity.

Overall, although the exact signaling mechanisms connecting microbiome activity, secondary Bas, and obesity have yet to be entirely described, it is clear that phylum-specific regulation of host BA metabolism has a direct and profound impact on the development of pathological adiposity and related complications in glucose and lipid metabolism.

2.4. *Role of the Diet in Shaping the Microbiome*

As research continues to corroborate the central importance of the microbiome in host health and pathological processes, modulating the microbiome to potentially rectify dysbiotic metabolic states has become a research area of great interest. Among the factors contributing to microbiome dynamics, it has become well established through mouse and human studies that diet can play a critical role in microbiome remodeling and dramatically alter its structure within a mere 24 h. Administration of a Western diet promotes restructuring of the distal gut microbial community such that a Mollicute lineage in the *Firmicutes*, normally present at low abundance in the mouse colon, expands dramatically to dominate this body habitat [83]. This effect may be largely due to the competitive metabolic advantage conferred upon these strains by an abundance of simple sugars, such as sucrose, allowing their expansion to dominate other microbial sub-populations [83]. In addition, a high-fat, obesogenic Western diet has been proven to significantly reduce bacterial diversity and richness in the GI tract of mice, an effect that is readily reversible upon reverting back to a normal chow diet [84]. This effect has also been replicated in humans transitioning between high-fiber and high-fat-and-simple-sugar diets, with the microbiome showing equally flexible functional and taxonomic profiles [14].

Interestingly, the deleterious effect of HFD was also demonstrated to be compounding in nature, as persistent microbial signatures during repeated cycles of HFD lead to enhanced metabolic derangements and accelerated weight gain after a period of normal feeding [85]. Expanding on this finding, work by Sonnenburg et al. has shown that such diet-driven changes in microbiota may span further than an individual's lifetime, inducing extinction of certain commensal strains across generations [86]. Restoration of diversity and reappearance of specific microbes in this context could only be achieved upon fecal microbial transplant (FMT) but not from diet switching.

Overall, these data suggest that the metabolic perturbances correlated with the poor Western nutrition may in fact be due to diet-induced insult to our gut microbiome. In light of this, modulating the microbiome via dietary pre and probiotics offers a unique therapeutic strategy that may not only serve to reintroduce beneficial strains, but also sustain restoration of a healthy microbial ecosystem. Compared to strategies currently used in treatment of obesity, including bariatric surgery, physical exercise, and pharmacotherapies, pre/probiotics offer a minimally invasive approach that curtails undesired collateral effects [87] and can be easily integrated into one's lifestyle via a functional-food based dietary modification. Thus, we will now consider the characteristics and physiological benefits of pre and probiotics, through a lens of commercial applications in functional food products.

3. Pre and Probiotics as Functional Food Therapies in Obesity and Metabolic Syndrome

Historically, pre and probiotics have been well-documented for their positive effects on gastrointestinal health [32,88]. Put simply, probiotics involve the direct delivery of live bacterial cells to the host, either in the form of artificial encapsulation or fermented food products, whereas prebiotics comprise dietary components that are utilized by and hence promote growth of resident gut microbes. A great amount of debate has surrounded stringent definitions for both terms, but over the previous decade a consensus has largely been reached regarding salient criteria. A 2014 statement released by the International Scientific Association for Probiotics and Prebiotics restricted the use of the word "probiotic" to "Live microorganisms that, when administered in adequate amounts, confer a health benefit on the host." [89]. In addition, Gibson et al. recently proposed a parsimonious definition of the term "prebiotic" as indigestible food ingredients fermented by gut microbes, that serve as "a substrate that is selectively utilized by host microorganisms conferring a health benefit" [90]. This definition also expanded on previous work to potentially include non-carbohydrate compounds (such as polyphenols and polyunsaturated fatty acids), and requires evidence that any beneficial health effects of a true prebiotic are in fact mediated by the microbiota [90].

Based on the salient criteria for their classification, both pre and probiotic ingredients provide an optimal target for the development of novel functional foods. Although the concept of "functional foods" is not precisely and consistently defined, some of its unique characteristics include being a conventional or everyday food that is consumed as part of the normal/usual diet, having a positive effect on target function(s) beyond nutritive value/basic nutrition, potentially reducing risk of disease, and having authorized and scientifically based health claims [91]. Thus, the marriage of functional foods with the potent physiological benefits of pre and probiotics offers a unique opportunity for microbiome-targeted dietary modification to thrive in the consumer marketplace.

Working from these delineations, the remainder of this review will examine the utility of pre and probiotic functional foods in obesity, including current evidence supporting therapeutic properties of pre and probiotics, the metabolic mechanisms underlying their benefits to both the microbiome and the host, and the current progress towards developing accessible pre and probiotic functional foods to target metabolic pathology.

3.1. Prebiotic Functional Foods in Obesity and Metabolic Syndrome

As aforementioned, prebiotic fibers serve as a useful metabolic substrate for intestinal microbes, which convert them via fermentation into SCFAs and other metabolites in the gut lumen. Dietary sources of prebiotics include asparagus, garlic, leeks, onions, bananas, Jerusalem artichoke, as well as chicory, wheat bran, and barley [92]. Some of the main classes of prebiotic fibers, which are generally distinguished based on source, degree of polymerization, and constituent moieties, are summarized in further detail in Table 1.

Table 1. An overview of the main classes of prebiotic fibers.

Prebiotic Description		Properties	Dietary Sources	References
Fructans	Inulin	DP = 2–60 units linear chain of fructose with β(2→1) linkages	Asparagus, sugar beet, garlic, chicory, onion, Jerusalem artichoke, wheat, honey, banana, barley, tomato and rye, blue agave, yacon root, leeks	Murari, 2014 [93]; Singh et al., 2017 [94]
	Fructo-oligosaccharide (FOS) * OR Oligofructo-saccharide (OFS)	DP < 10 units linear chain of fructose with β(2→1) linkages		

Table 1. *Cont.*

Prebiotic Description	Properties	Dietary Sources	References
Galacto-oligosaccharides (GOS)	DP = 2–9 units Chain of galactosyl residues and a terminal glucose linked by β-(1–2), β-(1–3), β-(1–4), or β-(1–6) glycosidic bonds	human milk cow's milk produced commercially from lactose by β-galactosidase	Contesini et al., 2019 [95]; Fischer and Kleinschmidt, 2018 [96]
Polydextrose (PDX)	Average DP of 12 (ranges from 2–120) Highly branched glucose polymer with various kinds of glycosidic bonds (primarily B(1→6))	Synthetic prebiotic, synthesized via polycondensation of glucose and sorbitol	DeCarmo et al., 2016 [97]; de Sousa, 2011 [98]
Xylooligosaccharides (XOS)	DP = 2–10 units xylose moeities linked by β-(1→4) glyosidic bonds	Bamboo shoots, fruits, vegetables, milk, honey and wheat bran produced commercially from xylan-containing lignocellulosic materials	Aachary and Prapulla, 2011 [99]; Jain and Kumar 2015 [100]
Cyclodextrins	Cyclic oligosaccharides of D-glucopyranose units linked by (α-1,4) glycosidic bonds	Water soluble glucans enzymatic digestion of starch	Jansook, Ogawa, and Loftsson, 2018 [101]; Singh et al., 2002 [102]
Lactulose	Disaccharide consisting of galactose and fructose moieties	Synthesized from isomerization of lactose	Alsheraji et al., 2013 [103]; Sitanggang, 2016 [104]
Triphala	Various polyphenolic compounds and complex carbohydrates	Polyherbal preparation, of *Terminalia bellerica*, *Terminalia chebula*, and *Emblica officinalis*	Westfall 2018 [105]; Tarasiuk et al., 2018 [106]

3.1.1. Anti-Obesogenic Effects of Prebiotic Fibers

Prebiotic fibers derived from the diet preferentially substantiate the growth of known commensal bacterial strains such as *Bifidobacterium* and various phyla of *Lactobacillus* [107,108]. Furthermore, through modulating intestinal pH prebiotics create a bactericidal environment for putative enteropathogens such as *Clostridium perfringens* and *Escherichia coli*, whose growth is attenuated by an acidic milieu [109]. Thus, consumption of more high fiber foods alongside naturally sourced prebiotic supplementation offers a unique dietary avenue for modulating gut microbial composition and metabolism, in order to reap the beneficial systemic effects on host health.

Numerous experimental studies have demonstrated the benefits of prebiotics in combatting obesity and metabolic abnormalities, through various mechanisms of action. Among others, there is growing evidence that prebiotic-based therapy attenuates obesity-associated systemic inflammation. Work by Cani et al. showed that oligofructose (OFS) restored intestinal *Bifidobacteria* in obese mice, a change in microbiota composition that was negatively correlated with both fat mass and inflammatory tone (as measured via metabolic endotoxemia and plasma cytokines) [110]. Further studies have shown that administration of a prebiotic blend of xylo-oligosaccharide (XOS) and inulin attenuates the pro-inflammatory effect of a high-fat diet, reducing serum LPS concentration and LPS-dependent IL-1B expression [111]. In human trials conducted by Dewulf et al., obese women treated with inulin/oligofructose prebiotics displayed greater proportions of *Bifidobacterium* and *Faecalibacterium*, an effect that coincided with reduced fat mass and serum LPS [112].

Although these and other studies present clear evidence of a positive "prebiotic effect" on inflammation, the mechanisms underlying these metabolic outcomes are incompletely understood. It has been proposed that the prebiotic-induced proliferation of commensal microbial strains positively alters the structure of the gut mucosa, leading to decreased translocation of bacterial endotoxin and attenuating activation of TLRs at the luminal surface [113,114]. This prebiotic effect may be further enhanced by increasing the endogenous production of intestinal glucagon like peptide 2 (GLP2), which is known to reinforce gut barrier function through upregulation of critical tight junction proteins in the epithelium [115].

The microbe-mediated effect of prebiotics on the gut epithelium is twofold: not only does it bolster mucosal barrier function and enteric immunity, but also stimulates hormone production in epithelial enteroendocrine cells to regulate hunger and satiety signaling. As aforementioned, in addition to providing an energy substrate for the host, SCFAs produced by gut bacteria are also active signaling molecules that can influence a variety of downstream metabolic effectors. The SCFA fermentation products of prebiotic fibers, particularly propionate, can bind to receptors on the surface of epithelial cells, promoting secretion of the anorexigenic peptides GLP1 and PYY and increasing satiety in the host [116]. Indeed, it has been repeatedly demonstrated in animal studies that feeding with prebiotic fibers promotes enteroendocrine L-cell differentiation and increase both luminal and plasma levels of PYY and GLP1 [39,117], which in turn reduces energy intake. In humans, supplementation with fructans-type prebiotics (16 g/d) has been shown to increase plasma PYY/GLP1, decrease hunger levels and attenuate glycemic response [118]. Similarly, a regime supplementing the diet of obese subjects with 21 g/d doses of inulin type fructans led to increased plasma PYY and suppressed production of ghrelin, markers that coincided with reduced food intake, fat mass, and body weight gain [119].

In addition to modulating immune function and energy intake, the anti-obesogenic effects of prebiotics also involve improvements to glucose and lipid metabolism as well as glycemic control. Recently, Nihei et al. reported that α-cyclodextrin administration increased the concentrations of lactic acid and SCFAs in obese mice, which was associated with altered expression of metabolic genes that regulate lipid homeostasis. Specifically, prebiotic treatment upregulated the gene expression of peroxisome proliferator-activated receptor (PPAR)γ and PPARα involved in adipocyte differentiation and energy expenditure, respectively, while downregulating that of sterol regulatory element-binding protein-1c (SREBP-1c) and fatty acid synthase, thereby reducing lipogenesis [120]. Similarly, Bomhof and Saha found that prebiotic OFS treatment elicited potent effects on the gut microbiota of diet-induced obese rats, thereby reducing adiposity and improving glycemic control as measured by reduced fasting insulin and increased insulin sensitivity [121]. In another study by Ahmadi et al., supplementation with sago and acorn-derived prebiotic fibers was also shown to prevent HFD-induced insulin resistance in mice, reportedly via the combined action of reducing enteric mucosal inflammation and exerting a modulatory effect on hypothalamic energy signaling [122].

Work in humans has corroborated prebiotic enhancement of glycemic control, in both the context of heathy and obese or diseased patients. Dehghan et al. demonstrated the hypoglycemic and anti-inflammatory effects of oligofructose-enriched inulin in patients with type 2 diabetes, where subjects showed marked reductions in fasting glucose, body weight, and inflammatory markers of endotoxemia [123]. These results have been corroborated by other studies in T2DM patient cohorts [124]. More recently, a study by Chambers et al. investigating the physiological activity of inulin-propionate esters demonstrated that 20 g/day prebiotic supplementation elicited marked improvements to insulin sensitivity and systemic inflammatory markers compared with cellulose-supplemented controls [125]. Interestingly, this effect was associated with elevated stool concentrations of propionate, further highlighting the important role of SCFAs in mediating the insulin-sensitizing effects of prebiotics [125].

A variety of mechanistic links have been proposed mediating the glycemic stabilizing effects of prebiotics, including adiponectin-mediated clearance of plasma free fatty acids (FFAs) [126,127] as well as the previously discussed systemic effects of SCFAs that enhance glucose metabolism and lower plasma FFA concentrations in humans [128,129]. Even in absence of a precisely defined mechanism of action, current research clearly supports the efficacity of prebiotic treatment in alleviating obesity-associated perturbations to glucose metabolism and lipid homeostasis.

3.1.2. Prebiotic Functional Foods for Targeting Obesity

In the modern Westernized diet, it is rare that consumption of fruits, vegetables, whole grains, and other high-fiber foods is sufficient to reap the benefits of their prebiotic components. Indeed, while many of the studies corroborating the physiological benefits of prebiotic fibers utilize doses between 5.5 and 20 g per day, depending on the substrate in question, average daily consumption of prebiotics like inulin and oligofructose has been estimated at 1–4 g in the US [130]. Thus, while foods naturally containing prebiotic fibers may be considered "functional" in their own right, extraction and synthesis of prebiotic fibers such as inulin, fructo-oligosaccharides (FOS), galacto-oligosaccharide (GOS), and Xylo-oligosaccharides (XOS) offers an appealing industrial strategy for enriching a broader range of commercial food products.

Isolation of prebiotics can be achieved via water extraction on plants such as chicory root (5%–15% inulin) and Jerusalem artichoke (up to 20% inulin). Alternatively, many prebiotic fibers can be produced on a large scale via enzymatic processing of simple and complex sugars [92]. For example, GOS is commercially synthesized from lactose via the action of β-galactosidases, whereas FOS can be manufactured from sucrose using a transfructosylation reaction or via enzymatic hydrolysis of inulin extract [131]. Novel synthetic prebiotics can also be manufactured at scale. These include lactulose, which produced from an alkali isomerization process that convert the glucose moiety of lactose to a fructose residue [103]. Importantly, these fibers maintain prebiotic activity over a range of pH and temperature values, as well as when exposed to Maillard reaction conditions, assuaging manufacturer concerns around prebiotic stability during processing and storage [132].

Incorporation of prebiotic functional ingredients into foods provides many advantages and some unique challenges. In addition to their functional, health promoting characteristics, prebiotics display a number of unique physiochemical properties that may potentially enhance food products beyond simply improving nutritional profiles. These properties include the ability to heighten the consumer sensory experience through modulating texture and mouthfeel. In this regard, textural modification capacity largely depends on the prebiotic fiber's degree of polymerization, which in turn alters its solubility and interaction with other food components in the structural network [133]. In many cases, prebiotic fibers in appropriate concentrations improve the textural evaluation and sensory qualities of foods, primarily due to their gelling properties that allow them to improve bulk, increase viscosity, and enhance overall body and mouthfeel [103]. This has been demonstrated in yogurts, where addition of GOS, polydextrose, and inulin resulted in more consistent, elastic, viscous, and firm products based on instrumental and sensory assessment [134]. Additionally, products supplemented with up to 6% inulin received higher preference ratings from consumers in terms of consistency and flavor [134].

These same texture-enhancing attributes can be extended to application of prebiotic fibers as fat substitutes. The most promising candidate in this regard is inulin, given its ability to form microcrystalline networks that retain moisture and simulate a fine, creamy texture with a mouth sensation similar to that of fat [135]. Furthermore, its solubility allows for incorporation into non-solid food products like spreads, dips, dressings, and drinks while maintaining emulsion and a spreadable consistency [103]. In solid products like meat and cheese, these properties provide a creamier, juicier mouthfeel even with significant reduction of fat content. Berizi et al. demonstrated that inulin could be substituted for up to 6% fat in emulsion type sausages, in combination with 12% water, which reduced overall energy content by 64% while providing similar sensory evaluation to the traditional product [136]. Similarly, Hennelly et al. found that up to 63% of the fat can be replaced by inulin in an imitation cheese product, without affecting the melting characteristics [137]. Comparable results have been obtained by substituting inulin in reduced-fat cream cheese, fresh cheeses, cheddar, and mozzarella cheese (see [138] for a comprehensive review). Finally, in the realm of bakery products, Laguna et al. were able to successfully replace 15% fat content in biscuits, while maintaining sensory acceptability and increasing crispness [139].

In addition to reduced fat products, FOS offers unique properties that make it a valuable tool to food manufacturers as a sugar substitute. Being 0.4–0.6 times sweeter than sucrose and possessing similar properties to simple syrups, these sweeteners provide all the above-mentioned benefits of prebiotic supplementation while offering a low-calorie substitute to a known obesogenic ingredient [140]. Studies using confectionary products such as cakes, cookies, and caramels have successfully replaced up to 60% sucrose without impinging upon overall sensory acceptance [141,142]. However, a potential drawback in this application is that to compensate for their reduced sweetness, prebiotics must be accompanied by more potent artificial sweeteners, which have controversial and largely unknown long-term health effects.

Thus, the benefit of prebiotic-enriched functional foods in combatting obesity is twofold. On one hand, prebiotic addition objectively enhances nutrient profile and nutritional value, by increasing dietary fiber content and promoting growth of commensal gut microbes. However, prebiotics also actively enhance physiochemical properties of the surrounding food matrix, allowing for reduction in fat, sugar, and energy content without depreciating product taste and texture. These effects are bolstered by an overall improved sensory experience for the consumer, promoting regular product consumption and dietary adherence. Indeed, while the regular intake of prebiotic fiber from natural sources is staggeringly low, simple addition of a prebiotic-enriched functional food, generally containing 2.5–6.5 g prebiotics per serving, may serve to double or triple this baseline amount and meet a threshold for beneficial effects with a single dietary modification.

Overall, based on the available evidence prebiotics show considerable efficacy not only in restructuring and stabilizing the host microbiome, but targeting many pathological mechanisms associated with the development and metabolic consequences of obesity (summarized in Figure 2). Furthermore, these benefits can be readily exploited through prebiotic enrichment of popular consumer foods, increasing chances of consistent consumption and substitution of other macronutrients to improve overall nutritional profile. In light of these results, prebiotic functional foods should be considered as a potential therapy for the treatment and prevention of obesity, both in the form of dietary modification and prebiotic-rich functional food ingredients that can be incorporated into extant dietary staples.

3.2. *Probiotic Functional Foods in Obesity and Metabolic Syndrome*

An alternate approach for restructuring the gut microbiota is the oral delivery of viable bacterial strains (probiotics), that can be integrated into the gut ecosystem. Probiotics can take the form of capsules containing desired concentrations of live bacterial cells, however, in the modern marketplace consumers have access to various food products enriched with probiotic microbiota as functional ingredients targeted to improve digestive health. In addition to incorporation into food products, probiotic bacteria can also be blended with prebiotic fibers to sustain their growth and activity. This combinatorial approach, termed "synbiotics", may serve to further enhance beneficial probiotic effects [143].

It is of important note that not all probiotics are created equal, and the benefits they confer upon the host are highly strain- and dose-specific. This extra dimension of control implies that although they may provide many of the same advantages as prebiotics, via similar mechanistic avenues, targeted probiotic treatments require enhanced understanding of microbiome–host interactions to ensure desirable metabolic outcomes. This trade-off warrants a separate discussion of the clinical evidence surrounding probiotic therapy, to examine the formulations and protocols that lead to optimal potency in treating obesity and related metabolic symptoms.

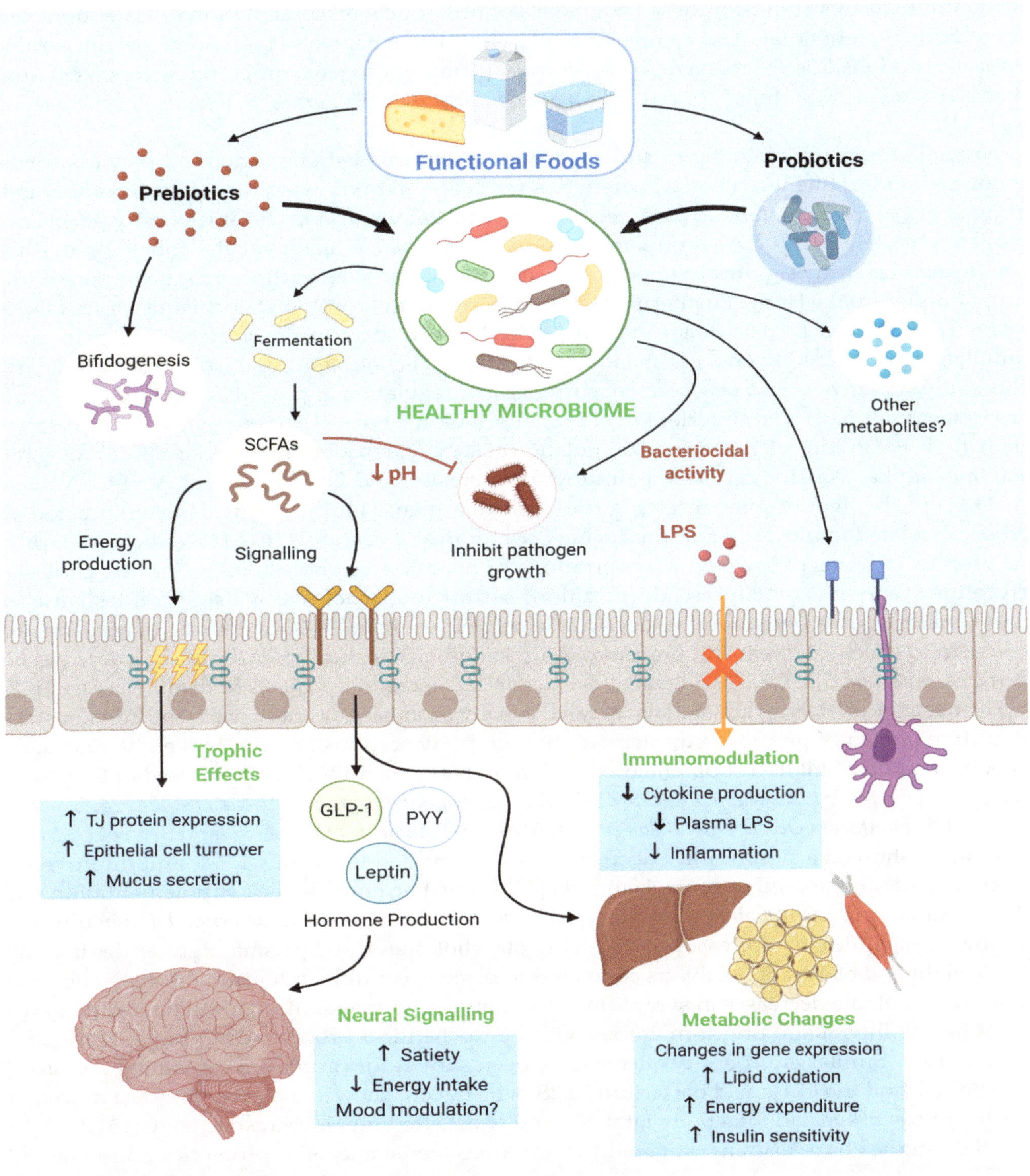

Figure 2. A summary of the mechanisms by which pre and probiotics delivered via functional foods initiate metabolic changes to combat development of obesity and metabolic syndrome. These mechanisms include the production of microbial metabolic products, noting short-chain fatty acids (SCFAs), a decrease in luminal pH, regulation of the immune system (modulating cytokine production), promoting satiety through gut–brain signaling and enhancing oxidative metabolism.

3.2.1. Clinical Evidence for Probiotic Therapy in Obesity

The most widely studied probiotic strains in humans and animals belong to the phyla *Lactobacillus* and *Bifidobacterium*. In a recent review compiling results from 72 animal studies and 15 human trials investigating various strains of these taxa, ≈85% of probiotic supplementation interventions led to reduced body weight or fat mass compared to placebo-treated controls [144]. Some specific strains of *Lactobacillus* and *Bifidobacterium* have shown consistent anti-obesogenic properties across most human and animal studies, including *L. casei, L. rhamnosus, L. gasseri, L. plantarum, B. infantis, B. longum*, and *B. breve* [144].

Animal studies of probiotic treatment derived from this list show marked benefits for both prevention and treatment of obesity, where this reduction in body weight is often accompanied by improvement of many metabolic parameters. Lee et al. demonstrated the anti-obesity effects of the conjugated linoleic acid (CLA)-producing strain *L. rhamnosus*, which over the course of an 8-week probiotic feeding study significantly reduced body weight and white adipose tissue in mice without altering energy intake [145]. Furthermore, mice treated with a probiotic consisting of *Lactobacillus curvatus HY7601* and *Lactobacillus plantarum KY1032* showed reduced body weight gain and fat accumulation, as well as lowered plasma insulin, leptin, total-cholesterol, and liver toxicity biomarkers. In this study, researchers also observed concurrent downregulation of pro-inflammatory genes (tumor necrosis factor alpha, TNFα; interleukin 6, IL6; interleukin 1 beta, IL1β; monocyte chemoattractant protein-1, MCP1) in adipose tissue and upregulation of fatty acid oxidation-related genes (PPAR-gamma coactivator alpha, PGC1α; carnitine palmitoyltransferase 1 and 2, CPT1/2; and Acyl-CoA oxidase 1, ACOX1) in the liver of mice receiving probiotic treatment [146]. Finally, hamsters treated with microencapsulated feruloyl esterase producing *Lactobacillus fermentum ATCC 11976* showed improved lipid profiles in terms of lowered concentrations of hepatic free cholesterol, esterified cholesterol, triglycerides, and phospholipids. In addition, serum total cholesterol, triglycerides, uric acid, and insulin resistance were found to decrease in treated animals [147]. Other microorganisms have also shown to effectively treat and prevent obesity in animals, including *Pediococcus pentosaceus LP28, Bacteroides uniformis CECT 7771, Akkermansia muciniphila*, and *Saccharomyces boulardii Biocodex* [148].

Further clinical trials in humans has revealed equally promising results, consistently demonstrating the positive impact of probiotic supplementation on body composition, body weight, and various metabolic markers. Children supplemented with a probiotic blend VSL#3 (composed of *Streptococcus thermophilus DSM24731, L. acidophilus DSM24735, L. delbrueckii subsp. Bulgaricus DSM24724, L. paracasei DSM24733, L. plantarum DSM24730, B. longum DSM24736, B. infantis DSM24737*, and *B. breve DSM24732*) for 4 months showed a significantly decreased BMI, increased levels of GLP-1, and improvements in liver adiposity compared to control subjects [149]. Furthermore, 8-week supplementation with a synbiotic containing *Lactobacillus acidophilus, Lactobacillus casei*, and *Bifidobacterium bifidum* plus inulin was shown to significantly decrease body weight, total cholesterol, and plasma triglycerides in a cohort of overweight and obese adult subjects compared to placebo controls. Interestingly, these effects were paralleled by notable decreases in symptoms of anxiety and depression in probiotic treated patients, suggesting the interaction of gut microbes with neurochemical processes that regulate mood and behavior [150]. Similar anti-obesity effects have been shown for probiotics containing *Lactobacillus gasseri BNR17* and the lactic acid bacterium LP28, which were shown to elicit significant decreases in visceral adipose tissue and total body fat, BMI, and waist circumference, respectively [151,152].

Other studies have also investigated the anti-obesogenic effects of probiotics administered as part of fermented food products. In a double-blind randomized controlled trial by Kadooka et al., obese subjects supplemented with fermented milk containing *Lactobacillus gasseri SBT2055* showed significant decreases in visceral fat, subcutaneous fat, and body weight, whereas controls experienced negligible change from baseline measures [153]. In a similar study using cheese supplemented with *Lactobacillus plantarum TENSIA*, obese hypertension patients showed significantly greater reductions to BMI compared to the placebo cheese group after 3 weeks of treatment, despite the fact that both groups were placed on identical calorie-restricted diets [154]. Finally, obese subjects consuming probiotic-enriched yoghurt (prepared with *S. thermophiles* and *L. bulgaricus* as starter culture, *B. lactis Bb-12* and inulin) had significantly reduced waist circumference and body fat percentage compared to those consuming plain yogurt, as well as lower triglyceride level and increased insulin sensitivity [155].

Similar work by Jones et al. demonstrated the efficacy of BSH-active *L. reuteri NCIMB 30242*-supplemented yoghurt for lowering LDL and total cholesterol in hypercholesterolaemic subjects, while increasing absorption of the fat soluble vitamin 25-hydroxyvitamin D [156,157].

Overall, these and other human clinical trials in both children [158] and adults [159,160] demonstrate that probiotic supplementation with various species of *Bifidobacterium, Lactobacillus* and other select taxa, either in isolation or as blended probiotics, elicit positive effects on obesity and associated metabolic pathophysiology. However, as aforementioned these results are highly dependent on the strains under study, the dosage used, and the duration of the intervention. In fact, some studies have found that certain strains such as *L. plantarum DSM 15,313* [161] and *Bifidobacterium animalis* subsp. *Lactis BB-12* [121] can increase weight gain in humans and animals, although concurrent improvements to glycemia and fasting insulin are also observed. This can potentially be attributed to the dual role of some microbial species in increasing energy harvest, a function that may be enhanced by artificial supplementation with select probiotic strains. Thus, while most research provides compelling evidence for the benefits of probiotics in treating obesity, further clinical and molecular studies are needed to further define the specific bacterial composition(s), dosage, and treatment period that will ensure and optimize anti-obesogenic effects.

3.2.2. Probiotic Functional Foods for Targeting Obesity

Numerous reviews have addressed and corroborate the direct benefits of probiotic administration in obesity, but few emphasize the importance of the food matrix as a delivery vehicle for probiotic cells. While some of the aforementioned studies utilize a food carrier and demonstrate its efficacity as a means of probiotic administration, most current literature considers the probiotic itself as a stand-alone functional ingredient such that delivery vehicle is irrelevant to experimental conclusions. Consequently, studies directly addressing the relative potency and clinical outcomes of isolated versus food-based probiotic treatments are sparse. In opposition to this view, however, some studies have shown that certain probiotic strains are effective in treating adiposity only in combination with certain food components but not in isolation, suggesting these ingredients play an active role in mediating their physiological benefits [162].

The ability of a probiotic strain to cope with stressors including encapsulated storage, temperature, oxygen, and a harsh gastrointestinal environment is important in not only the selection process of appropriate strains but devising a strategy to ensure their survival in the host. Faced with this challenge functional foods offer a unique opportunity to facilitate delivery and enhance potency, by interacting with probiotic ingredients in numerous ways. These benefits include inducing changes in cell viability and physiological status of the probiotic, providing complementary active ingredients and fermentation substrates such as fiber, and improving the likelihood of regular patient consumption through product palatability and incorporation into the diet.

Numerous studies support the advantages of a food-based delivery matrix for probiotic formulations over direct administration of isolated bacterial cells. Commonly, efficacious doses of probiotics range between 100 million and 10 billion CFU/day, which translates into cell levels of $\approx$1–100 million CFU/g of food, depending on serving size [143]. By far the most investigated food product in this regard is milk and its derivative dairy products, which are known to exert antimicrobial, immunomodulatory, and prebiotic properties that could effectively complement probiotic functions in the gut [143]. Furthermore, under simulated gastric conditions, dairy-based products such as fermented milk seem to outperform freeze-dried capsules [163] and saline solution [164] in terms of bacterial survival. Finally, in a recent review correcting for dosage and initial microbe concentration across studies, it was found that probiotics integrated into dairy-based food matrices show increased survival in human subjects compared to lyophilized probiotic powder or capsule delivery [165].

In addition to dairy, research suggests that many cereals, such as malt, barley, and wheat, support growth and resistance of probiotic bacteria in stressful conditions, thus offering an alternative probiotic product for individuals with restricted dietary needs [166]. The survival and stability of probiotic strains has also been shown in fermentable vegetable beverages, fruit juices, and peanut butter, among other food items [165].

Finally, perhaps the most promising approach to developing effective probiotic functional foods is addition of complementary prebiotic ingredients such as inulin and FOS, in what could be considered a synbiotic food product. This approach has been shown to improve probiotic survival in food products, presumably through provision of metabolic substrates that facilitate GIT transit [165]. For example, Speranza et al. recently formulated a novel synbiotic cream cheese with addition of lactulose and FOS, which was found to prolong cultivability of the probiotic strains *B. animalis* subsp. *lactis DSM 10140* and *L. reuteri DSM 20016* during storage and gastric conditions compared to probiotic addition alone. Not only did the synbiotic product maintain probiotic cell viability above recommended levels for 28 days, but addition of these functional ingredients did not introduce any adverse effects to the product's sensory acceptability [167]. Similarly, Oliveira et al. demonstrated the prebiotic potential of 4% inulin-enriched skim milk, fermented by co-cultures and pure cultures of *Bifidobacterium lactis* and various strains of *Lactobascillus*. The addition of inulin exerted a superior bifidogenic effect and enhanced probiotic survival during storage compared to regular fermented milk, in addition to improving the product's acidification kinetics and increasing apparent viscosity [168]. This effect has also been replicated in specifically formulated synbiotic cheese [169], yogurt [170], and ice cream [171], all of which optimize probiotic viability during storage compared to their unenriched counterparts.

Although many food carriers may contain some amount of fermentable substrate to sustain bacterial growth, the prebiotic component of these "complementary" synbiotics may not necessarily register any ecological advantage to the probiotic strain in question. Addition of strain-specific prebiotic fibers, as seen in the examples above, offers a "synergistic" approach, such that prebiotic ingredients are added to a food formulation with the exact purpose of supporting the growth of the probiotic strain [172]. Indeed, some investigations showing that the chain length of fructans is an important criterion to determine which bacteria can ferment them, meaning that specific probiotic strains may thrive in presence of some prebiotic fibers but not others [173]. Thus, in addition to providing nutrients that are beneficial to host health, including protein, fiber, vitamins, and minerals, probiotic-enriched functional foods can also offer a synbiotic environment that facilitates GIT colonization and may serve to augment anti-obesogenic effects.

Although this and other research provides a strong incentive to further investigate probiotic "functional foods" as an enhanced method of probiotic delivery, few studies have directly addressed the in vivo differences in bacterial viability and clinical outcomes conferred by a viable food matrix. Thus, the focus of future work should not only be centered around the physiological effects of probiotic supplementation in combatting obesity, but how functional food delivery vehicles can be optimized to improve microbial viability, stable colonization, and long-term dietary adherence.

4. Conclusion and Future Directions

In light of the current obesity epidemic plaguing much of Western society, there is a call for sustainable, accessible, and efficient treatments to combat this public health crisis. Although the etiology of obesity is multi-factorial and incredibly complex, recent research strongly implicates gut dysbiosis as a key contributor to its development and associated metabolic abnormalities. It thus follows that modulation of the gut microbiome to restore a stable, coherent metabolic state has become a research area of great interest in recent years.

Overall, the scope of the current literature provides overwhelming evidence for the benefits of pre and probiotic foods and their potential as a therapeutic avenue for treating obesity and metabolic syndrome. Such treatments, incorporating fermentable carbohydrates and/or strains of *Lactobacillus*, *Bifidobacterium*, and other select taxa, not only mediate improvements to body weight and adiposity but exert many positive effects on metabolic parameters such as glycemic control, systemic inflammation, and energy intake. However, gross generalizations of these results are to be interpreted with caution, as some studies suggest that certain bacterial species of these same genera may be ineffective or even deleterious for obese patients. Furthermore, an egregious lack of consistency in sample size, dose parameters, treatment duration, and drug delivery method hinders comparative analysis across studies, impinging upon the cycle of innovation that could allow pre and probiotic treatment to reach its full therapeutic potential.

In the face of these challenges, we propose a roadmap for the continued investigation of pre and probiotic treatment in obesity and metabolic syndrome, that hinges on the following set of recommendations:

1. A standardized clinical protocol for assessing the effectiveness of novel pre and probiotic formulations;
2. Further studies to expand current knowledge of microbiome–host interactions and how pre/probiotics can be used to modulate this dynamic relationship;
3. Direct investigation into the use of effective carriers and functional foods in order to optimize probiotic's effects on body weight;
4. Collaboration with manufacturers to improve production strategies for pre/probiotic foods and further incorporation of pre/probiotic functional ingredients into consumer products.

Using these recommendations to guide further experimentation, we can hope to better understand the subtle taxonomic and metabolomic microbiome alterations that contribute to development of obesity and related metabolic diseases. This knowledge, in turn, will allow future research to harness the potential of pre/probiotics in prevention and treatment of these ailments, and to develop integrative functional food solutions that are accessible to society at large.

5. Limitations of Pre and Probiotic Therapies

Although available data suggests a significant therapeutic potential of probiotics in obesity, many barriers remain to be overcome before probiotic treatment is endorsed in medical practice. Currently the United States Food and Drug Administration (US FDA) has approved a select list probiotic microorganisms, which are known to be considered as safe, for commercial use in food and in probiotic supplements [174]. However, the FDA has not approved any claims for probiotics that relate them to a reduction in the risk of disease or as a viable treatment for extant medical conditions [175]. Indeed, in addition to the numerous health benefits of probiotics there are risks and uncertainties associated with their use. Numerous reports have connected probiotic use to deleterious effects including sepsis, immunoreactivity, and gene transfer resulting in pathogenic antibiotic resistance [175,176]. These risks are of highest concern with respect to vulnerable groups including the elderly, critically ill, and immunocompromised, making probiotic use in the context of pathology especially prone to complications. Furthermore, the highly strain-specific effects of probiotic supplementation makes it especially susceptible to pleiotropic or unanticipated metabolic outcomes [175]. As such, there is an egregious lack of consensus in the literature and the field regarding the appropriate formulation, dose, and treatment schedule that will maximize patient outcome while minimizing collateral effects.

Overall, in order to be regulated at the level of a pharmaceutical or biological product, much further work remains to be done in order to ensure probiotic therapies meet standards of safety, purity, and potency appropriate for medical applications. By further understanding the mechanisms underlying both the benefits and detriments of probiotics in host health, there is opportunity to generate safe, targeted treatment methods that maximize the potential of probiotics in combatting metabolic pathology.

Author Contributions: Conceptualization: M.G. and S.P.; Data curation: M.G.; Funding acquisition: S.P.; Methodology: M.G.; K.A. and S.P.; Project administration: S.P.; Resources: S.P.; Software: M.G. and K.A.; Validation: S.P.; Visualization: K.A. and M.G.; Writing—original draft: M.G.; Writing—review and editing M.G., K.A., S.P. All authors have read and agreed to the published version of the manuscript.

References

1. James, P.T.; Rigby, N.; Leach, R. The obesity epidemic, metabolic syndrome and future prevention strategies. *Eur. J. Cardiovasc. Prev. Rehabil.* **2004**, *11*, 3–8. [CrossRef] [PubMed]
2. Fernandez, M.L. The Metabolic Syndrome. *Nutr. Rev.* **2007**, *65* (Suppl. 1), S30–S34. [CrossRef]
3. Stein, C.J.; Colditz, G.A. The Epidemic of Obesity. *J. Clin. Endocrinol. Metab.* **2004**, *89*, 2522–2525. [CrossRef] [PubMed]
4. Saklayen, M.G. The Global Epidemic of the Metabolic Syndrome. *Curr Hypertens Rep* **2018**, *20*, 12. [CrossRef]
5. Wahba, I.M.; Mak, R.H. Obesity and Obesity-Initiated Metabolic Syndrome: Mechanistic Links to Chronic Kidney Disease. *Clin. J. Am. Soc. Nephrol.* **2007**, *2*, 550. [CrossRef] [PubMed]
6. Haffner, S.; Taegtmeyer, H. Epidemic Obesity and the Metabolic Syndrome. *Circulation* **2003**, *108*, 1541–1545. [CrossRef] [PubMed]
7. Bäckhed, F.; Ley, R.E.; Sonnenburg, J.L.; Peterson, D.A.; Gordon, J.I. Host-Bacterial Mutualism in the Human Intestine. *Science* **2005**, *307*, 1915. [CrossRef]
8. Dinan, T.G.; Cryan, J.F. Brain–gut–microbiota axis—Mood, metabolism and behaviour. *Nat. Rev. Gastroenterol. Hepatol.* **2017**, *14*, 69–70. [CrossRef]
9. Turnbaugh, P.J.; Ley, R.E.; Mahowald, M.A.; Magrini, V.; Mardis, E.R.; Gordon, J.I. An obesity-associated gut microbiome with increased capacity for energy harvest. *Nature* **2006**, *444*, 1027–1031. [CrossRef]
10. Nehra, V.; Allen, J.M.; Mailing, L.J.; Kashyap, P.C.; Woods, J.A. Gut Microbiota: Modulation of Host Physiology in Obesity. *Physiology* **2016**, *31*, 327–335. [CrossRef]
11. Khan, M.J.; Gerasimidis, K.; Edwards, C.A.; Shaikh, M.G. Role of Gut Microbiota in the Aetiology of Obesity: Proposed Mechanisms and Review of the Literature. *J. Obes.* **2016**, *2016*, 7353642. [CrossRef] [PubMed]
12. Agustí, A.; García-Pardo, M.P.; López-Almela, I.; Campillo, I.; Maes, M.; Romaní-Pérez, M.; Sanz, Y. Interplay Between the Gut-Brain Axis, Obesity and Cognitive Function. *Front. Neurosci.* **2018**, *12*, 155. [CrossRef] [PubMed]
13. Zhang, C.; Zhang, M.; Wang, S.; Han, R.; Cao, Y.; Hua, W.; Mao, Y.; Zhang, X.; Pang, X.; Wei, C.; et al. Interactions between gut microbiota, host genetics and diet relevant to development of metabolic syndromes in mice. *ISME J.* **2010**, *4*, 232–241. [CrossRef] [PubMed]
14. David, L.A.; Maurice, C.F.; Carmody, R.N.; Gootenberg, D.B.; Button, J.E.; Wolfe, B.E.; Ling, A.V.; Devlin, A.S.; Varma, Y.; Fischbach, M.A.; et al. Diet rapidly and reproducibly alters the human gut microbiome. *Nature* **2014**, *505*, 559–563. [CrossRef]
15. Bäckhed, F.; Ding, H.; Wang, T.; Hooper, L.V.; Koh, G.Y.; Nagy, A.; Semenkovich, C.F.; Gordon, J.I. The gut microbiota as an environmental factor that regulates fat storage. *Proc. Natl. Acad. Sci. USA* **2004**, *101*, 15718. [CrossRef]
16. Ridaura, V.K.; Faith, J.J.; Rey, F.E.; Cheng, J.; Duncan, A.E.; Kau, A.L.; Griffin, N.W.; Lombard, V.; Henrissat, B.; Bain, J.R.; et al. Gut Microbiota from Twins Discordant for Obesity Modulate Metabolism in Mice. *Science* **2013**, *341*, 1241214. [CrossRef]
17. Ley, R.E.; Turnbaugh, P.J.; Klein, S.; Gordon, J.I. Human gut microbes associated with obesity. *Nature* **2006**, *444*, 1022–1023. [CrossRef]
18. Ley, R.E.; Bäckhed, F.; Turnbaugh, P.; Lozupone, C.A.; Knight, R.D.; Gordon, J.I. Obesity alters gut microbial ecology. *Proc. Natl. Acad. Sci. USA* **2005**, *102*, 11070. [CrossRef]
19. Nadal, I.; Santacruz, A.; Marcos, A.; Warnberg, J.; Garagorri, M.; Moreno, L.A.; Martin-Matillas, M.; Campoy, C.; Martí, A.; Moleres, A.; et al. Shifts in clostridia, bacteroides and immunoglobulin-coating fecal bacteria associated with weight loss in obese adolescents. *Int. J. Obes.* **2009**, *33*, 758–767. [CrossRef]
20. Remely, M.; Tesar, I.; Hippe, B.; Gnauer, S.; Rust, P.; Haslberger, A.G. Gut microbiota composition correlates with changes in body fat content due to weight loss. *Benef. Microbes* **2015**, *6*, 431–439. [CrossRef]
21. Sze, M.A.; Schloss, P.D. Looking for a Signal in the Noise: Revisiting Obesity and the Microbiome. *MBio* **2016**, *7*, e01018-16. [CrossRef] [PubMed]
22. Le Chatelier, E.; Nielsen, T.; Qin, J.; Prifti, E.; Hildebrand, F.; Falony, G.; Almeida, M.; Arumugam, M.; Batto, J.-M.; Kennedy, S.; et al. Richness of human gut microbiome correlates with metabolic markers. *Nature* **2013**, *500*, 541–546. [CrossRef] [PubMed]
23. Turnbaugh, P.J.; Hamady, M.; Yatsunenko, T.; Cantarel, B.L.; Duncan, A.; Ley, R.E.; Sogin, M.L.; Jones, W.J.; Roe, B.A.; Affourtit, J.P.; et al. A core gut microbiome in obese and lean twins. *Nature* **2009**, *457*, 480–484. [CrossRef] [PubMed]

24. Canfora, E.E.; Meex, R.C.R.; Venema, K.; Blaak, E.E. Gut microbial metabolites in obesity, NAFLD and T2DM. *Nat. Rev. Endocrinol.* **2019**, *15*, 261–273. [CrossRef]
25. Roediger, W.E.W. Utilization of Nutrients by Isolated Epithelial Cells of the Rat Colon. *Gastroenterology* **1982**, *83*, 424–429. [CrossRef]
26. Bergman, E.N. Energy contributions of volatile fatty acids from the gastrointestinal tract in various species. *Physiol. Rev.* **1990**, *70*, 567–590, (0031-9333 (Print)). [CrossRef]
27. Den Besten, G.; Lange, K.; Havinga, R.; van Dijk, T.H.; Gerding, A.; van Eunen, K.; Müller, M.; Groen, A.K.; Hooiveld, G.J.; Bakker, B.M.; et al. Gut-derived short-chain fatty acids are vividly assimilated into host carbohydrates and lipids. *Am. J. Physiol.-Gastrointest. Liver Physiol.* **2013**, *305*, G900–G910. [CrossRef]
28. Høverstad, T.; Midtvedt, T. Short-Chain Fatty Acids in Germfree Mice and Rats. *J. Nutr.* **1986**, *116*, 1772–1776. [CrossRef]
29. Wostmann, B.S.; Larkin, C.; Moriarty, A.; Bruckner-Kardoss, E. Dietary intake, energy metabolism, and excretory losses of adult male germfree Wistar rats. *Lab Anim Sci* **1983**, *33*, 46–50.
30. Fernandes, J.; Su, W.; Rahat-Rozenbloom, S.; Wolever, T.M.S.; Comelli, E.M. Adiposity, gut microbiota and faecal short chain fatty acids are linked in adult humans. *Nutr. Diabetes* **2014**, *4*, e121. [CrossRef]
31. Schwiertz, A.; Taras, D.; Schäfer, K.; Beijer, S.; Bos, N.A.; Donus, C.; Hardt, P.D. Microbiota and SCFA in Lean and Overweight Healthy Subjects. *Obesity* **2010**, *18*, 190–195. [CrossRef] [PubMed]
32. Gogineni, V.; Morrow, L.; Malesker, M.; Gregory, P. Probiotics: History and Evolution. *J. Anc. Dis. Prev. Remedies* **2013**, *1*, 1–7. [CrossRef]
33. Belobrajdic, D.P.; King, R.A.; Christophersen, C.T.; Bird, A.R. Dietary resistant starch dose-dependently reduces adiposity in obesity-prone and obesity-resistant male rats. *Nutr. Metab.* **2012**, *9*, 93. [CrossRef]
34. Samuel, B.S.; Shaito, A.; Motoike, T.; Rey, F.E.; Backhed, F.; Manchester, J.K.; Hammer, R.E.; Williams, S.C.; Crowley, J.; Yanagisawa, M.; et al. Effects of the gut microbiota on host adiposity are modulated by the short-chain fatty-acid binding G protein-coupled receptor, Gpr41. *Proc. Natl. Acad. Sci. USA* **2008**, *105*, 16767. [CrossRef] [PubMed]
35. De Vadder, F.; Kovatcheva-Datchary, P.; Goncalves, D.; Vinera, J.; Zitoun, C.; Duchampt, A.; Bäckhed, F.; Mithieux, G. Microbiota-Generated Metabolites Promote Metabolic Benefits via Gut-Brain Neural Circuits. *Cell* **2014**, *156*, 84–96. [CrossRef]
36. Tolhurst, G.; Heffron, H.; Lam, Y.S.; Parker, H.E.; Habib, A.M.; Diakogiannaki, E.; Cameron, J.; Grosse, J.; Reimann, F.; Gribble, F.M. Short-Chain Fatty Acids Stimulate Glucagon-Like Peptide-1 Secretion via the G-Protein–Coupled Receptor FFAR2. *Diabetes* **2012**, *61*, 364. [CrossRef]
37. Zaibi, M.S.; Stocker, C.J.; O'Dowd, J.; Davies, A.; Bellahcene, M.; Cawthorne, M.A.; Brown, A.J.H.; Smith, D.M.; Arch, J.R.S. Roles of GPR41 and GPR43 in leptin secretory responses of murine adipocytes to short chain fatty acids. *FEBS Lett.* **2010**, *584*, 2381–2386. [CrossRef]
38. Forbes, S.; Stafford, S.; Coope, G.; Heffron, H.; Real, K.; Newman, R.; Davenport, R.; Barnes, M.; Grosse, J.; Cox, H. Selective FFA2 Agonism Appears to Act via Intestinal PYY to Reduce Transit and Food Intake but Does Not Improve Glucose Tolerance in Mouse Models. *Diabetes* **2015**, *64*, 3763. [CrossRef]
39. Zhou, J.; Martin, R.J.; Tulley, R.T.; Raggio, A.M.; McCutcheon, K.L.; Shen, L.; Danna, S.C.; Tripathy, S.; Hegsted, M.; Keenan, M.J. Dietary resistant starch upregulates total GLP-1 and PYY in a sustained day-long manner through fermentation in rodents. *Am. J. Physiol.-Endocrinol. Metab.* **2008**, *295*, E1160–E1166. [CrossRef]
40. Chambers, E.S.; Viardot, A.; Psichas, A.; Morrison, D.J.; Murphy, K.G.; Zac-Varghese, S.E.K.; MacDougall, K.; Preston, T.; Tedford, C.; Finlayson, G.S.; et al. Effects of targeted delivery of propionate to the human colon on appetite regulation, body weight maintenance and adiposity in overweight adults. *Gut* **2015**, *64*, 1744. [CrossRef]
41. Frost, G.; Sleeth, M.L.; Sahuri-Arisoylu, M.; Lizarbe, B.; Cerdan, S.; Brody, L.; Anastasovska, J.; Ghourab, S.; Hankir, M.; Zhang, S.; et al. The short-chain fatty acid acetate reduces appetite via a central homeostatic mechanism. *Nat. Commun.* **2014**, *5*, 3611. [CrossRef] [PubMed]
42. Li, Z.; Yi, C.-X.; Katiraei, S.; Kooijman, S.; Zhou, E.; Chung, C.K.; Gao, Y.; van den Heuvel, J.K.; Meijer, O.C.; Berbée, J.F.P.; et al. Butyrate reduces appetite and activates brown adipose tissue via the gut-brain neural circuit. *Gut* **2018**, *67*, 1269. [CrossRef] [PubMed]

43. Goswami, C.; Iwasaki, Y.; Yada, T. Short-chain fatty acids suppress food intake by activating vagal afferent neurons. *J. Nutr. Biochem.* **2018**, *57*, 130–135. [CrossRef] [PubMed]
44. Gao, Z.; Yin, J.; Zhang, J.; Ward, R.E.; Martin, R.J.; Lefevre, M.; Cefalu, W.T.; Ye, J. Butyrate Improves Insulin Sensitivity and Increases Energy Expenditure in Mice. *Diabetes* **2009**, *58*, 1509. [CrossRef] [PubMed]
45. Sahuri-Arisoylu, M.; Brody, L.P.; Parkinson, J.R.; Parkes, H.; Navaratnam, N.; Miller, A.D.; Thomas, E.L.; Frost, G.; Bell, J.D. Reprogramming of hepatic fat accumulation and 'browning' of adipose tissue by the short-chain fatty acid acetate. *Int. J. Obes.* **2016**, *40*, 955–963. [CrossRef] [PubMed]
46. Kondo, T.; Kishi, M.; Fushimi, T.; Kaga, T. Acetic Acid Upregulates the Expression of Genes for Fatty Acid Oxidation Enzymes in Liver To Suppress Body Fat Accumulation. *J. Agric. Food Chem.* **2009**, *57*, 5982–5986. [CrossRef]
47. Den Besten, G.; Bleeker, A.; Gerding, A.; van Eunen, K.; Havinga, R.; van Dijk, T.H.; Oosterveer, M.H.; Jonker, J.W.; Groen, A.K.; Reijngoud, D.-J.; et al. Short-Chain Fatty Acids Protect Against High-Fat Diet–Induced Obesity via a PPARγ-Dependent Switch From Lipogenesis to Fat Oxidation. *Diabetes* **2015**, *64*, 2398. [CrossRef]
48. Canfora, E.E.; van der Beek, C.M.; Jocken, J.W.E.; Goossens, G.H.; Holst, J.J.; Olde Damink, S.W.M.; Lenaerts, K.; Dejong, C.H.C.; Blaak, E.E. Colonic infusions of short-chain fatty acid mixtures promote energy metabolism in overweight/obese men: A randomized crossover trial. *Sci. Rep.* **2017**, *7*, 2360. [CrossRef]
49. Van der Beek, C.M.; Canfora, E.E.; Lenaerts, K.; Troost, F.J.; Olde Damink, S.W.; Holst, J.J.; Masclee, A.A.; Dejong, C.H.; Blaak, E.E. Distal, not proximal, colonic acetate infusions promote fat oxidation and improve metabolic markers in overweight/obese men. *Clin. Sci.* **2016**, *130*, 2073–2082. [CrossRef]
50. Chambers, E.S.; Byrne, C.S.; Aspey, K.; Chen, Y.; Khan, S.; Morrison, D.J.; Frost, G. Acute oral sodium propionate supplementation raises resting energy expenditure and lipid oxidation in fasted humans. *DiabetesObes. Metab.* **2018**, *20*, 1034–1039. [CrossRef]
51. Choi, J.; Joseph, L.; Pilote, L. Obesity and C-reactive protein in various populations: A systematic review and meta-analysis. *Obes. Rev.* **2013**, *14*, 232–244. [CrossRef]
52. Bahceci, M.; Gokalp, D.; Bahceci, S.; Tuzcu, A.; Atmaca, S.; Arikan, S. The correlation between adiposity and adiponectin, tumor necrosis factor α, interleukin-6 and high sensitivity C-reactive protein levels. Is adipocyte size associated with inflammation in adults? *J. Endocrinol. Investig.* **2007**, *30*, 210–214. [CrossRef] [PubMed]
53. Hotamisligil, G.S. Inflammation and metabolic disorders. *Nature* **2006**, *444*, 860–867. [CrossRef] [PubMed]
54. Yuan, M.; Konstantopoulos, N.; Lee, J.; Hansen, L.; Li, Z.-W.; Karin, M.; Shoelson, S.E. Reversal of Obesity- and Diet-Induced Insulin Resistance with Salicylates or Targeted Disruption of Ikkβ. *Science* **2001**, *293*, 1673. [PubMed]
55. Osborn, O.; Olefsky, J.M. The cellular and signaling networks linking the immune system and metabolism in disease. *Nat. Med.* **2012**, *18*, 363–374. [CrossRef]
56. Ukena, S.N.; Singh, A.; Dringenberg, U.; Engelhardt, R.; Seidler, U.; Hansen, W.; Bleich, A.; Bruder, D.; Franzke, A.; Rogler, G.; et al. Probiotic Escherichia coli Nissle 1917 inhibits leaky gut by enhancing mucosal integrity. *PLoS ONE* **2007**, *2*, e1308. [CrossRef]
57. Pearson, J.; Brownlee, I. The Interaction of Large Bowel Microflora with the Colonic Mucus Barrier. *Int. J. Inflamm.* **2010**, *2010*, 321426. [CrossRef]
58. Cani, P.D.; Bibiloni, R.; Knauf, C.; Waget, A.; Neyrinck, A.M.; Delzenne, N.M.; Burcelin, R. Changes in Gut Microbiota Control Metabolic Endotoxemia-Induced Inflammation in High-Fat Diet–Induced Obesity and Diabetes in Mice. *Diabetes* **2008**, *57*, 1470. [CrossRef]
59. Creely, S.J.; McTernan, P.G.; Kusminski, C.M.; Fisher, F.M.; Da Silva, N.F.; Khanolkar, M.; Evans, M.; Harte, A.L.; Kumar, S. Lipopolysaccharide activates an innate immune system response in human adipose tissue in obesity and type 2 diabetes. *Am. J. Physiol.-Endocrinol. Metab.* **2007**, *292*, E740–E747. [CrossRef]
60. Clemente-Postigo, M.; Oliva-Olivera, W.; Coin-Aragüez, L.; Ramos-Molina, B.; Giraldez-Perez, R.M.; Lhamyani, S.; Alcaide-Torres, J.; Perez-Martinez, P.; El Bekay, R.; Cardona, F.; et al. Metabolic endotoxemia promotes adipose dysfunction and inflammation in human obesity. *Am. J. Physiol. -Endocrinol. Metab.* **2018**, *316*, E319–E332. [CrossRef]
61. Harte, A.L.; Varma, M.C.; Tripathi, G.; McGee, K.C.; Al-Daghri, N.M.; Al-Attas, O.S.; Sabico, S.; O'Hare, J.P.; Ceriello, A.; Saravanan, P.; et al. High fat intake leads to acute postprandial exposure to circulating endotoxin in type 2 diabetic subjects. *Diabetes Care* **2012**, *35*, 375–382. [CrossRef] [PubMed]

62. Cani, P.D.; Amar, J.; Iglesias, M.A.; Poggi, M.; Knauf, C.; Bastelica, D.; Neyrinck, A.M.; Fava, F.; Tuohy, K.M.; Chabo, C.; et al. Metabolic Endotoxemia Initiates Obesity and Insulin Resistance. *Diabetes* **2007**, *56*, 1761. [CrossRef] [PubMed]
63. Kim, K.-A.; Gu, W.; Lee, I.-A.; Joh, E.-H.; Kim, D.-H. High fat diet-induced gut microbiota exacerbates inflammation and obesity in mice via the TLR4 signaling pathway. *PLoS ONE* **2012**, *7*, e47713. [CrossRef] [PubMed]
64. Vallianou, N.; Stratigou, T.; Christodoulatos, G.S.; Dalamaga, M. Understanding the Role of the Gut Microbiome and Microbial Metabolites in Obesity and Obesity-Associated Metabolic Disorders: Current Evidence and Perspectives. *Curr. Obes. Rep.* **2019**, *8*, 317–332. [CrossRef] [PubMed]
65. Guarner, F.; Malagelada, J.-R. Gut flora in health and disease. *Lancet* **2003**, *361*, 512–519. [CrossRef]
66. Everard, A.; Belzer, C.; Geurts, L.; Ouwerkerk, J.P.; Druart, C.; Bindels, L.B.; Guiot, Y.; Derrien, M.; Muccioli, G.G.; Delzenne, N.M.; et al. Cross-talk between Akkermansia muciniphila and intestinal epithelium controls diet-induced obesity. *Proc. Natl. Acad. Sci. USA* **2013**, *110*, 9066–9071. [CrossRef]
67. Ewaschuk, J.B.; Diaz, H.; Meddings, L.; Diederichs, B.; Dmytrash, A.; Backer, J.; Looijer-van Langen, M.; Madsen, K.L. Secreted bioactive factors from Bifidobacterium infantis enhance epithelial cell barrier function. *Am. J. Physiol.-Gastrointest. Liver Physiol.* **2008**, *295*, G1025–G1034. [CrossRef]
68. Shen, T.Y.; Qin, H.L.; Gao, Z.G.; Fan, X.B.; Hang, X.M.; Jiang, Y.Q. Influences of enteral nutrition combined with probiotics on gut microflora and barrier function of rats with abdominal infection. *World J. Gastroenterol.* **2006**, *12*, 4352, (1007-9327 (Print)). [CrossRef]
69. Hamer, H.M.; Jonkers, D.; Venema, K.; Vanhoutvin, S.; Troost, F.J.; Brummer, R.J. Review article: The role of butyrate on colonic function. *Aliment. Pharmacol. Ther.* **2008**, *27*, 104–119. [CrossRef]
70. Topping, D.L.; Clifton, P.M. Short-Chain Fatty Acids and Human Colonic Function: Roles of Resistant Starch and Nonstarch Polysaccharides. *Physiol. Rev.* **2001**, *81*, 1031–1064. [CrossRef]
71. Vinolo, M.A.; Rodrigues, H.G.; Nachbar, R.T.; Curi, R. Regulation of inflammation by short chain fatty acids. *Nutrients* **2011**, *3*, 858–876. [CrossRef] [PubMed]
72. Ma, H.; Patti, M.E. Bile acids, obesity, and the metabolic syndrome. *Best Pract. Res. Clin. Gastroenterol.* **2014**, *28*, 573–583. [CrossRef] [PubMed]
73. Joyce, S.A.; Gahan, C.G. Disease-associated changes in bile acid profiles and links to altered gut microbiota. *Dig. Dis.* **2017**, *35*, 169–177. [CrossRef] [PubMed]
74. Lin, H.; An, Y.; Tang, H.; Wang, Y. Alterations of Bile Acids and Gut Microbiota in Obesity Induced by High Fat Diet in Rat Model. *J. Agric. Food Chem.* **2019**, *67*, 3624–3632. [CrossRef] [PubMed]
75. Islam, K.B.M.S.; Fukiya, S.; Hagio, M.; Fujii, N.; Ishizuka, S.; Ooka, T.; Ogura, Y.; Hayashi, T.; Yokota, A. Bile Acid Is a Host Factor That Regulates the Composition of the Cecal Microbiota in Rats. *Gastroenterology* **2011**, *141*, 1773–1781. [CrossRef]
76. Tremaroli, V.; Bäckhed, F. Functional interactions between the gut microbiota and host metabolism. *Nature* **2012**, *489*, 242–249. [CrossRef]
77. Kim, I.; Ahn, S.H.; Inagaki, T.; Choi, M.; Ito, S.; Guo, G.L.; Kliewer, S.A.; Gonzalez, F.J. Differential regulation of bile acid homeostasis by the farnesoid X receptor in liver and intestine. *J. Lipid Res.* **2007**, *48*, 2664–2672, (0022-2275 (Print)). [CrossRef]
78. Sayin, S.I.; Wahlström, A.; Felin, J.; Jäntti, S.; Marschall, H.U.; Bamberg, K.; Angelin, B.; Hyötyläinen, T.; Orešič, M.; Bäckhed, F. Gut Microbiota Regulates Bile Acid Metabolism by Reducing the Levels of Tauro-beta-muricholic Acid, a Naturally Occurring FXR Antagonist. *Cell Metab.* **2013**, *17*, 225–235. [CrossRef]
79. Cicione, C.; Degirolamo, C.; Moschetta, A. Emerging role of fibroblast growth factors 15/19 and 21 as metabolic integrators in the liver. *Hepatology* **2012**, *56*, 2404–2411. [CrossRef]
80. Joyce, S.A.; MacSharry, J.; Casey, P.G.; Kinsella, M.; Murphy, E.F.; Shanahan, F.; Hill, C.; Gahan, C.G.M. Regulation of host weight gain and lipid metabolism by bacterial bile acid modification in the gut. *Proc. Natl. Acad. Sci. USA* **2014**, *111*, 7421–7426. [CrossRef]
81. Parséus, A.; Sommer, N.; Sommer, F.; Caesar, R.; Molinaro, A.; Ståhlman, M.; Greiner, T.U.; Perkins, R.; Bäckhed, F. Microbiota-induced obesity requires farnesoid X receptor. *Gut* **2017**, *66*, 429–437. [CrossRef] [PubMed]
82. Yao, L.; Seaton, S.C.; Ndousse-Fetter, S.; Adhikari, A.A.; DiBenedetto, N.; Mina, A.I.; Banks, A.S.; Bry, L.; Devlin, A.S.J.E. A selective gut bacterial bile salt hydrolase alters host metabolism. *Elife* **2018**, *7*, e37182. [CrossRef] [PubMed]

83. Turnbaugh, P.J.; Bäckhed, F.; Fulton, L.; Gordon, J.I. Diet-Induced Obesity Is Linked to Marked but Reversible Alterations in the Mouse Distal Gut Microbiome. *Cell Host Microbe* **2008**, *3*, 213–223. [CrossRef] [PubMed]
84. Zhang, C.; Zhang, M.; Pang, X.; Zhao, Y.; Wang, L.; Zhao, L. Structural resilience of the gut microbiota in adult mice under high-fat dietary perturbations. *ISME J.* **2012**, *6*, 1848–1857. [CrossRef]
85. Thaiss, C.A.; Itav, S.; Rothschild, D.; Meijer, M.T.; Levy, M.; Moresi, C.; Dohnalová, L.; Braverman, S.; Rozin, S.; Malitsky, S.; et al. Persistent microbiome alterations modulate the rate of post-dieting weight regain. *Nature* **2016**, *540*, 544–551. [CrossRef]
86. Sonnenburg, E.D.; Smits, S.A.; Tikhonov, M.; Higginbottom, S.K.; Wingreen, N.S.; Sonnenburg, J.L. Diet-induced extinctions in the gut microbiota compound over generations. *Nature* **2016**, *529*, 212–215. [CrossRef]
87. Kumar, S.; Kelly, A.S. Review of Childhood Obesity: From Epidemiology, Etiology, and Comorbidities to Clinical Assessment and Treatment. In *Mayo Clinic Proceedings*; Elsevier: Amsterdam, The Netherlands, 2017; pp. 251–265.
88. Gasbarrini, G.; Bonvicini, F.; Gramenzi, A. Probiotics history. *J. Clin. Gastroenterol.* **2016**, *50*, S116–S119. [CrossRef]
89. Hill, C.; Guarner, F.; Reid, G.; Gibson, G.R.; Merenstein, D.J.; Pot, B.; Morelli, L.; Canani, R.B.; Flint, H.J.; Salminen, S. Expert consensus document: The International Scientific Association for Probiotics and Prebiotics consensus statement on the scope and appropriate use of the term probiotic. *Nat. Rev. Gastroenterol. Hepatol.* **2014**, *11*, 506–514. [CrossRef]
90. Gibson, G.R.; Hutkins, R.; Sanders, M.E.; Prescott, S.L.; Reimer, R.A.; Salminen, S.J.; Scott, K.; Stanton, C.; Swanson, K.S.; Cani, P.D.; et al. Expert consensus document: The International Scientific Association for Probiotics and Prebiotics (ISAPP) consensus statement on the definition and scope of prebiotics. *Nat. Rev. Gastroenterol. Hepatol.* **2017**, *14*, 491–502. [CrossRef]
91. Tufarelli, V.; Laudadio, V. An overview on the functional food concept: Prospectives and applied researches in probiotics, prebiotics and synbiotics. *J. Exp. Biol. Agric. Sci.* **2016**, *6*, 3.
92. Florowska, A.; Krygier, K.; Florowski, T.; Dłużewska, E. Prebiotics as functional food ingredients preventing diet-related diseases. *Food Funct.* **2016**, *7*, 2147–2155. [CrossRef] [PubMed]
93. Murari, S. Fructooligosaccharides-type prebiotic: A Review. *J. Pharm. Res.* **2014**, *8*, 321–330.
94. Singh, S.P.; Jadaun, J.S.; Narnoliya, L.K.; Pandey, A. Prebiotic Oligosaccharides: Special Focus on Fructooligosaccharides, Its Biosynthesis and Bioactivity. *Appl. Biochem. Biotechnol.* **2017**, *183*, 613–635. [CrossRef] [PubMed]
95. Contesini, F.J.; de Lima, E.A.; Mandelli, F.; Borin, G.P.; Alves, R.F.; Terrasan, C.R.F. Carbohydrate Active Enzymes Applied in the Production of Functional Oligosaccharides. In *Encyclopedia of Food Chemistry*; Melton, L., Shahidi, F., Varelis, P., Eds.; Academic Press: Oxford, UK, 2019; pp. 30–34.
96. Fischer, C.; Kleinschmidt, T. Combination of two β-galactosidases during the synthesis of galactooligosaccharides may enhance yield and structural diversity. *Biochem. Biophys. Res. Commun.* **2018**, *506*, 211–215. [CrossRef] [PubMed]
97. Do Carmo, M.M.R.; Walker, J.C.L.; Novello, D.; Caselato, V.M.; Sgarbieri, V.C.; Ouwehand, A.C.; Andreollo, N.A.; Hiane, P.A.; Dos Santos, E.F.J.N. Polydextrose: Physiological function, and effects on health. *Nutrients* **2016**, *8*, 553. [CrossRef]
98. Sousa, V.R.M.C.D.; Santos, E.F.D.; Sgarbieri, V.C. The Importance of Prebiotics in Functional Foods and Clinical Practice. *Food Nutr. Sci.* **2011**, *2*, 4. [CrossRef]
99. Aachary, A.A.; Prapulla, S.G.J.; Safety, F. Xylooligosaccharides (XOS) as an emerging prebiotic: Microbial synthesis, utilization, structural characterization, bioactive properties, and applications. *Compr. Rev. Food Sci. Food Saf.* **2011**, *10*, 2–16. [CrossRef]
100. Jain, I.; Kumar, V.; Satyanarayana, T. Xylooligosaccharides: An economical prebiotic from agroresidues and their health benefits. *Indian J. Exp. Biol.* **2015**, *53*, 131–142.
101. Jansook, P.; Ogawa, N.; Loftsson, T. Cyclodextrins: Structure, physicochemical properties and pharmaceutical applications. *Int. J. Pharm.* **2018**, *535*, 272–284. [CrossRef]
102. Singh, M.; Sharma, R.; Banerjee, U.C. Biotechnological applications of cyclodextrins. *Biotechnol. Adv.* **2002**, *20*, 341–359. [CrossRef]

103. Al-Sheraji, S.H.; Ismail, A.; Manap, M.Y.; Mustafa, S.; Yusof, R.M.; Hassan, F.A. Prebiotics as functional foods: A review. *J. Funct. Foods* **2013**, *5*, 1542–1553. [CrossRef]
104. Sitanggang, A.B.; Drews, A.; Kraume, M. Recent advances on prebiotic lactulose production. *World J. Microbiol. Biotechnol.* **2016**, *32*, 1–10. [CrossRef] [PubMed]
105. Westfall, S.; Lomis, N.; Prakash, S. A polyphenol-rich prebiotic in combination with a novel probiotic formulation alleviates markers of obesity and diabetes in Drosophila. *J. Funct. Foods* **2018**, *48*, 374–386. [CrossRef]
106. Tarasiuk, A.; Mosińska, P.; Fichna, J. Triphala: Current applications and new perspectives on the treatment of functional gastrointestinal disorders. *Chin. Med.* **2018**, *13*, 39. [CrossRef] [PubMed]
107. Roberfroid, M.; Gibson, G.R.; Hoyles, L.; McCartney, A.L.; Rastall, R.; Rowland, I.; Wolvers, D.; Watzl, B.; Szajewska, H.; Stahl, B.J. Prebiotic effects: Metabolic and health benefits. *Br. J. Nutr.* **2010**, *104*, S1–S63. [CrossRef]
108. Gibson, G.R.; Beatty, E.R.; Wang, X.; Cummings, J.H. Selective stimulation of bifidobacteria in the human colon by oligofructose and inulin. *Gastroenterology* **1995**, *108*, 975–982. [CrossRef]
109. Kaur, N.; Gupta, A.K. Applications of inulin and oligofructose in health and nutrition. *J. Biosci.* **2002**, *27*, 703–714, (0250-5991 (Print)). [CrossRef]
110. Cani, P.D.; Neyrinck, A.M.; Fava, F.; Knauf, C.; Burcelin, R.G.; Tuohy, K.M.; Gibson, G.R.; Delzenne, N.M. Selective increases of bifidobacteria in gut microflora improve high-fat-diet-induced diabetes in mice through a mechanism associated with endotoxaemia. *Diabetologia* **2007**, *50*, 2374–2383. [CrossRef]
111. Lecerf, J.-M.; Dépeint, F.; Clerc, E.; Dugenet, Y.; Niamba, C.N.; Rhazi, L.; Cayzeele, A.; Abdelnour, G.; Jaruga, A.; Younes, H.; et al. Xylo-oligosaccharide (XOS) in combination with inulin modulates both the intestinal environment and immune status in healthy subjects, while XOS alone only shows prebiotic properties. *Br. J. Nutr.* **2012**, *108*, 1847–1858. [CrossRef]
112. Dewulf, E.M.; Cani, P.D.; Claus, S.P.; Fuentes, S.; Puylaert, P.G.B.; Neyrinck, A.M.; Bindels, L.B.; de Vos, W.M.; Gibson, G.R.; Thissen, J.-P.; et al. Insight into the prebiotic concept: Lessons from an exploratory, double blind intervention study with inulin-type fructans in obese women. *Gut* **2013**, *62*, 1112. [CrossRef]
113. Peterson, C.T.; Sharma, V.; Elmén, L.; Peterson, S.N. Immune homeostasis, dysbiosis and therapeutic modulation of the gut microbiota. *Clin. Exp. Immunol.* **2015**, *179*, 363–377. [CrossRef] [PubMed]
114. Langlands, S.J.; Hopkins, M.J.; Coleman, N.; Cummings, J.H. Prebiotic carbohydrates modify the mucosa associated microflora of the human large bowel. *Gut* **2004**, *53*, 1610–1616, (0017-5749 (Print)). [CrossRef] [PubMed]
115. Cani, P.D.; Possemiers, S.; Van de Wiele, T.; Guiot, Y.; Everard, A.; Rottier, O.; Geurts, L.; Naslain, D.; Neyrinck, A.; Lambert, D.M.; et al. Changes in gut microbiota control inflammation in obese mice through a mechanism involving GLP-2-driven improvement of gut permeability. *Gut* **2009**, *58*, 1091. [CrossRef]
116. Posovszky, C.; Wabitsch, M. Regulation of Appetite, Satiation, and Body Weight by Enteroendocrine Cells. Part 2: Therapeutic Potential of Enteroendocrine Cells in the Treatment of Obesity. *Horm. Res. Paediatr.* **2015**, *83*, 11–18. [CrossRef]
117. Cani, P.D.; Hoste, S.; Guiot, Y.; Delzenne, N.M. Dietary non-digestible carbohydrates promote L-cell differentiation in the proximal colon of rats. *Br. J. Nutr.* **2007**, *98*, 32–37. [CrossRef] [PubMed]
118. Cani, P.D.; Lecourt, E.; Dewulf, E.M.; Sohet, F.M.; Pachikian, B.D.; Naslain, D.; De Backer, F.; Neyrinck, A.M.; Delzenne, N.M. Gut microbiota fermentation of prebiotics increases satietogenic and incretin gut peptide production with consequences for appetite sensation and glucose response after a meal. *Am. J. Clin. Nutr.* **2009**, *90*, 1236–1243. [CrossRef] [PubMed]
119. Parnell, J.A.; Reimer, R.A. Weight loss during oligofructose supplementation is associated with decreased ghrelin and increased peptide YY in overweight and obese adults. *Am. J. Clin. Nutr.* **2009**, *89*, 1751–1759. [CrossRef] [PubMed]
120. Nihei, N.; Okamoto, H.; Furune, T.; Ikuta, N.; Sasaki, K.; Rimbach, G.; Yoshikawa, Y.; Terao, K. Dietary α-cyclodextrin modifies gut microbiota and reduces fat accumulation in high-fat-diet-fed obese mice. *BioFactors* **2018**, *44*, 336–347. [CrossRef]
121. Bomhof, M.R.; Saha, D.C.; Reid, D.T.; Paul, H.A.; Reimer, R.A. Combined effects of oligofructose and Bifidobacterium animalis on gut microbiota and glycemia in obese rats. *Obesity* **2014**, *22*, 763–771. [CrossRef]
122. Ahmadi, S.; Nagpal, R.; Wang, S.; Gagliano, J.; Kitzman, D.W.; Soleimanian-Zad, S.; Sheikh-Zeinoddin, M.;

Read, R.; Yadav, H. Prebiotics from acorn and sago prevent high-fat-diet-induced insulin resistance via microbiome–gut–brain axis modulation. *J. Nutr. Biochem.* **2019**, *67*, 1–13. [CrossRef]

123. Dehghan, P.; Pourghassem Gargari, B.; Asghari Jafar-abadi, M. Oligofructose-enriched inulin improves some inflammatory markers and metabolic endotoxemia in women with type 2 diabetes mellitus: A randomized controlled clinical trial. *Nutrition* **2014**, *30*, 418–423. [CrossRef] [PubMed]
124. Pourghassem Gargari, B.; Dehghan, P.; Aliasgharzadeh, A.; Asghari Jafar-abadi, M. Effects of High Performance Inulin Supplementation on Glycemic Control and Antioxidant Status in Women with Type 2 Diabetes. *Diabetes Metab. J.* **2013**, *37*, 140–148. [CrossRef] [PubMed]
125. Chambers, E.S.; Byrne, C.S.; Morrison, D.J.; Murphy, K.G.; Preston, T.; Tedford, C.; Garcia-Perez, I.; Fountana, S.; Serrano-Contreras, J.I.; Holmes, E.; et al. Dietary supplementation with inulin-propionate ester or inulin improves insulin sensitivity in adults with overweight and obesity with distinct effects on the gut microbiota, plasma metabolome and systemic inflammatory responses: A randomised cross-over trial. *Gut* **2019**, *68*, 1430.
126. Tschritter, O.; Fritsche, A.; Thamer, C.; Haap, M.; Shirkavand, F.; Rahe, S.; Staiger, H.; Maerker, E.; Häring, H.; Stumvoll, M. Plasma Adiponectin Concentrations Predict Insulin Sensitivity of Both Glucose and Lipid Metabolism. *Diabetes* **2003**, *52*, 239. [CrossRef]
127. Alligier, M.; Dewulf, E.M.; Salazar, N.; Mairal, A.; Neyrinck, A.M.; Cani, P.D.; Langin, D.; Delzenne, N.M. Positive interaction between prebiotics and thiazolidinedione treatment on adiposity in diet-induced obese mice. *Obesity* **2014**, *22*, 1653–1661. [CrossRef] [PubMed]
128. Thorburn, A.; Muir, J.; Proietto, J. Carbohydrate fermentation decreases hepatic glucose output in healthy subjects. *Metabolism* **1993**, *42*, 780–785. [CrossRef]
129. Berggren, A.M.; Nyman, E.M.G.L.; Lundquist, I.; Björck, I.M.E. Influence of orally and rectally administered propionate on cholesterol and glucose metabolism in obese rats. *Br. J. Nutr.* **1996**, *76*, 287–294. [CrossRef]
130. Roberfroid, M.B. Prebiotics and probiotics: Are they functional foods? *Am. J. Clin. Nutr.* **2000**, *71*, 1682S–1687S. [CrossRef]
131. Martins, G.N.; Ureta, M.M.; Tymczyszyn, E.E.; Castilho, P.C.; Gomez-Zavaglia, A. Technological Aspects of the Production of Fructo and Galacto-Oligosaccharides. *Enzymatic Synthesis and Hydrolysis.* **2019**, 6.
132. Huebner, J.; Wehling, R.L.; Parkhurst, A.; Hutkins, R.W. Effect of processing conditions on the prebiotic activity of commercial prebiotics. *Int. Dairy J.* **2008**, *18*, 287–293. [CrossRef]
133. Guimarães, J.T.; Balthazar, C.F.; Silva, R.; Rocha, R.S.; Graça, J.S.; Esmerino, E.A.; Silva, M.r.C.; Sant'Ana, A.S.; Duarte, M.C.K.H.; Freitas, M.Q.; et al. Impact of probiotics and prebiotics on food texture. *Curr. Opin. Food Sci.* **2020**, *33*, 38–44. [CrossRef]
134. Costa, M.F.; Pimentel, T.C.; Guimaraes, J.T.; Balthazar, C.F.; Rocha, R.S.; Cavalcanti, R.N.; Esmerino, E.A.; Freitas, M.Q.; Raices, R.S.L.; Silva, M.C.; et al. Impact of prebiotics on the rheological characteristics and volatile compounds of Greek yogurt. *LWT Food Sci. Technol.* **2019**, *105*, 371–376. [CrossRef]
135. Rodriguez Furlán, L.; Campderros, M. The combined effects of Stevia and sucralose as sugar substitute and inulin as fat mimetic on the physicochemical properties of sugar-free reduced-fat dairy dessert. *Int. J. Gastron. Food Sci.* **2017**, *10*, 16–23. [CrossRef]
136. Berizi, E.; Shekarforoush, S.S.; Mohammadinezhad, S.; Hosseinzadeh, S.; Farahnaki, A. The use of inulin as fat replacer and its effect on texture and sensory properties of emulsion type sausages. *Iran. J. Vet. Res.* **2017**, *18*, 253–257.
137. Hennelly, P.J.; Dunne, P.G.; O'Sullivan, M.; O'Riordan, E.D. Textural, rheological and microstructural properties of imitation cheese containing inulin. *J. Food Eng.* **2006**, *75*, 388–395. [CrossRef]
138. Karimi, R.; Azizi, M.H.; Ghasemlou, M.; Vaziri, M. Application of inulin in cheese as prebiotic, fat replacer and texturizer: A review. *Carbohydr. Polym.* **2015**, *119*, 85–100. [CrossRef]
139. Laguna, L.; Primo-Martín, C.; Varela, P.; Salvador, A.; Sanz, T. HPMC and inulin as fat replacers in biscuits: Sensory and instrumental evaluation. *LWT Food Sci. Technol.* **2014**, *56*, 494–501. [CrossRef]
140. Bali, V.; Panesar, P.S.; Bera, M.B.; Panesar, R.J. Fructo-oligosaccharides: Production, purification and potential applications. *Crit. Rev. Food Sci. Nutr.* **2015**, *55*, 1475–1490. [CrossRef]
141. Handa, C.; Goomer, S.; Siddhu, A. Physicochemical properties and sensory evaluation of fructoligosaccharide enriched cookies. *J. Food Sci. Technol.* **2012**, *49*, 192–199. [CrossRef]
142. Protonotariou, S.V.; Karali, E.; Evageliou, V.; Yanniotis, S.; Mandala, I. Rheological and sensory attributes of

cream caramel desserts containing fructooligosaccharides as substitute sweeteners. *Int. J. Food Sci. Technol.* **2013** *48*, 663–669. [CrossRef]

143. Sanders, M.E.; Marco, M.L. Food Formats for Effective Delivery of Probiotics. *Annu. Rev. Food Sci. Technol.* **2010**, *1*, 65–85. [CrossRef] [PubMed]
144. Ejtahed, H.-S.; Angoorani, P.; Soroush, A.-R.; Atlasi, R.; Hasani-Ranjbar, S.; Mortazavian, A.M.; Larijani, B. Probiotics supplementation for the obesity management; A systematic review of animal studies and clinical trials. *J. Funct. Foods* **2019**, *52*, 228–242. [CrossRef]
145. Lee, H.-Y.; Park, J.-H.; Seok, S.-H.; Baek, M.-W.; Kim, D.-J.; Lee, K.-E.; Paek, K.-S.; Lee, Y.; Park, J.-H. Human originated bacteria, Lactobacillus rhamnosus PL60, produce conjugated linoleic acid and show anti-obesity effects in diet-induced obese mice. *Biochim. Et Biophys. Acta (Bba) Mol. Cell Biol. Lipids* **2006**, *1761*, 736–744. [CrossRef] [PubMed]
146. Park, D.-Y.; Ahn, Y.-T.; Park, S.-H.; Huh, C.-S.; Yoo, S.-R.; Yu, R.; Sung, M.-K.; McGregor, R.A.; Choi, M.-S. Supplementation of Lactobacillus curvatus HY7601 and Lactobacillus plantarum KY1032 in diet-induced obese mice is associated with gut microbial changes and reduction in obesity. *PLoS ONE* **2013**, *8*, e59470. [CrossRef]
147. Bhathena, J.; Martoni, C.; Kulamarva, A.; Tomaro-Duchesneau, C.; Malhotra, M.; Paul, A.; Urbanska, A.M.; Prakash, S. Oral Probiotic Microcapsule Formulation Ameliorates Non-Alcoholic Fatty Liver Disease in Bio F1B Golden Syrian Hamsters. *PLoS ONE* **2013**, *8*, e58394. [CrossRef]
148. Cerdó, T.; García-Santos, J.A.; GBermúdez, M.; Campoy, C. The Role of Probiotics and Prebiotics in the Prevention and Treatment of Obesity. *Nutrients* **2019**, *11*, 635. [CrossRef]
149. Alisi, A.; Bedogni, G.; Baviera, G.; Giorgio, V.; Porro, E.; Paris, C.; Giammaria, P.; Reali, L.; Anania, F.; Nobili, V. Randomised clinical trial: The beneficial effects of VSL#3 in obese children with non-alcoholic steatohepatitis. *Aliment. Pharmacol. Ther.* **2014**, *39*, 1276–1285.
150. Hadi, A.; Sepandi, M.; Marx, W.; Moradi, S.; Parastouei, K. Clinical and psychological responses to synbiotic supplementation in obese or overweight adults: A randomized clinical trial. *Complementary Ther. Med.* **2019**, *47*, 102216. [CrossRef]
151. Kim, J.; Yun, J.M.; Kim, M.K.; Kwon, O.; Cho, B. Lactobacillus gasseri BNR17 Supplementation Reduces the Visceral Fat Accumulation and Waist Circumference in Obese Adults: A Randomized, Double-Blind, Placebo-Controlled Trial. *J. Med. Food* **2018**, *21*, 454–461. [CrossRef]
152. Higashikawa, F.; Noda, M.; Awaya, T.; Danshiitsoodol, N.; Matoba, Y.; Kumagai, T.; Sugiyama, M.J. Antiobesity effect of Pediococcus pentosaceus LP28 on overweight subjects: A randomized, double-blind, placebo-controlled clinical trial. *Eur. J. Clin. Nutr.* **2016**, *70*, 582–587. [CrossRef]
153. Kadooka, Y.; Sato, M.; Imaizumi, K.; Ogawa, A.; Ikuyama, K.; Akai, Y.; Okano, M.; Kagoshima, M.; Tsuchida, T. Regulation of abdominal adiposity by probiotics (Lactobacillus gasseri SBT2055) in adults with obese tendencies in a randomized controlled trial. *Eur. J. Clin. Nutr.* **2010**, *64*, 636–643. [CrossRef] [PubMed]
154. Sharafedtinov, K.K.; Plotnikova, O.A.; Alexeeva, R.I.; Sentsova, T.B.; Songisepp, E.; Stsepetova, J.; Smidt, I.; Mikelsaar, M. Hypocaloric diet supplemented with probiotic cheese improves body mass index and blood pressure indices of obese hypertensive patients–a randomized double-blind placebo-controlled pilot study. *Nutr. J.* **2013**, *12*, 138. [CrossRef] [PubMed]
155. Mohammadi-Sartang, M.; Bellissimo, N.; Totosy de Zepetnek, J.O.; Brett, N.R.; Mazloomi, S.M.; Fararouie, M.; Bedeltavana, A.; Famouri, M.; Mazloom, Z. The effect of daily fortified yogurt consumption on weight loss in adults with metabolic syndrome: A 10-week randomized controlled trial. *Nutr. Metab. Cardiovasc. Dis.* **2018**, *28*, 565–574. [CrossRef]
156. Jones, M.L.; Martoni, C.J.; Prakash, S. Oral Supplementation With *Probiotic* L. reuteri NCIMB 30242 Increases Mean Circulating 25-Hydroxyvitamin D: A Post Hoc Analysis of a Randomized Controlled Trial. *J. Clin. Endocrinol. Metab.* **2013**, *98*, 2944–2951. [CrossRef] [PubMed]
157. Jones, M.L.; Martoni, C.J.; Parent, M.; Prakash, S. Cholesterol-lowering efficacy of a microencapsulated bile salt hydrolase-active Lactobacillus reuteri NCIMB 30242 yoghurt formulation in hypercholesterolaemic adults. *Br. J. Nutr.* **2012**, *107*, 1505–1513. [CrossRef] [PubMed]
158. Sanchis-Chordà, J.; del Pulgar, E.M.G.; Carrasco-Luna, J.; Benítez-Páez, A.; Sanz, Y.; Codoñer-Franch, P.J. Bifidobacterium pseudocatenulatum CECT 7765 supplementation improves inflammatory status in insulin-resistant obese children. *Eur. J. Nutr.* **2019**, *58*, 2789–2800. [CrossRef]

159. Pedret, A.; Valls, R.M.; Calderón-Pérez, L.; Llauradó, E.; Companys, J.; Pla-Pagà, L.; Moragas, A.; Martín-Luján, F.; Ortega, Y.; Giralt, M.J. Effects of daily consumption of the probiotic *Bifidobacterium animalis* subsp. *lactis* CECT 8145 on anthropometric adiposity biomarkers in abdominally obese subjects: A randomized controlled trial. *Int. J. Obes.* **2019**, *43*, 1863–1868. [CrossRef]
160. Minami, J.; Iwabuchi, N.; Tanaka, M.; Yamauchi, K.; Xiao, J.Z.; Abe, F.; Sakane, N. Effects of Bifidobacterium breve B-3 on body fat reductions in pre-obese adults: A randomized, double-blind, placebo-controlled trial. *Biosci. Microbiota Food Health* **2018**. (2186-6953 (Print)). [CrossRef]
161. Andersson, U.; Bränning, C.; Ahrné, S.; Molin, G.; Alenfall, J.; Önning, G.; Nyman, M.; Holm, C.J.B.M. Probiotics lower plasma glucose in the high-fat fed C57BL/6J mouse. *Benef. Microbes* **2010**, *1*, 189–196. [CrossRef]
162. Ali, A.A.; Velasquez, M.T.; Hansen, C.T.; Mohamed, A.I.; Bhathena, S.J. Effects of soybean isoflavones, probiotics, and their interactions on lipid metabolism and endocrine system in an animal model of obesity and diabetes. *J. Nutr. Biochem.* **2004**, *15*, 583–590, (0955-2863 (Print)). [CrossRef]
163. Fredua-Agyeman, M.; Gaisford, S. Comparative survival of commercial probiotic formulations: Tests in biorelevant gastric fluids and real-time measurements using microcalorimetry. *Benef. Microbes* **2015**, *6*, 141–151. [CrossRef]
164. Wang, J.; Zhong, Z.; Zhang, W.; Bao, Q.; Wei, A.; Meng, H.; Zhang, H. Comparative analysis of the gene expression profile of probiotic Lactobacillus casei Zhang with and without fermented milk as a vehicle during transit in a simulated gastrointestinal tract. *Res. Microbiol.* **2012**, *163*, 357–365. [CrossRef] [PubMed]
165. Flach, J.; van der Waal, M.B.; van den Nieuwboer, M.; Claassen, E.; Larsen, O.F.A. The underexposed role of food matrices in probiotic products: Reviewing the relationship between carrier matrices and product parameters. *Crit. Rev. Food Sci. Nutr.* **2018**, *58*, 2570–2584. [CrossRef] [PubMed]
166. Shori, A.B. Influence of food matrix on the viability of probiotic bacteria: A review based on dairy and non-dairy beverages. *Food Biosci.* **2016**, *13*, 1–8. [CrossRef]
167. Speranza, B.; Campaniello, D.; Monacis, N.; Bevilacqua, A.; Sinigaglia, M.; Corbo, M.R. Functional cream cheese supplemented with *Bifidobacterium animalis* subsp. *lactis* DSM 10140 and *Lactobacillus reuteri* DSM 20016 and prebiotics. *Food Microbiol.* **2018**, *72*, 16–22. [CrossRef] [PubMed]
168. De Souza Oliveira, R.P.; Perego, P.; de Oliveira, M.N.; Converti, A. Effect of inulin as prebiotic and synbiotic interactions between probiotics to improve fermented milk firmness. *J. Food Eng.* **2011**, *107*, 36–40. [CrossRef]
169. Angiolillo, L.; Conte, A.; Faccia, M.; Zambrini, A.V.; Del Nobile, M.A. A new method to produce synbiotic Fiordilatte cheese. *Innov. Food Sci. Emerg. Technol.* **2014**, *22*, 180–187. [CrossRef]
170. Donkor, O.N.; Henriksson, A.; Vasiljevic, T.; Shah, N.P. Effect of acidification on the activity of probiotics in yoghurt during cold storage. *Int. Dairy J.* **2006**, *16*, 1181–1189. [CrossRef]
171. Parussolo, G.; Busatto, R.T.; Schmitt, J.; Pauletto, R.; Schons, P.F.; Ries, E.F. Synbiotic ice cream containing yacon flour and Lactobacillus acidophylus NCFM. *LWT Food Sci. Technol.* **2017**, *82*, 192–198. [CrossRef]
172. Krumbeck, J.A.; Walter, J.; Hutkins, R.W. Synbiotics for Improved Human Health: Recent Developments, Challenges, and Opportunities. *Annu. Rev. Food Sci. Technol.* **2018**, *9*, 451–479. [CrossRef]
173. Scott, K.P.; Martin, J.C.; Duncan, S.H.; Flint, H.J. Prebiotic stimulation of human colonic butyrate-producing bacteria and bifidobacteria, in vitro. *Fems Microbiol. Ecol.* **2014**, *87*, 30–40. [CrossRef] [PubMed]
174. Bhadoria, P.; Mahapatra, S.C. Prospects, technological aspects and limitations of probiotics—A worldwide review. *Eur. J. Food Res. Rev.* **2001**, *1*, 23–42.
175. Ayichew, T.; Belete, A.; Alebachew, T.; Tsehaye, H.; Berhanu, H.; Minwuyelet, A. Bacterial Probiotics their Importances and Limitations: A Review. *J. Nutr. Health Sci.* **2017**, *4*, 202.
176. Boyle, R.J.; Robins-Browne, R.M.; Tang, M.L.K. Probiotic use in clinical practice: What are the risks? *Am. J. Clin. Nutr.* **2006**, *83*, 1256–1264. [CrossRef] [PubMed]

3

Probiotics, Prebiotics and Synbiotics—A Promising Strategy in Prevention and Treatment of Cardiovascular Diseases?

Beata Olas

Department of General Biochemistry, Faculty of Biology and Environmental Protection, University of Lodz, Pomorska 141/3, 90-236 Lodz, Poland; beata.olas@biol.uni.lodz.pl

Abstract: Recent evidence suggests that probiotics, prebiotics and synbiotics may serve as important dietary components in the prevention (especially) and treatment of cardiovascular diseases (CVD), but the recommendations for their use are often based on brief reports and small clinical studies. This review evaluates the current literature on the correlation between CVD and probiotics, prebiotics and synbiotics. Although research on probiotics, prebiotics and synbiotics has grown exponentially in recent years, particularly regarding the effect of probiotics on CVD, their mechanisms have not been clearly defined. It has been proposed that probiotics lower cholesterol levels, and may protect against CVD, by increasing bile salt synthesis and bile acid deconjugation. Similar effects have also been observed for prebiotics and synbiotics; however, probiotics also appear to have anti-oxidative, anti-platelet and anti-inflammatory properties. Importantly, probiotics not only have demonstrated effects in vitro and in animal models, but also in humans, where supplementation with probiotics decreases the risk factors of CVD. In addition, the properties of commercial probiotics, prebiotics and synbiotics remain undetermined, and further experimental research is needed before these substances can be used in the prevention and treatment of CVD. In particular, well-designed clinical trials are required to determine the influence of probiotics on trimethylamine-N-oxide (TMAO), which is believed to be a marker of CVDs, and to clarify the long-term effects, and action, of probiotic, prebiotic and synbiotic supplementation in combination with drug therapy (for example, aspirin). However, while it cannot be unequivocally stated whether such supplementation yields benefits in the prevention and treatment of CVDs, it is important to note that clinical studies performed to date have not identified any side-effects to use.

Keywords: probiotic; prebiotic; synbiotic; cardiovascular disease

---

1. Introduction

Cardiovascular diseases (CVD) are conditions that involve the heart or blood vessels, the most well-known being coronary artery diseases (angina and myocardial infarction), stroke, hypertensive heart diseases, cardiomyopathy, venous thrombosis, arrhythmia and thromboembolic disease. The underlying mechanisms vary depending on the disease. For example, coronary artery disease, peripheral artery disease, and stroke involve atherosclerosis [1,2]. They may be associated with various lifestyle factors such as poor diet or smoking, and are characterized by high blood pressure, high cholesterol levels, obesity and hyperactivation of blood platelets [1]. CVDs are believed to have been responsible for about 18 million deaths worldwide (about 32%) in 2015 [2].

CVD management does not necessarily require therapeutic intervention or prophylaxis. For example, it is known that a diet high in fruits and vegetables can decrease the risk of CVD via various mechanisms, including reducing plasma cholesterol level and inhibiting blood platelet activation. However, such dietary modification can also result in changes in the microbial and metabolic composition of the intestines, which themselves are known to be characteristic of a range of physiological and pathological states, including CVD; the composition of the gut microbiota has been found to be associated with atherogenesis, thrombosis, chronic heart conditions and arterial hypertension [3–7], and this correlation has also been noted in a recent meta-analysis [8].

Dietary supplements, often termed functional foods, can bestow beneficial effects against various risk factors associated with cardiovascular diseases. However, little, if anything, is known about the role of probiotic, prebiotic and symbiotic supplements as important dietary components in the prevention and treatment of CVD. For example, in a review paper, Vascquez et al. [9] indicated that probiotics may decrease the production of reactive oxygen species, and reduce oxidative stress. Nevertheless, some brief reports and small clinical studies have been conducted, and these may nevertheless offer new directions in treatment; in addition, the body of research regarding these supplements, particularly concerning the effect of probiotics on cardiovascular diseases, has recently grown exponentially. For example, 201 articles were published during 2014–2020, and 63 were published on "probiotics and cardiovascular diseases" during 2009–2013 (PubMed June, 2020). Therefore, the aim of this review is to discuss the roles of probiotics, prebiotics and synbiotics in the prevention and treatment of cardiovascular diseases based on data from journals recorded in international databases, including *inter alia* PubMed and Scopus.

2. Probiotics

Belief in the beneficial effects of certain types of bacteria on the human body dates back to ancient times. It is known that Plinius the Elder advocated drinking beverages made from fermented milk to alleviate stomach troubles [10].

The term *probiotic* is derived from the Greek *pro bios*, meaning *for life*. It was introduced in 1965 by Lilly and Stillwell, who identified a probiotic as "an organism or substance that affects the balance of intestinal microflora". In 1989, Fuller saw the benefits of probiotics and described them as a "live, microbiological food supplement" [10]. In 2002, the Food and Agriculture Organization/World Health Organization (WHO) defined probiotics as "live micro-organisms which when present in adequate amounts, confer benefits to the body of the host" [11].

In the early twentieth century, research on probiotics chiefly focused on the species of *Lactobacillus* found in dairy products, for example *Lactobacillus casei* (the first probiotic strain isolated in Japan), and on its Western equivalent *Lactobacillus acidophilus*. In 1970, Ilyich Metchnikoff (who is usually considered the founder of probiotics) reported that the quantity of *Lactobacilli* in the gastrointestinal tract has an influence on the health of the host [12]. *Lactobacillus* is one of the main genera of probiotic microorganisms with a long history of safe use; it is recognized by the US Food and Drug Administration (FDA) for consumption, and is approved for use in dairy products [10,13].

Probiotic bacteria are constantly present in humans and are naturally present in the digestive tract and the mouth; they are consumed around the world along with traditional food products. They have also been widely used to preserve the freshness of foods such as salami, cheese, soy sauce or sauerkraut for hundreds, or even thousands, of years [10].

Probiotics are believed to adhere to intestinal epithelial cells, preventing the development of harmful microorganisms by producing anti-bacterial substances including bacteriocins and organic acids. The quantitative share of bacteria in the digestive tract is variable, with the number of *Bifidobacteria* in the human colon ranging from 8×10^4 to 2.5×10^{13} cells (mean 1.6×10^{10} cells), and the number *Lactobacillus* bacteria ranging from 4×10^4 to 3.2×10^{12} (mean 4×10^9 cells). Twelve species of *Bifidobacteria* are known to occur in humans, particularly *B. longum*, *B. pseudolongum*, *B. animalis* and *B. bifidum*; *Bifidobacteria* is one of the first genera of microorganisms to colonize the sterile digestive tracts of newborns, and is believed to constitute the largest group of intestinal microflora, representing up to 95% of the total microbial population during breast feeding [10].

WHO regulations state that the number of living cells in probiotic foods at the time of human consumption may not be lower than 10^6 cells per 1 mL or 1 g of product, while the therapeutic dose is 10^8–10^9 cells in 1 mL or 1 g of product. Given that the microorganism must remain viable and should not be killed by passing through the gastrointestinal tract, the probiotic must be resistant to the action of gastric juice and bile salts. After passing through this chemical barrier, probiotics should adhere to the surface of the intestine, where their health-promoting functions can be realized. In addition, if probiotic microorganisms do not colonize the intestine, the repeated consumption of probiotic products may be necessary [10].

Probiotics can enhance the nonspecific cellular immune response through the activation of natural killer cells, macrophages and the release of various cytokines. They can also improve the gut mucosal immune system by increasing the number of IgA(+) cells [14,15]. In addition, probiotics can also aid the process of digestion and the breakdown of lactose, improve the absorption of minerals such as calcium, zinc, iron and manganese, and improve the synthesis of many vitamins, including thiamin, riboflavin, niacin, pantothenic acid and vitamin K. Probiotics play an important role in the treatment of various diseases, such as hepatic disease, diarrhea and gastroenteritis. Probiotics have also been shown to have anti-proliferative, pro-apoptotic and anti-oxidative properties [14,15].

Probiotics and CVDs

Probiotics may support the prevention and treatment of some cardiovascular diseases by reducing elevated cholesterol levels [10,16,17]. Unfortunately, most studies on the effects of probiotics on cardiovascular diseases have been performed in vitro. While some in vivo studies have examined the effect of probiotic supplementation on risk factors of CVDs in people and animals, the number of commercial probiotic supplements is too limited to unequivocally demonstrate that such probiotics have a beneficial effect on the cardiovascular system.

Probiotics may reduce cholesterol levels by several mechanisms [18]. Most *Bifidobacteria* bacteria demonstrate higher cholilogl̈icin hydrolase activity than other microorganisms. This enzyme hydrolyzes the amide bonds conjugated with taurine or glycine in bile acids, resulting in the release of primary bile acids; these are easily precipitated at low pH, resulting in their expulsion from the gastrointestinal tract. As these are not reabsorbed from the intestine, they must be replaced by bile produced in the liver from blood cholesterol. Alternatively, *Bifidobacteria*-driven cholesterol assimilation, or precipitation in the acidic environment of the gut, can also reduce plasma cholesterol level by slowing its absorption from food into the blood [10].

A recent meta-analysis by Mo et al. [19] indicated that the use of probiotics significantly lowers total cholesterol and low-density lipoprotein (LDL) cholesterol in hypercholesterolemic adults. Niamah et al. [20] also note that soy milk fermented (3 mL/day) by a probiotic starter (Log.11.1 cfu/mL) consisting of *S. thermophilis*, *L. acidophilus* LA-5 and *B. bifidum* BG-12 decreases the level of cholesterol and triglyceride compared with control.

Malik et al. [21] report that *L. plantarum* 299v (Lp299v) supplementation improves vascular endothelial function and reduces inflammatory biomarkers in men with stable coronary artery disease. In this experiment, twenty men with stable coronary artery disease consumed a drink containing 20 billion colony-forming units (cfu) of Lp299v per day for six weeks. Vascular endothelial function was measured by brachial artery flow-mediated dilation, and endothelial vasodilation was measured by video microscopy. It was also found that the administered probiotics can regulate the genes responsible for the intestinal transport of cholesterol (including *ABCG8*, *ABCG5* and *NPC1L1*), as well as some genes responsible for the homeostasis of cholesterol in the liver, including those controlling the production of 3-hydroxy-3-methylglutaryl-coenzyme A reductase (HMGCR) [21].

A recent study by Lew et al. [22] found *L. plantarum* DR7 to exert cholesterol-lowering properties via AMPK phosphorylation, resulting in the reduced expression of HMGCR. Nguyen et al. [23] also suggest that the probiotic *L. plantarum* PH40 may also possess cholesterol-lowering properties. Wang et al. [24]

reported that the four-week administration of *L. acidophilus* (10^9 cfu/mL) improves lipid-regulating activity in hypercholesterolemic rats, together with one of statin—rosuvastatin (10 mg/kg).

Systematic inflammation is commonly observed among CVDs, as are many risk factors, such as hypertension [25]. Oxidative stress is also known to play a role in the course of CVDs [24]. *Lactobacillus* and *Bifidobacterium* have been found to inhibit lipid peroxidation and ROS production, and hence may slow or even halt the development of CVDs and other oxidative stress-related diseases [26–28].

Yadav et al. [29] reported that the consumption of probiotic *L. fermentum* MTCC: 5898-fermented milk not only attenuated dyslipidemia, but also reduced oxidative stress and inflammation in male rats fed a cholesterol-enriched diet. Oxidative stress was measured by the activity of various anti-oxidative enzymes, such as catalase, superoxide dismutase and glutathione peroxidase, and the level of thiobarbituric acid reactive substances (TBARS) in the liver and kidney—a marker of lipid peroxidation. Inflammation, measured by the expression of inflammatory cytokines, including tumor necrosis factor-alpha (TNF-α) and interleukin-6 (IL-6), was also influenced at the genetic level. The study examined the effect of 90-day probiotic supplementation among male Wistar rats. The rats were divided into three groups: one was fed a standard diet (Group 1), another fed a cholesterol-enriched diet (Group 2), and another fed a cholesterol-enriched diet together with 2 mL MTCC: 5898-fermented milk (2×10^9 cfu) per day (Group 3). The probiotic-fermented milk was prepared by inoculating 1% of activated *L. fermentum* MTCC: 5898 (in skimmed milk) into fresh milk (2.5% fat), which was then incubated at 37 °C for 18 h before feeding.

Tenorio-Jimenez et al. [30] report that the 12-week administration of a daily dose of 5×10^9 cfu *L. reuteri* V3401 in capsules was associated with lower levels of inflammation biomarkers, such as TNF-α, IL-6, IL-8 and soluble intercellular adhesion molecule-1 (sICAM-1), in obese adults aged 18 to 65 years with metabolic syndrome, as well as with a reduced risk of CVD. Szulinska et al. [31] also observed that supplementation with the multispecies probiotic Ecologic® Barrier modified both the functional and biochemical parameters of vascular dysfunction in a group of 81 obese postmenopausal Caucasian women. The subjects were assigned to three groups: (1) placebo, (2) those receiving a low dose (2.5×10^9 cfu per day), and (3) those receiving a high dose (1×10^{10} cfu per day). The supplement was administered for 12 weeks. The authors note that the low and high doses decrease systolic blood pressure and serum vascular endothelial growth factor (VEGF), TNF-α and IL-6. Other clinical trials have also found probiotic use to be associated with a moderate or significant reduction in blood pressure among both healthy and obese participants [32–36]. The anti-hypertensive action of probiotics is believed to act via several mechanisms, including regulating the renin–angiotensin system [36].

The hyperactivation of blood platelets also plays a key role in thrombotic disorders. Although pharmacological strategies are available, such as those based on aspirin and its derivatives, these treatments are often accompanied by side-effects and complications that outweigh their benefits. In addition, blood platelet function is strongly influenced by diet, including the consumption of fruit and vegetables [37,38]. Although the precise roles played by probiotics in the modulation of hemostasis and its various elements, such as blood platelet function, are generally not well documented, a few in vitro and in vivo studies have nevertheless examined their effects on various elements of hemostasis, such as platelet activation. For example, Schreiber et al. reported that *L. reuteri* reduces P-selectin expression on the platelet surface and decreases blood platelet–endothelial cell interactions in rats treated with dextran sodium sulfate (DSS) [39]. In addition, Haro and Medina [40] also indicated that the oral administration of probiotic *L. casei* CRL431 may be a promising candidate for the prevention of thrombotic complications associated with pneumococcal pneumonia, especially in at-risk patients. It was found that the oral administration of CRL431 in a respiratory pneumococcal infection model in mice reduces blood platelet activation, measured by various parameters, including P-selectin expression, and modulates antithrombin levels within the normal range. These findings may indicate that *L. casei* may also influence the coagulation system [40]. In addition, in vitro experiments found no significant difference in the levels of blood platelet activation markers, such as ADP-induced platelet aggregation, between resting platelets and samples incubated with *L. rhamnosus* HN001 and *B. lactis*

HN019. The authors suggest that these probiotic strains do not appear to participate in the pathogenesis of thrombotic disorders [41].

It is likely that inflammatory processes play an important role in the pathogenesis and progression of atherosclerosis, as elevated levels of proinflammatory cytokines have been observed in patients with atherosclerosis [42]. However, although some studies have demonstrated that probiotics can decrease the production of pro-inflammatory cytokines, their underlying mechanism remains unclear [7].

A recent study by Majewska et al. [43] found probiotic supplementation (Ecologic® BARIER, containing 2.5×10^9 cfu/g; for 12 weeks) to inhibit the inflammation process, reduce oxidative stress, and decrease the concentration of homocysteine in obese women ($n = 50$; aged 45–70 years).

3. Prebiotics

Prebiotics contain no microorganisms—only substances which stimulate their growth. These do not undergo digestion; therefore, they reach the intestinal lumen unchanged, where they can then act. For food ingredients to be considered prebiotics, they must meet certain criteria: they must be resistant to the actions of stomach acids, bile salts and other hydrolyzing enzymes in the intestine, have a known chemical structure, provide a substrate for one or more strains of beneficial bacteria, stimulate the growth and activity of the desired groups of bacteria in the digestive tract, and possess proven health benefits [10,44].

Prebiotics can be obtained from various sources, including breast milk, soybeans and raw oats [10,45]. However, the most popular prebiotics are the oligosaccharides contained in plants, such as asparagus, artichokes, chicory and onions [10]. Oligosaccharides may benefit the gastrointestinal tract via fermentation and the proliferation of desirable bacterial species. For example, fructo-oligosaccharide promotes the growth of bifidobacteria in vivo. Oligofructose and inulin also increase the population of colonic bifidobacteria [46,47]. Hsu et al. [48] observed that xylo-oligosaccharides and fructo-oligosaccharides affect the intestinal microbiota and precancerous development of colonic lesions in rats. Nowadays, probiotics are often added as supplements to dairy products, meat products and beverages, such as health drinks. Recently, Cherry et al. [49] reported that seaweed may be a good source of polysaccharide components, which may act as prebiotics.

Prebiotics and CVDs

Parnell and Reiner [50] reported that probiotic supplementation lowers total serum cholesterol in a hypercholesterolemic rat model. In this experiment, rats were administered one of three diets supplemented with 0, 10 or 20% prebiotic fiber for 10 weeks. Both doses of prebiotic fiber reduced serum cholesterol concentrations by about 25%. In addition, this change was correlated with an increase in caeca digesta, as well as the up-regulation of genes involved in cholesterol biosynthesis and bile production. In addition, the obese rats with 10% prebiotic supplementation demonstrated an approximately 40% reduction in triacylglycerol accumulation in the liver (Table 1).

Obesity is often associated with the progression of CVDs. However, both probiotic and prebiotic supplementation have been reported to have anti-obesogenic effects in various clinical trials (Table 1) [51–55].

The role of prebiotics in preventing and treating hypertension is reviewed in greater detail by Ghaffari and Roshanravan [56].

4. Synbiotics

A synbiotic is a combination of probiotics and prebiotics, typically oligosaccharides or inulin, which demonstrate an additive action and are used to restore normal bacterial flora [10].

Synbiotics and CVDs

A number of studies have found synbiotics to demonstrate promising hypercholesterolemic properties [57–60]. For example, Mofid et al. [60] reported that the regular intake of synbiotic yoghurts reduces the risk of CVDs among hypercholesterolemic patients.

Haghighat et al. [59] noted that 12-week synbiotic supplementation reduces the concentration of intracellular adhesion molecule type 1 (ICAM-1), which is a risk factor for cardiovascular diseases in hemodialysis patients. The study included three groups of subjects: synbiotic, probiotic and placebo. Those in the synbiotic group received 15 g of prebiotic (three different fiber types: 5 g fructo-oligosaccharides, 5 g galacto-oligosaccharides and 5 g inulin) and 5 g probiotic powder (Bioflora®) containing *L. acidophilus* strain T16, *B. bifidum* strain BIA-6, *B. lactis* strain BIA-6, and *B. longum* strain LAF-5 (2.7×10^7 cfu/g each) in sachets. The probiotic group received 5 g probiotics, as in the synbiotic group, with 15 g of maltodextrin powder in sachets. The placebo group received 20 g of maltodextrin powder in sachets.

It has been found that a synbiotic containing *L. acidophilus* ATCC 4962 reduces total cholesterol, triacylglycerol, and LDL-cholesterol in hypercholesterolemic pigs, probably in the form of cholesterol esters, via the interrelated pathways of lipid transporters, including high-density lipoprotein (HDL), LDL and very low-density lipoprotein (VLDL). In this experiment, three commercially available prebiotics were used: mannitol, fructo-oligosacharides and inulin. The pigs on the symbiotic diet were supplemented with powdered *L. acidophilus* ATCC 4962 (1 g/pig per day), mannitol (1.56 g/pig per day), fructo-oligosacharides (1.25 g/pig per day) and inulin (2.2 g/pig per day). The animals were also given dietary fat (5 and 15%) (Table 1). In addition, it was found that the synbiotic reduces the deformation of erythrocytes via improved membrane permeability and fluidity [57,58].

5. The Effects of Probiotics, Prebiotics and Synbiotics on TMAO Levels

Trimethylamine-N-oxide ($(CH_3)_3NO$; TMAO) is an organic compound produced from choline, phosphatidylcholine, and carnitine precursors. These are converted into an intermediate compound, trimethylamine (TMA), by members of the gut microbiota, such as Acinetobacter; TMA is in turn oxidized into TMAO by the action of hepatic flavin monooxygenases (FMOs) [61]. As such, the consumption of carnitine-containing food products, such as some energy drinks and dietary supplements, results in increased TMAO levels in the blood [62].

However, the nature of the relationship between TMAO levels and CVDs remains unclear. Wilson et al. proposed that a high concentration of TMAO in the blood may be correlated with an increased risk of CVDs [63]. TMAO has also been indicated as a marker of cardiovascular events [64], and has been observed to influence the metabolism of cholesterol in the liver in the intestinal and artery walls. Hazen reported an increased deposition of cholesterol in peripheral cells, such as those in artery walls, in the presence of TMAO, together with the decreased removal of cholesterol [65]. In addition, carnitine intake and a high plasma concentration of TMAO have been found to correlate with low aortic lesions in ApoE -/- transgenic mice expressing cholesterol ester transfer protein (CETP) [66]. Ufnal et al. [67] and Tilg [68] suggest that TMAO may be involved in the etiology of hypertension and thrombosis, and in the regulation of arterial blood pressure. A review by Kanitsoraphan et al. [69] suggests that the concentration of TMAO could be incorporated into existing risk stratification tools, and could lead to novel prevention and treatment.

A recent study by Hardin et al. [70] described a possible mechanism connecting TMAO and the enhancement of atherosclerotic factors. They proposed that increased TMAO concentrations in plasma promoted the upregulation of macrophage scavenger receptors, which promote the recruitment of macrophages and associated inflammation. Being unable to properly metabolize the lipids inside them, the accumulated macrophages produce foamy cells. The resulting inflammation, foamy cell production and accumulation of macrophages promote the development of atherosclerosis and other CVDs. Leustean et al. [71] described other mechanisms of TMAO action in CVDs, including blood platelet aggregation and decreases in nitric oxide level (Figure 1).

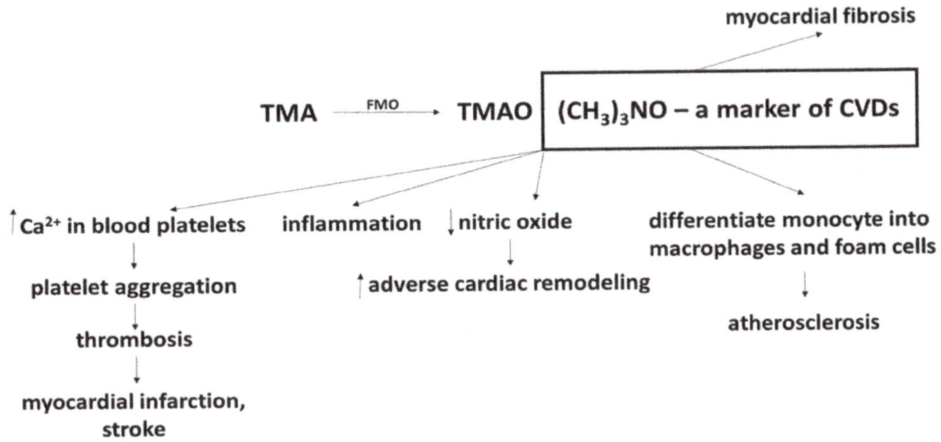

Figure 1. Effect of trimethylamine-N-oxide (TMAO) on cardiovascular diseases (CVDs) (modified) [70] More details in text.

Preliminary results suggest that antibiotic therapy may suppress TMAO levels, but the long-term stability of such therapy remains unknown [64]. It has been proposed that probiotic treatment may prevent the development of CVDs following TMAO accumulation (Figure 2). However, Malik et al. [21] noted that supplementation with a drink containing *L. plantarum* 299v (Lp299v), 20 billion cfu daily for six weeks, did not significantly change plasma TMAO concentrations in a group of 20 men aged 40–75 years with stable coronary artery disease. Tripolt et al. [72] also noted that supplementation with *L. casei* Shirota (6.5 × 109 cfu, daily) three times for 12 weeks does not change TMAO levels in subjects with metabolic syndrome. Similar results were observed by Boutagy et al. [73] in a study of nineteen non-obese subjects who consumed a mix of various probiotics (900 billion live bacteria) for four weeks.

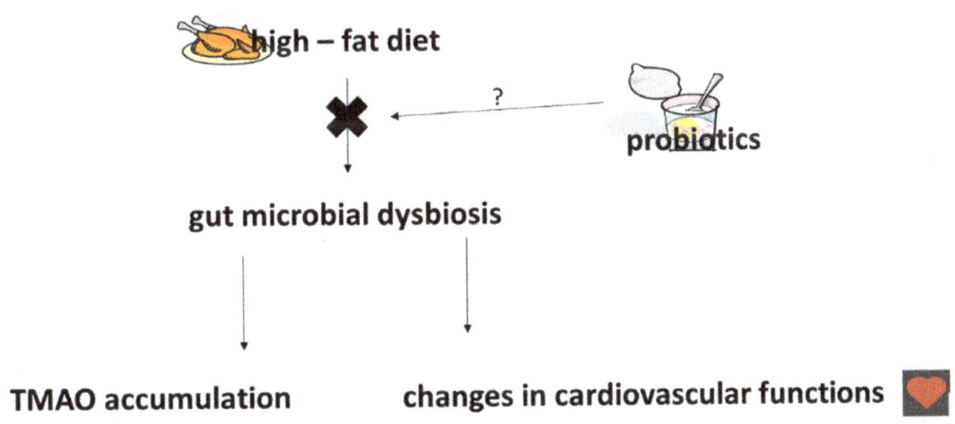

Figure 2. Effect of probiotics on trimethylamine-N-oxide (TMAO) accumulation and changes in cardiovascular functions. More details in text (modified) [69].

In contrast, Qui et al. [74] observed that *L. plantarum* ZDYO4 inhibits the development of TMAO-induced atherosclerosis in ApoE-/- 1.3% choline-fed mice, compared to controls. Tenore et al. [75] reported a decrease in TMAO level among a group of 90 individuals with CVD risk factors, including high total cholesterol and LDL levels, following the consumption of lactofermented annurca apple puree (125 g/day for 16 weeks). Each dose contained approximately 3×10^8 cfu *L. rhamnosus* LRH11 and *L. plantarum* SGL07.

Liu et al. reported that the consumption of probiotic-fermented purple sweet potato yoghurt may reverse congestive heart failure induced by hypertension; this was proposed to occur via the attenuation of cardiomyocyte apoptosis by the inhibition of Fas receptor-dependent apoptotic pathways [76]. It has also been indicated that the probiotic *B. animalis* subsp. *lactis* LKM512 may decrease TMA levels in healthy volunteers [77], and that probiotics may play an important role in atherosclerosis by modulating TMAO concentration [78].

Table 1. The effect of probiotics, prebiotics, and synbiotics on various risk factors of cardiovascular diseases (*in vivo* model).

Probiotic/Prebiotic/Synbiotic Consumption	Dose (Per Day)	Days/Weeks	Subjects	Risk Factors of Cardiovascular Diseases	Ref.
Probiotic					
L. plantarum 299v	20 billion cfu	6 weeks	Patients with stable coronary artery disease (people)	Reducing inflammatory biomarkers. No effect on trimethylamine-N-oxide (TMAO) level	[21]
L. plantarum PH04	10^7 cfu	14 days	Male mice fed a high-cholesterol diet containing 10% *w/v* skim milk and 10% *w/v* cream	Lowering total cholesterol and triglycerides	[23]
L. reuteri V3401	5×10^9 cfu	12 weeks	Obese adults (people) with metabolic syndrome	Reducing inflammation	[30]
Multispecies probiotic Ecologic® Barrier	2.5×10^9 cfu; 1×10^{10} cfu	12 weeks	Obese postmenopausal Caucasian women	Decreasing systolic blood pressure and inflammation	[31]
Multispecies probiotic Ecologic® Barrier	2.5×10^9 cfu	12 weeks	Obese women	Decreasing homocysteine	[43]
L. acidophilus	10^9 cfu/mL	4 weeks	Hypercholesterolemic rats	Lowering total cholesterol and low-density lipoprotein (LDL)	[24]
L. fermentum MTCC:5898-fermented milk	2×10^9 cfu	90 days		Reducing dyslipidemia, oxidative stress and inflammation	[29]
L. rhamnosus LRH11 and *L. plantarum* SGL07	3×10^8 cfu	16 weeks	People with CVDs risks	Reducing plasma trimethylamine-N-oxide (TMAO) level	[75]
B. animalis subsp. *lactis* LKM512	No described	12 weeks	Healthy people	Reducing plasma trimethylamine-N-oxide (TMAO) level	[77]
L. casei Shirota	6.5×10^9 cfu	12 weeks	Subjects with metabolic syndrome	No effect on trimethylamine-N-oxide (TMAO) level	[72]
S. thermophilis, *L. acidophilus* LA-5 and *B. bifidum* BG-12	No described (3 mL/day)	4 weeks	Healthy animals	Lowering cholesterol and triglyceride	[20]
Prebiotic					
Prebiotic fiber	10 or 20%	10 weeks	Obese hyperlipidemic rats	Lowering total serum cholesterol and triacylglycerol	[50]
Oligofructose	8 g/day	16 weeks	Overweight and obese children aged 7–12 years	Decreasing body weight	[53]
Oligofructose	21 g/day	12 weeks	Overweight and obese adults	Decreasing body weight	[51]
Synbiotic					
Prebiotic (three different fiber types: 5 g fructooligosaccharides, 5 g galactooligosaccharides and 5 g inulin) and probiotic powder (Bioflora®) containing *L. acidophilus* strain T16, *B. bifidum* strain BIA-6, *B. lactis* strain BIA-6, and *B. longum* strain LAF-5	15 g of prebiotic and 5 g probiotic in sachet	12 weeks	Hemodialysis patients	Reducing the concentration of intracellular adhesion molecule type 1	[59]
Synbiotic containing *L. acidophilus* ATCC 4962, and three commercially available prebiotics (mannitol, fructooligosacharides and inulin)	*L. acidophilus* ATCC 4962 (1 g/pig per day), mannitol (1.56 g/pig per day), fructooligosacharides (1.25 g/pig per day) and inulin (2.2 g/pig per day)	8 weeks	Hypercholesterolemic pigs	Reducing total cholesterol, triacylglycerol, low-density lipoprotein (LDL)-cholesterol	[57,58]

A recent study by Montrucchio et al. [79] found serum TMAO concentrations in people living with HIV (PLWH) to be correlated with higher cardiovascular risk and atherosclerosis, and to not be affected by high-dose probiotic supplementation—no change in TMAO concentration was observed after six months of probiotic supplementation. The study included 175 participants, with TMAO concentrations of about 165 ng/mL (Table 1). More information about the reduction of TMAO level by probiotics has been described in a review by Din et al. [58].

6. The Effects of Probiotics, Prebiotics and Synbiotics on Uric Acid Levels

Valdivielso et al. reported the existence of a correlation between the occurrence of chronic kidney disease (CKD) and CVDs, including atherosclerosis; they also noted that the progression of atherosclerosis appeared to be related to CKD progression, as well as to a higher uric acid level [80]. An increased level of uric acid in serum has been associated with the presence of CKD and CVDs due to various molecular mechanisms, such as oxidative stress and inflammation. Conversely, certain antioxidants, such as phenolic compounds, may decrease uric acid level [81]. It has been suggested that probiotics, prebiotic and synbiotics, i.e., a combination of probiotics and prebiotics, may also change the level of uric acid. For example, Rossi et al. [82] reported that a synbiotic intervention based on the administration of 15 g of prebiotics (including a combination of three different types of fibers), and 90 billion cfu from nine different strains of *Lactobacillus*, *Streptococcus* and *Bifidobacteria*, daily for three weeks, may influence the outcome of CVDs and CKDs. The authors also suggested that this mixture of pre- and probiotics may reduce the levels of various toxins, including indoxyl sulphate (IS) and p-cresyl sulphate (PCS) [80]. Like TMAO, IS and PCS have been identified as proatherogenic risk factors [83].

Al-Okbi et al. [84] also noted that a combination of encapsulated probiotic (*B. bifidum*, *L. delbrueckii*, and *S. thremophilus*) and green tea alcohol extract reduces the level of uric acid in rats with hepatorenal syndrome. Wang et al. [85] reported that supplementation with *Lactobacillus* DM9218 decreases serum uric acid in fructose-fed mice; the authors suggested that it may protect against high-fructose-induced liver damage and retinol uric acid accumulation by degrading inosine. The uric acid level was also significantly reduced in non-dialysis patients with CKD who received probiotics [86]. Moreover, the eight-week consumption of *L. gasseri* PA-3 yoghurt was found to decrease the level of serum uric acid in 25 patients [87].

However, Haghighat et al. reported that daily synbiotic supplementation for 12 weeks with sachets containing 15 g of prebiotics and 5 g of probiotic (2.7×10^7 cfu) did not appear to influence uric acid level in a group of 75 hemodialysis patients [58]. Garcia-Arrayo et al. [88] found that five-week probiotic supplementation with *L. acidophilus* KB27 (5 billion cfu/daily) and *L. rhamnosus* KB79 (5 billion cfu/daily) elevates uric acid extraction in rats; it was also found to increase oxonic acid- induced intrarenal accumulation, which is known to stimulate hyperuricemia and renal damage. Firouzi and Haghighatdoost [89] reported elevated uric acid levels in healthy people ($n = 437$) who consumed probiotics, prebiotics and synbiotics, compared with a placebo group.

7. Conclusions

Although it has been proposed that probiotic consumption may bestow anti-hypertensive properties and be associated with improved serum lipid profiles [57,58,90,91], these postulated benefits were based on an in vitro model. More recent in vivo trials indicate that the consumption of probiotics, prebiotics or a combination of the two, i.e., synbiotics, may assist in the prevention and treatment of cardiovascular diseases; however, few studies have examined the role of probiotics in this regard, and their precise medicinal and prophylactic doses for humans remain unknown (Table 1). It is also very difficult to demonstrate the specific correlation, relationship and synergic relationships between probiotics, prebiotics and synbiotics in the prevention and treatment of CVD. However, Liong et al. [57,59] and Haghighat et al. [59] indicated that probiotics, prebiotics and synbiotics may offer promise in the prevention and treatment of CVD; for example, a synbiotic containing *L. acidophilus*

ATCC 4962 and three commercially available prebiotics (mannitol, fructooligosacharides and inulin) has been found to reduce total cholesterol, triacylglycerol and LDL-cholesterol levels (Table 1). Moreover, other authors [21] describe the role of probiotics in patients with stable coronary artery disease. On the other hand, their role in patients with other CVDs, including stroke, cardiomyopathy, and carditis, is not known.

In addition, the mechanisms of action of probiotics, prebiotics and synbiotics remain poorly defined. Probiotics are believed to modulate various factors which may play an important role in CVDs (Figure 3). Similarly to prebiotics and synbiotics, they may lower cholesterol levels by increasing bile salt synthesis and bile acid deconjugation, and may offer protection from cardiovascular diseases. Moreover, probiotics have been found to have anti-oxidative, anti-platelet and anti-inflammatory properties (Figure 3). However, further experimental research, particularly well-designed clinical studies, are needed before these substances can effectively be used in the prevention and treatment of CVD. Finally, no studies have yet evaluated the effect of their use on CVDs in combination with classical therapy, for example aspirin; therefore, although no side-effects have been reported in clinical studies to date, it cannot be unequivocally stated whether probiotic, prebiotic and synbiotic use represents an effective strategy for the prevention and treatment of CVDs.

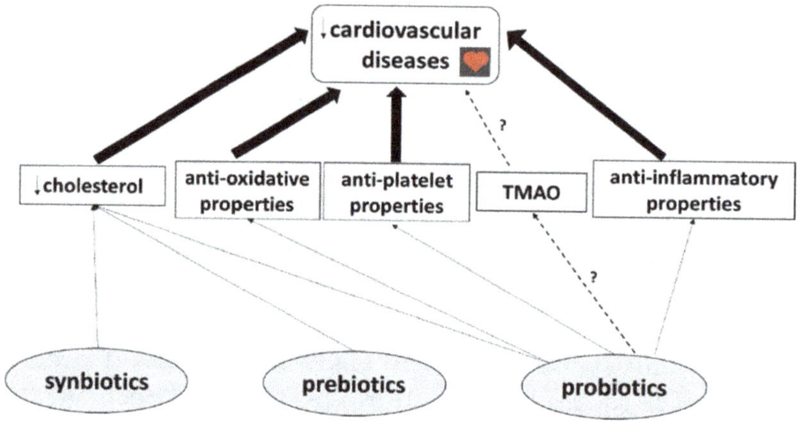

Figure 3. The effect of probiotics, prebiotics and synbiotics on cardiovascular disease. Probiotics lower the level of cholesterol by increasing bile salt synthesis and bile acid deconjugation. Probiotics also have anti-oxidative, anti-platelet and anti-inflammatory properties, and hence may offer protection from cardiovascular diseases. One proposed model of preventing the CVD-induced accumulation of TMAO may be probiotic supplementation. However, prebiotics and synbiotics may also decrease the level of total cholesterol and offer similar protection from cardiovascular disease. More details in text.

Abbreviations

cfu—colony-forming units; CKD—chronic kidney disease; FDA—Food and Drug Administration; FMO—flavin monooxygenases; HDL—high-density lipoprotein; IS—indoxyl sulphate; LDL—low-density lipoprotein; PCS—p-cresyl sulphate; TMA—trimethylamine; TMAO—trimethylamine-N-oxide; WHO—World Health Organization; VLDL—very low-density lipoprotein.

References

1. Shanthi, M.; Pekka, P.; Bo, N. *Global Atlas on Cardiovascular Diseases Prevention and Control*; World Health Organization in collaboration with the World Heart Federation and the World Stroke Organization: Geneva, Switzerland, 2011; pp. 3–18.
2. GBD. Mortality and Causes of Death Collaborators. 2013. Available online: https://doi.org/10.1016/S0140-6736(14)61682-2 (accessed on 17 December 2014).

3. Katsi, V.; Didagelos, M.; Skevofilax, S.; Armenis, I.; Kartalis, A.; Vlachopoulos, C.; Karvounis, H.; Tousoulis, D. Gut microbiota—Gut dysbiosis—Arterial hypertension: New horizons. *Curr. Hyperten. Rev.* **2018**, *12*, 1–14.
4. Pimenta, F.S.; Luaces-Regueira, M.; Ton, A.M.M.; Campagnaro, B.P.; Campos-Toimil, M.; Pereira, T.M.C.; Vasquez, E.C. Mechanisms of action of kefir in chronic cardiovascular and metabolic diseases. *Cell. Physiol. Biochem.* **2018**, *48*, 1901–1914. [CrossRef] [PubMed]
5. Rezac, S.; Kok, C.R.; Herrmann, M.; Hutkins, R. Fermented foods as a dietary source of live organisms. *Front. Microbiol.* **2018**, *9*, 1–29. [CrossRef] [PubMed]
6. Weis, M. Impact of the gut microbiome in cardiovascular and autoimmune diseases. *Clin. Sci.* **2018**, *132*, 2387–2389. [CrossRef]
7. O'Morain, V.L.; Ramji, D.P. The potential of probiotics in the prevention and treatment of atherosclerosis. *Mol. Nutr. Food Res.* **2020**, *64*, 1–15. [CrossRef]
8. Deng, X.; Ma, J.; Song, M.; Jin, Y.; Ge, W.; Guo, C. Effects of products designed to modulate the gut microbiota on hyperlipidaemia. *Eur. J. Nutr.* **2018**, *1*, 1–15. [CrossRef]
9. Vasquez, E.C.; Pereira, T.M.C.; Peotta, V.A.; Baldo, M.P.; Campos-Toimil, M. Probiotics as beneficial dietary supplements to prevent and treat cardiovascular diseases: Uncovering their impact on oxidative stress. *Oxid. Med. Cell. Longev.* **2019**, *7*, 1–12. [CrossRef]
10. Pandey, K.R.; Naik, S.R.; Vakil, B.V. Probiotics, prebiotics and synbiotics—A review. *J. Food Sci. Technol.* **2010**, *52*, 7577–7587. [CrossRef]
11. *Guildelines for the Evaluation of Probiotics in Food*; Joint FAO/WHO Working Group on Drafting Guidelines for the Evaluation of Probiotics in Food: London, ON, Canada, 2002.
12. Metchnikoff, E. Sur la lute des cellules de l'organisme centre l'invasion des microbes. *Ann. Inst. Pasteur.* **1887**, *1*, 321.
13. Khalesi, S.; Bellissimo, N.; Vandelanotte, C.; Williview, S.; Stanley, D.; Irwin, C. A review of probiotic supplementation in healthy adults: Helpful or hype? *Eur. J. Clin. Nutr.* **2018**, *26*, 1–16. [CrossRef]
14. Oberreuther-Moschner, D.L.; Jahreis, G.; Rechkemmer, G.; Pool-Zobel, B.L. Dietary intervention with the probiotics *Lactobacillus acidophilus* 145 and *Bifidobacterium longum* 913 modulates the potential of human faecal water to induce damage in HT29clone19A cells. *Br. J. Nutr.* **2004**, *91*, 925–932. [CrossRef] [PubMed]
15. Nowak, A.; Paliwoda, A.; Blasiak, J. Anti-proliferative, pro-apoptotic and anti-oxidative activity of *Lactobacillus* and *Bifidobacterium* strains: A review of mechanism and therapeutic perspectives. *Crit. Rev. Food. Sci. Nutr.* **2018**, *1*, 1–12. [CrossRef] [PubMed]
16. Sudha, M.R.; Chauhan, P.; Dixit, K.; Babu, S.; Jamil, K. Probiotics as complementary therapy for hypercholesterolemia. *Biol. Med.* **2009**, *1*, 1–13.
17. Bronzato, S.; Durante, A. Dietary supplements and cardiovascular diseases. *Inter. J. Cardiovas. Dis.* **2018**, *9*, 1–10.
18. Gadelha, C.J.M.U.; Bezerra, A.N. Effects of probiotics on the lipid profile: Systematic review. *J. Vasc. Bras.* **2019**, *9*, 1–18.
19. Mo, R.; Zhang, X.; Yang, Y. Effect of probiotics on lipid profiles in hypercholesterolaemic adults: A meta-analysis of randomized controlled trials. *Med. Clin.* **2018**, *19*, 1–12.
20. Niamah, A.K.; Sahi, A.A.; Al-Sharifi, A.S.N. Effect of feeding soy milk fermented by probiotic bacteria on some blood criteria and weight of experimental animals. *Prob. Antimicrob. Proteins* **2017**, *9*, 284–291. [CrossRef]
21. Malik, M.; Suboc, T.M.; Tyagi, S.; Salzman, N.; Wang, J.; Ying, R.; Tanner, M.J.; Kakarla, M.; Baker, J.E.; Widlansky, M.E. *Lactobacillus plantarum* 299v supplementation improves vascular endothelial function and reduces inflammatory biomarkers in med with stable coronary artery disease. *Circ. Res.* **2018**, *123*, 1091–1102. [CrossRef]
22. Lew, L.C.; Choi, S.B.; Khoo, B.Y.; Sreenivasan, S.; Ong, K.L.; Liong, M.T. *Lactobacillus plantarum* DR7 reduces cholesterol via phosphorylation of AMPK that down-regulated the mRNA expression of HMG-CoA reductase. *Kor. J. Food Sci. Animal Res.* **2018**, *38*, 350–361.
23. Nguyen, T.D.T.; Kang, J.H.; Lee, M.S. Characterization of *Lactobacillus plantarum* PH04, a potential probiotic bacterium with cholesterol-lowering effects. *Inter. J. Food Microbiol.* **2007**, *113*, 358–361. [CrossRef]
24. Wang, L.; Zhou, B.; Zhou, X.; Wang, Y.; Wang, H.; Jia, S.; Zhang, Z.; Chu, C.; Mu, J. Combined lowering effects of rosuvastatin and *L. acidophilus* on cholesterol levels in rat. *J. Microbiol. Biotechnol.* **2019**, *29*, 473–481. [CrossRef] [PubMed]

25. Del Pinto, R.; Pietropaoli, D.; Monaco, A.; Desideri, G.; Ferri, C.; Grassi, D. Non-pharmacological strategies against systemic inflammation: Molecular basis and clinical evidence. *Curr. Pharm. Des.* **2020**, *3*, 1–20.
26. Lin, M.Y.; Chang, F.J. Antioxidative effect of intestinal bacteria *Bifidobacterium longum* ATCC 15708 and *Lactobacillus acidophilus* ATCC 4356. *Dig. Dis. Sci.* **2000**, *45*, 1617–1622. [CrossRef] [PubMed]
27. El-Adawi, H.I.; Khalil, M.A.; El-Sheekh, M.M.; El-Deeb, N.M.; Hussein, M.Z. Cytotoxicity assay and antioxidant activities of the lactic acid bacterial strains. *Afric. J. Microbiol. Res.* **2012**, *6*, 1700–1712.
28. Zhong, C.; Qu, C.; Wang, B.; Liang, B.S.; Zeng, B. Probiotics for preventing and treating intestinal bacterial overgrowth: A meta-analysis and systematic review of current evidence. *J. Clin. Gastroenterol.* **2017**, *51*, 300–311. [CrossRef]
29. Yadav, R.; Khan, S.H.; Mada, S.B.; Meena, S.; Kapila, R.; Kaila, S. Consumption of probiotic *Lactobacillus fermentum* MTCC: 5898-fermented milk attenuates dyslipidemia, oxidative stress, and inflammation in male rats fed on cholesterol-enriched diet. *Probiotics Antimicro. Protein* **2018**, *1*, 1–10. [CrossRef]
30. Tenorio-Jimenez, C.; Martinez-Rmirez, M.J.; Tercero-Lozano, M.; Arraiza-Irigoyen, C.; Del Castillo-Codes, I.; Olza, J.; Plaza-Diaz, J.; Fontana, L.; Migueles, J.H.; Olivares, M.; et al. Evaluation of the effect of *Lactobacillus reuteri* V3401 on biomarkers of inflammation, cardiovascular risk and liver steatosis in obese adults with metabolic syndrome: A randomized clinical trial (PROSIR). *BMC Compl. Alter. Med.* **2018**, *18*, 1–8. [CrossRef]
31. Szulinska, M.; Loniewski, I.; Skrypnik, K.; Sobieska, M.; Korybalska, K.; Suliburska, J.; Bogdanska, P. Multispecies probiotic supplementation favorably affects vascular function and reduces arterial stiffness in obese postmenopausal women- A 12-week placebo-controlled and randomized clinical study. *Nutrients* **2018**, *10*, 1672. [CrossRef]
32. Agerholm-Larsen, L.; Raben, A.; Haulvik, N.; Hansen, A.S.; Manders, M.; Astrup, A. Effect of 8 week intake of probiotic milk products on risk factors for cardiovascular diseases. *Eur. J. Clin. Nutr.* **2000**, *54*, 288–297. [CrossRef]
33. Mizushima, S.; Ohshige, K.; Watanabe, J.; Kimura, M.; Kodowski, T.; Nakamurs, Y.; Tochikubo, O.; Ueshima, H. Randomized controlled trial of sour milk on blood pressure in bordeline hypertensive men. *Am. J. Hypertens* **2004**, *17*, 701–706. [CrossRef]
34. Aoyagi, Y.; Park, S.; Matsubara, S.; Honda, Y.; Amamoto, R.; Kushiro, A.; Miyazaki, K.; Shephard, R.J. Habitual intake of fermented milk products containing *Lactobacillus casei* strain Shirota and a reduced risk of hypertension in older people. *Benef. Microbes* **2017**, *8*, 23–29. [CrossRef] [PubMed]
35. Naruszewicz, M.; Johansson, M.L.; Zapolska-Downar, D.; Bukowska, H. Effect of *Lactobacillus plantarum* 299v on cardiovascular disease risk factors in smokers. *Microbiome* **2017**, *5*, 14–20. [CrossRef] [PubMed]
36. Matsumoto, T. Potential benefits of garlic and other dietary supplements for the management of hypertension. Review. *Exp. Ther. Med.* **2020**, *19*, 1479–1484.
37. Olas, B. Dietary supplements with antiplatelet activity: A solution for everyone? *Adv. Nutr.* **2018**, *9*, 51–57. [CrossRef] [PubMed]
38. Olas, B. Anti-aggregatory potential of selected vegetables—Promising dietary components for the prevention and treatment of cardiovascular disease. *Adv. Nutr.* **2019**, *10*, 280–290. [CrossRef]
39. Schreiber, O.; Petersson, J.; Phillipson, M.; Perry, M.; Ross, S.; Holm, L. *Lactobacillus reuteri* prevents colitis by reducing P-selectin-associated leukocyte- and platelet-endothelial cell interactions. *Am. J. Physiol. Gastrointest. Liver Physiol.* **2009**, *296*, G534–G542. [CrossRef]
40. Haro, C.; Medina, M. *Lactobacillus casei* CRL 431 improves endothelial and platelet functionality in a pneumococcal infection model. *Benef. Microbes* **2019**, *10*, 533–541. [CrossRef]
41. Zhou, J.S.; Rutherfurd, K.J.; Gill, H.S. Inability of probiotic bacterial strains *Lactobacillus rhamnosus* HN001 and *Bifidobacterium lactis* HN019 to induce human platelet aggregation I vitro. *J. Food Protect.* **2005**, *68*, 2459–2464. [CrossRef]
42. Libby, P. History of discovery: Inflammation in atherosclerosis. *Arterioscler. Thromb. Vasc. Biol.* **2012**, *32*, 2045–2051. [CrossRef]
43. Majewska, K.; Kregielska-Narożna, M.; Jakubowski, K.; Szulinska, M.; Bogdanski, P. The multispecies probiotic effectively reduces homocysteine concentration in obese women: A randomized double-blind placebo-controlled study. *J. Clin. Med.* **2020**, *4*, 1–11.
44. Kuo, S.M. The interplay between fiber and the intestinal microbiome in the inflammatory response. *Adv. Nutr.* **2013**, *4*, 16–28. [CrossRef] [PubMed]

45. Pokusaeva, K.; Fitzgerald, G.F.; van Sinderen, D. Carbohydrate metabolism in Bifidobacteria. *Genes Nutr.* **2011**, *6*, 285–306. [CrossRef] [PubMed]
46. Hidaka, H.; Eida, T.; Takizawa, T.; Tokunage, T.; Tashiro, Y. Effects of fructooligosacharides on intestinal flora and human health. *Bifidobact. Microflora* **1986**, *5*, 37–50. [CrossRef]
47. Hidaka, H.; Tashiro, Y.; Eida, T. Proliferation of bifidobacteria by oligosaccharides and their useful effects on human health. *Bifidobact. Microflora* **1991**, *10*, 65–79. [CrossRef]
48. Hsu, C.K.; Liao, J.W.; Chung, Y.C.; Hsieh, C.P.M.; Chan, Y.C. Xylooligosaccharides and fructooligosaccharides affect the intestinal microbiota and precancerous colonic lesion development in rats. *J. Nutr.* **2004**, *134*, 1523–1528. [CrossRef]
49. Cherry, P.; Vadav, S.; Strain, C.R.; Allsopp, P.J.; McSorley, E.M.; Ross, R.P.; Stanton, C. Probiotics from seaweeeds: An ocean of opportunity? *Marine Drugs* **2019**, *17*, 327. [CrossRef] [PubMed]
50. Parnell, J.A.; Reimer, R.A. Effect of prebiotic fibre supplementation on hepatic gene expression and serum lipids: A dose-response study in JCR:LA-cp rats. *Br. J. Nutr.* **2010**, *103*, 1177–1184. [CrossRef]
51. Parnell, J.A.; Reamer, R.A. Weight loss during oligofructose supplementation is associated with decreased ghrelin and increased peptide YY in overweight and obese adults. *Am. J. Clin. Nutr.* **2009**, *89*, 1751–1759. [CrossRef]
52. Hume, M.P.; Nicolucci, A.C.; Reimer, R.A. Prebiotic supplementation improves appetite control in children with overweight and obesity: A randomized controlled trial. *Am. J. Clin. Nutr.* **2017**, *105*, 790–799. [CrossRef]
53. Nicolucci, A.C.; Hume, M.P.; Martinez, I.; Mayengbam, S.; Walter, J.; Reimer, R.A. Prebiotics reduce body fat and alter intestinal microbiota in children who are overweight or with obesity. *Gastroenterology* **2017**, *153*, 711–722. [CrossRef]
54. Reimer, R.A.; Willis, H.J.; Tunnicliffe, J.M.; Park, H.; Madsen, K.L.; Sot-Vaca, A. Inulin-type fructans and whey protein both modulate appetite but only fructans alter gut microbiota in adults with overweight/obesity: A randomized controlled trial. *Mol. Nutr. Food Res.* **2017**, *61*, 1–17. [CrossRef] [PubMed]
55. Kim, B.; Choi, H.N.; Yim, J.E. Effect of diet on the gut microbiota associated with obesity. *J. Obesity Metab. Synd.* **2019**, *28*, 216–224. [CrossRef] [PubMed]
56. Ghaffari, S.; Roshanravan, N. The role of nutraceuticals in prevention and treatment of hypertension: An updated review of the literature. *Food Res. Int.* **2020**, *128*, 1–12. [CrossRef] [PubMed]
57. Liong, M.T. Probiotics: A critical review of their potential role as antihypertenstives, immune modulators, hypocholesterolemics, and perimenopausal treatments. *Nutr. Rev.* **2007**, *65*, 316–328. [CrossRef] [PubMed]
58. Liong, M.T.; Dunshea, F.R.; Shah, N.P. Effects of a symbiotic containing *Lactobacillus acidophilus* ATCC 4962 on plasma lipid profiles and morphology of erythrocytes in hypercholesterolemic pigs on high- and low-fat diets. *Br. J. Nutr.* **2007**, *98*, 736–744. [CrossRef] [PubMed]
59. Haghighat, N.; Mohammadshahi, M.; Shayanpour, S.; Haghighizadeh, M.H. Effect of symbiotic and probiotic supplementation on serum levels of endothelial cell adhesion molecules in hemodialysis patients: A randomized control study. *Probiotics Antimicro. Proteins* **2018**, *1*, 1–9.
60. Mofid, V.; Izadi, A.; Majtehedi, S.Y.; Khemoat, L. Therapeutic and nutritional effects of synbiotic yogurts in children and adults: A clinical review. *Probiotics Antimicrob. Proteins* **2019**, *10*, 1–17. [CrossRef]
61. Din, A.U.; Hassan, A.; Zhu, Y.; Yin, T.; Gregersen, H.; Wang, G. Amelioration of TMAO through probiotics and its potential role in atherosclerosis. *Appl. Microbiol. Biotechnol.* **2019**, *103*, 9217–9228. [CrossRef]
62. Janeiro, M.H.; Ramirez, M.J.; Milago, F.I.; Martinez, J.A.; Solas, M. Implication of trimethylamine N-oxide (TMAO) in disease: Potential biomarker or new therapeutic target. *Nutrients* **2018**, *10*, 1398. [CrossRef]
63. Wilson, T.W.H.; Wang, Z.; Levison, B.S.; Koeth, R.A.; Britt, E.B.; Fu, X.; Wu, Y.; Hazen, S.L. Intestinal microbial metabolism of phosphatidylcholine and cardiovascular risk. *N. Eng. J. Med.* **2013**, *368*, 1575–1584.
64. Moludi, J.; Alizadeh, M.; Yagin, N.L.; Pasdar, Y.; Nachvak, S.M.; Abdollahzad, H.; Tabaei, A.S. New insights on atherosclerosis: Endcananabinoid systems with gut microbiota. *J. Cardiovasc. Thorac. Res.* **2018**, *10*, 129–137. [CrossRef] [PubMed]
65. Hazen, S. *New Research on Red Meat and Heart Disease*; The Diane Rehm Show (Transcript); WAMU 88.5 American University Radio: Washington, DC, USA, 2013.
66. Collins, H.L.; Drazul-Schrader, D.; Sulpizio, A.C.; Koster, P.D.; Williamson, Y.; Adelman, S.J.; Owen, K.; Sanli, T.; Bellamine, A. L-Carnitine intake and high trimethylamine N-oxide plasma levels correlate with low aortic lesions in ApoE−/− transgenic mice expressing CETP. *Atherosclerosis* **2006**, *244*, 29–37. [CrossRef] [PubMed]

67. Ufnal, M.; Jazwiec, R.; Dadlez, M.; Drapala, A.; Sikora, M.; Skrzypecki, J. Trimethylamine-N-oxide: A carnitine-derived metabolite that prolongs the hypertensive effect of angiotensin II in rats. *Canad. J. Cardiol.* **2014**, *30*, 1700–1705. [CrossRef] [PubMed]
68. Tilg, H. A gut feeling about thrombosis. *N. Eng. J. Med.* **2016**, *374*, 2494–2496. [CrossRef]
69. Kanitsoraphan, C.; Rattanawong, P.; Charensri, S.; Vichai, S. Trimethylamine N-oxide and risk of cardiovascular disease and mortality. *Curr. Nutr. Rep.* **2018**, *7*, 2017–2213. [CrossRef] [PubMed]
70. Hardin, S.J.; Homme, R.; George, A.K.; Tyagi, S.C. Diet-induced chronic syndrome, metabolically transformed trimethylamine-N-oxide, and the cardiovascular functions. *Rev. Cardiovasc. Med.* **2019**, *20*, 121–128. [PubMed]
71. Leustean, A.M.; Ciocoiu, M.; Sava, A.; Costea, C.F.; Floria, M.; Tarniceriu, C.C.; Tanase, D.M. Implication of the intestinal microbiota in dignosisng the progression of diabetes and the presence of cardiovascular disease. *J. Diab. Res.* **2018**, 1–9. [CrossRef]
72. Tripolt, N.J.; Leber, B.; Triebl, A.; Kofeler, H.; Stadlbauer, V.; Sourij, H. Effect of Lactobacillus casei Shirota supplementation on trimethylamine-N-oxide levels in patients with metabolic syndrome: An open-label, randomized study. *Atherosclerosis* **2015**, *242*, 141–144. [CrossRef]
73. Boutagy, N.E.; Neilson, A.P.; Ostergerg, K.L.; Smithson, A.T.; England, T.R.; Davy, B.M.; Hulver, M.W.; Davy, K.P. Probiotic supplementation and trimethylamine-N-oxide production following a high-fat diet. *Obesity* **2015**, *23*, 2357–2363. [CrossRef]
74. Qui, L.; Tao, X.; Xiong, H.; Yu, J.; Wei, H. Lactobacillus plantarum ZDY04 exhibits a strain-specific property of lowering TMAO via the modulation of gut microbiota in mice. *Food Funct.* **2018**, *9*, 4299–4309.
75. Tenore, G.C.; Caruso, D.; Buonamo, G.; D'Avino, M.; Ciampaglia, R.; Maisto, M.; Schsano, C.; Bochino, B.; Novellino, E. Lactofermented annurca apple puree as a functional food indicated for the control of plasma lipid an oxidative amine levels: Results from a randomized clinical trial. *Nutrients* **2019**, *11*, 122. [CrossRef] [PubMed]
76. Liu, W.C.; Yang, M.C.; Wu, Y.Y.; Chen, P.H.; Hsu, C.M.; Chen, L.W. Lactobacillus plantarum revers diabetes-induced Fmo3 and iCAM expression in mice through enteric dysbiosis-related c-Jun NH2-terminal kinase pathways. *PLoS ONE* **2018**, *13*, e0196511.
77. Matsumoto, M.; Kitada, Y.; Shimomura, Y.; Naito, Y. Bifidobacterium animalis subsp. lactis LKM512 reduces levels of intestinal trimethylamine produced by intestinal microbiota in healthy volunteers: A double-blind, placebo-controlled study. *J. Funct. Food* **2017**, *36*, 94–101. [CrossRef]
78. Bogiatzi, C.; Gloor, G.; Allen-Vercoe, E.; Reid, G.; Wong, R.G.; Urquhart, B.L.; Dinculescu, V.; Reutz, K.N.; Velenosi, T.J.; Pignanelli, M.; et al. Metabolic products of the intestinal microbiome and extremes of atherosclerosis. *Atherosclerosis* **2018**, *273*, 91–97. [CrossRef] [PubMed]
79. Montrucchio, C.; De Nicolo, A.; D'Ettorre, G.; D'Ascenzo, F.; Lazzaro, A.; Fettoni, M.; D'Avolio, A.; Bonora, S.; Celani, L.; Di Perri, G.; et al. Serum trimethylamine-N-oxide concentrations in people living with HIV and the effect of probiotic supplementation. *Int. J. Antimicrob. Agents* **2020**, *55*, 1–10. [CrossRef] [PubMed]
80. Vadivielso, J.M.; Rodriquez-Puyol, D.; Pascual, J.; Barrios, C.; Bermudez-Lopez, M.; Sanchez-Nino, M.D.; Perez-Fernandez, M.; Ortiz, A. Atherosclerosis in chronic kidney disease: More, less, or just different? *Arterioscler. Thromb. Vasc. Biol.* **2019**, *10*, 1938–1966. [CrossRef]
81. Roumeliotis, S.; Roumeliotis, A.; Dounousi, E.; Eleftheriadis, T.; Liakopoulos, V. Dietary antioxidant supplements and uric acid in chronic kidney disease: A review. *Nutrients* **2019**, *11*, 1911. [CrossRef]
82. Rossi, M.; Johnson, D.W.; Morrison, M.; Pascoe, E.; Coombes, J.S.; Forbes, J.M.; McWhinney, B.C.; Ungerer, J.P.J.; Dimeski, G.; Campbell, K.L. SYNbiotics easing renal failure by improving gut microbiology (SYNERGY): A protocol of placebo-controlled randomized cross-over trial. *BMC Neprol.* **2014**, *15*, 1–10. [CrossRef]
83. Brown, J.M.; Hazen, S.L. Metaorganismal nutrient metabolism as a basis of cardiovascular disease. *Curr. Opin. Lipidol.* **2014**, *25*, 48–53. [CrossRef]
84. Al-Okbi, S.Y.; Mohamed, D.A.; Hamed, T.E.S.; Khalek, A.B.A.E.; Mohammed, S.E. Role of probiotic mixture with and without green tea extract in prevention of hepatorenal syndrome in rat model. *Pak. J. Biol. Sci.* **2019**, *22*, 21–27.
85. Wang, H.; Mei, L.; Deng, Y.; Liu, Y.; Wei, X.; Liu, M.; Zhou, J.; Ma, H.; Zheng, P.; Yuan, J.; et al. *Lactobacillus brevis* DM9218 ameliorates fructose-induced hyperuricemia through inosine degradation and manipulation of intestinal dysbiosis. *Nutrition* **2019**, *62*, 63–73. [CrossRef] [PubMed]
86. Tao, S.; Tao, S.; Cheng, Y.; Liu, J.; Ma, L.; Fu, P. Effects of probiotic supplements on the progression of chronic kidney disease: A meta-analysis. *Nephrology* **2019**, *24*, 1122–1130. [CrossRef] [PubMed]

87. Yamanaka, H.; Taniguchi, A.; Tsubai, H.; Kano, H.; Asami, Y. Hypouricaemic effects of yoghurt containing *Lactobacillus gasseri* PA-3 in patients with hyperuricaemia and/or gout: A randomized, double-blind, placebo-controlled study. *Mod. Rhematol.* **2019**, *29*, 146–150. [CrossRef] [PubMed]
88. Garcia-Arrayo, F.E.; Ganzaga, G.; Munoz-Jimenez, I.; Blas-Marron, M.G.; Silverio, O.; Tapia, E.; Soto, V.; Ranganathan, N.; Ranganathan, P.; Vyas, U.; et al. Probiotic supplements prevented oxonic acid-induced hyperuricemia and renal damage. *PLoS ONE* **2018**, *24*, e0202901.
89. Firouzi, S.; Haghighatdoost, F. The effects of prebiotic, probiotic, and synbiotic supplementation on blood parameters of renal function: A systematic review and meta-analysis of clinical trials. *Nutrition* **2018**, *51*, 104–113. [CrossRef]
90. Chi, C.; Li, C.; Wu, D.; Buys, N.; Wang, W.; Fan, H.; Sun, J. Effects of probiotics on patients with hypertension: A systematic review and meta-analysis. *Curr. Hypertens Rep.* **2020**, *21*, 1–12. [CrossRef]
91. Shah, B.R.; Li, B.; Al Sabbah, H.; Xu, W.; Mraz, J. Effects of prebiotic dietary fibers and probiotics on human health: With special focus on recent advancement in their encapsulated formulations. *Trends Food Sci. Technol.* **2020**, *102*, 178–192. [CrossRef]

4

Para-Probiotics for Preterm Neonates—The Next Frontier

Girish Deshpande [1,2], Gayatri Athalye-Jape [3] and Sanjay Patole [3,*]

1. Department of Neonatology, Nepean Hospital, Kingswood, NSW 2747, Australia; girish.deshpande@health.nsw.gov.au
2. Sydney Medical School Nepean, University of Sydney, Kingswood, NSW 2747, Australia
3. Department of Neonatology, King Edward Memorial Hospital for Women, Perth, WA 6008, Australia; gayatri.jape@health.wa.gov.au

* Correspondence: sanjay.patole@health.wa.gov.au

Abstract: Current evidence supports the use of probiotics in preterm neonates for prevention of necrotizing enterocolitis, mortality and late onset sepsis. Despite the strong evidence, the uptake of this intervention has not been universal due to concerns including probiotic sepsis, pro-inflammatory response and transmission of antibiotic resistance. Critically ill extremely preterm neonates with potentially compromised gut integrity are at higher risk of probiotic sepsis due to translocation. In most countries, probiotics are sold as food supplements with poor quality control. The traditional definition of probiotics as "live microorganisms" has been challenged as many experts have questioned the importance of viability in the context of the beneficial effects of probiotics. Paraprobiotics (ghost probiotics), are defined as non-viable microbial cells (intact or broken) or crude cell extracts (i.e., with complex chemical composition), which, when administered (orally or topically) in adequate amounts, confer a benefit on the human or animal consumer. Current evidence indicates that paraprobiotics could be safe alternatives to probiotics in preterm neonates. High-quality pre-clinical and clinical studies including adequately powered randomised controlled trials (RCTs) are warranted in preterm neonates to explore this new frontier.

Keywords: infant; newborn; probiotics; review; sepsis

---

1. Introduction

Despite the recent advances in technology and progress in research, necrotising enterocolitis (NEC), mortality, late onset sepsis (LOS), and long-term neurodevelopmental impairment (NDI) continue to remain a major health burden in preterm neonates [1,2]. NEC continues to be major gastrointestinal emergency in ~7% of preterm very low birth weight (VLBW: Birth weight < 1500 g) neonates. Mortality is high, up to 20 to 30%, with the highest rate among neonates requiring surgery [3–6]. The morbidity of definite (≥Stage II) NEC is significant and includes prolonged hospitalisation, recurrent infections, long-term dependence on parenteral nutrition, and survival with intestinal failure, and long-term NDI, especially in extremely low birth weight (ELBW: Birth weight < 1000 g) neonates needing surgery for the illness [7]. Stey et al. have estimated the cost of treatment of one case of NEC requiring surgery, close to $400,000 [8].

The World Health Organisation (WHO) defines probiotics as "live microorganisms which when administered in adequate amounts confer a health benefit on the host." [9]. Bacteria such as bifidobacteria, and lactobacilli, and non-pathogenic fungi such as Saccharomyces, are the most common type of microorganisms used as probiotics. The mechanisms for the benefits of probiotics include gut barrier enhancement, immune response modulation (e.g., TLR4 receptor, nuclear factor-B, inflammatory cytokines), and competitive inhibition of gut colonisation by pathogens [10,11].

Systematic reviews of randomised controlled trials (RCTs) have shown that prophylactic administration of enteral probiotics significantly reduces the risk of ≥Stage II NEC, mortality, LOS and the time to full enteral feeding in preterm VLBW neonates [12,13]. Many developed countries including Australia, Canada, Finland, Denmark, and Germany, are currently using probiotics as standard practice for prevention of NEC in preterm VLBW neonates [14–18]. A systematic review of observational studies has confirmed the benefits of enteral probiotics in preterm neonates [19].

Despite the various systematic reviews of RCTs and 'before vs. after' routine use studies (Non-RCTs) reporting significant benefits of probiotics in reducing the risk of ≥Stage II NEC, LOS, all-cause mortality, and feeding intolerance, the uptake of this intervention has been relatively slow, and not universal. The reasons for this slow uptake include the concerns about probiotic sepsis, development and transmission of antibiotic resistance, possibility of an exaggerated pro-inflammatory response, and non-availability of or difficulties in accessing high quality, safe and effective products [20]. In most countries, probiotics are sold as food supplements with poor quality control. The death of a preterm neonate from a contaminated probiotic product that was used in a large RCT by Jacobs et al., has highlighted the issue of poor quality control for probiotic products [21,22].

The risk of probiotic translocation and sepsis is higher; especially in critically ill and/or extremely preterm neonates (e.g., suspected/proven sepsis or NEC) with potentially compromised gut integrity [14,23–26]. Although none of the RCTs have reported probiotic sepsis, there are reports of the administered probiotic causing serious infections such as septicemia, pneumonia and meningitis [24–29]. Kopp et al. reported that *L. rhamnosus* GG (LGG) supplementation during pregnancy and early infancy did not reduce the incidence or severity of atopic dermatitis in children, but was associated with an increased rate of recurrent episodes of wheezing bronchitis [30]. It is important to note that probiotic strains may express virulence factors or acquire antibiotic resistance genes via horizontal gene transfer [31]. However, advances in technology have allowed the removal of plasmid for antibiotic resistance from maternal strain [32]. Zheng et al. have emphasised the importance of broader screening of antibiotic resistance in commercially manufactured probiotic supplements. They recommend techniques such as computational simulations, live imaging and functional genomics to study the evolutionary behaviour, adaptations and dynamics of commercially manufactured probiotic for optimising their safety [33].

2. Para-probiotics

Probiotic products contain a mix of live and dead cells; however, the population of dead cells at any given time during the shelf life of such products is virtually unknown [34–36]. The dead cell preparations from probiotics have been fractionated and various cellular components and metabolites have been shown to produce a range of biological responses [34]. Taverniti et al. propose the term 'paraprobiotic' (ghost probiotics), to define non-viable microbial cells (intact or broken) or crude cell extracts (i.e., with complex chemical composition), which, when administered (orally or topically) in adequate amounts, confer a benefit on the human or animal consumer [37].

Several methods of inactivation of probiotics have been studied including the use of heat, chemicals (e.g., formalin), gamma or ultraviolet rays, and sonication. Different methods of inactivation may affect structural components of the cell differently, and influence its immunomodulatory activity [37]. Heat treatment seems to be the method of choice for inactivation of probiotic strains in majority of studies [37,38].

3. Mechanisms of Action of Para-probiotics

The mechanisms of action of heat-inactivated/killed probiotics are poorly understood. A variety of biological responses have been reported after administering killed (mostly heat-killed) probiotics to various mammalian and avian species [37]. Animal studies in gastrostomy-fed infant rats show that live and heat-killed *L. rhamnosus GG* decreases LPS-induced pro-inflammatory mediators and increases anti-inflammatory mediators [39]. Bloise et al. reported similar results on human placental trophoblast cells [40]. Studies in epithelial cells and in an infant formula-fed rodent model suggest that killed microbes may be as effective as live microbes in modulating additional inflammatory stimuli [41,42]. Other potential mechanisms of action of killed/inactivated probiotics include adhesive properties of BoPA a cell surface lipoprotein identified in *Bifidobacterium (B.) bifidum* and anti-inflammatory effects of *L. acidophilus* and *L. plantarum* [37,43]. Other killed probiotics with beneficial immunomodulatory responses in laboratory settings include *L. rhamnosus GG, L. plantarum* L-137, *B. breve, Escherichia coli Nissle* 1917, *B. bifidum, L. acidophilus, L. helveticus, B. bifidum* and *L. casei.* [37]. Sakai et al. reported that killed *Enterococcus faecalis* (EC-12) prevented vancomycin-resistant enterococci colonization in the cecum of newly hatched chicks [44]. Reduced capacity for mucosal adhesion is a potential adverse effect of heat inactivation of a probiotic strain. However, contrary to the expectation, strain *P. freundereichii* has been shown to have an increased ability for adhesion after heat inactivation [45]. Reduced ability to exert an anti-inflammatory effect after heat inactivation is another concern. However, heat-inactivated strains *L. casei* strain Shirota or *L. fermentum* MS15 [46] have been shown to modulate inflammatory response by regulating IL-10, human B-defensin and other pro-inflammatory cytokines and *B. breve* and *B. bifidum* have improved ability to increase the secretion of IL-10, an anti-inflammatory cytokine [47].

Adams and Kataria et al. have also explored the field of non-viable versus viable probiotic strains. Adams reviewed the 'probiotic paradox', and beneficial biological responses of live and dead probiotic bacteria [34]. Enhanced safety and longer shelf life were considered as the advantages of 'dead' probiotic bacteria. Dead probiotics had various biological responses including anti-inflammatory effects, attenuation of colitis, reduction of IL-8 production, stimulation of gut immune system, and stimulation of IL-6 production, in pre-clinical studies [34]. Kataria et al. summarised the mechanisms of action of "dead" probiotics or their components, and reported that dead microbes could modulate anti-inflammatory effects as effectively as live probiotics [20].

4. Which Probiotic Species Can Be Used in Their Heat-Inactivated form as Para-probiotics?

The *Lactobacillus* and *Bifidobacterium* species are commonly used probiotics. Emerging evidence indicates that strains of both *Lactobacillus* [45,48,49] and *Bifidobacterium* [50–54] species are capable of beneficial effects in their heat-inactivated form. The case of *B. breve* M-16V is worth noting, as this probiotic strain is being used routinely in preterm infants for prevention of NEC [55]. Sugahara et al. have investigated the differences between live and heat-killed *B. breve* M-16V, in the regulation of immune function, intestinal metabolism and intestinal gene expression using gnotobiotic mouse model and omics approaches [50]. Both live and heat-killed forms of *B. breve* M-16V showed immune-modulating effects that suppressed pro-inflammatory cytokine production in spleen cells and affected intestinal metabolism. However, live strains exhibited more significant effects in the regulation of intestinal metabolism and intestinal gene expression involved in nutrient metabolism [50]. Athalye-Jape et al. have reported a strain specific systematic review of RCTs and non-RCTs of *B. breve* M-16V in preterm infants [55]. A total of 5 RCTs (n = 482) and 4 non-RCTs (n = 2496) were included. Data from the 3 small RCTs (n = 386) reporting on clinically important outcomes was inadequate to derive firm conclusions [18,56,57]. Meta-analysis of data from non-RCTs showed significant benefits on LOS, mortality, and the postnatal age at full feeds. There were no *B. breve* M-16V related adverse effects [55]. The findings reported by Sugahara et al., and Athalye-Jape et al. suggest that inactivated *B. breve* M-16V may be a suitable paraprobiotic strain for assessment in clinical trials [50,55]. Research on other paraprobiotics (developed from other probiotic strains that have been shown to be effective in RCTs and/or non-RCTs) is important to study their safety and efficacy against placebo and/or probiotics in preterm VLBW neonates.

5. Clinical and Pre-Clinical Studies of Para-probiotics

Lahtinen has recently reviewed the pre-clinical and clinical studies on live versus inactivated probiotics [35]. Clinical studies comparing non-viable versus viable probiotic strains for various conditions (e.g., diarrhoea, irritable bowel syndrome, eradication of H. pylori, cow's milk protein intolerance) were few, and showed comparable, high or lower efficacy of non-viable versus viable probiotics. Small sample sizes, lack of a placebo group, and use of non-standardised strains were some of the limitations of these studies. Findings from various preclinical studies included the following: (1) Viable and non-viable lactobacilli had equal ability for adherence to gut mucosa [58], and heat-killing and protease treatments impaired the mucus adherent property [59]; (2) Heat-killing changed the intestinal location of the bacteria. Live bacteria were seen in Peyer's patches and lamina propria whereas most heat-killed bacteria were in the lumen and cleared rapidly [60]; (3) Heat-killed lactobacilli inhibited pathogen adhesion to the gut mucosa by competitive exclusion [61]; (4) Inactivated lactobacilli enhanced gut epithelial barrier [62]; (5) Non-viable probiotic components such as cell wall extracts [63], lipoteichoic acid [64], bacterial DNA [65,66], and surface (S)-layer proteins [67] can have immunomodulatory effects by various mechanisms including increased salivary IgA production [68], modulation of host T-cell responses [69] and gene expression [70]; (6) Live and inactivated probiotics had comparable effects on innate immunity [71–73]; (7) Live as well as killed *B. lactis* HN019 enhanced phagocytic responses in peripheral blood cells; however, only viable bacteria increased the phagocytic activity of peritoneal cells [74]; (8) As for adaptive immunity, many studies favoured live over non-viable bacteria [60,75–78], but some showed that both forms had similar effects on the phenotype and functions of human myeloid dendritic cells [79]. Overall, the evidence from pre-clinical and clinical studies suggested that "in some situations, depending on the mechanism of action, probiotic effects are not dependent on cell viability". The need for clinical studies and consideration of the differences in the effects of dormant (during storage), inactivated and live bacteria was emphasised [80].

6. Systematic Review of Studies of Modified Probiotics for Prevention and Treatment of Various Diseases

Zorzela et al. have reported a systematic review of trials of dead bacteria/yeasts ('Modified microbes') inactivated by heating/sonication of probiotic strains, for prevention ($n = 14$) or treatment ($n = 26$) of various diseases, mainly in adults and children [38]. The trials compared modified microbes with either placebo (44%) or the same probiotic strain (39%) or standard treatment (17%). Compared with probiotics, the modified microbes were not significantly more or less effective in 86% of prevention and 69% of treatment trials. Meta-analysis of data from 5 RCTs showed significant benefits of modified L. acidophilus (Standard mean difference: −0.81, 95% CI: −1.44, −0.17) as an adjuvant in treatment of acute diarrhoea; however, there was significant heterogeneity ($I^2 = 86\%$). The incidence of adverse events was comparable for modified microbes, probiotics and other controls but many trials did not report adequate data on safety. Overall, there was some evidence that modified microbes may be useful for few conditions. The limitations of this review include the heterogeneity of methodology and the tested strains in the included studies and their small sample sizes [38].

In summary, current evidence indicates that paraprobiotics could be safe alternatives to probiotics in preterm neonates. High quality pre-clinical as well as clinical studies including adequately powered RCTs are warranted in preterm neonates to explore this new frontier. A cluster RCT design is appropriate to avoid the issue of cross-contamination. A non-inferiority design will be acceptable for this purpose. However, deciding the clinically acceptable margin of inferiority will be an important issue considering the effect size for benefits of probiotics for NEC, all-cause mortality, late onset sepsis, and time to full feeding in preterm infants. Considering that effects of probiotic strains are 'strain-specific', rigorous assessment of specific effects of different paraprobiotic strains are important. This issue is also relevant when a mixture of strains is used. Assessment of the effects of added prebiotic oligosaccharides is another important issue. Finally, the significance of the utility of paraprobiotics beyond the preterm neonatal population cannot be ignored.

References

1. Glass, H.C.; Costarino, A.T.; Stayer, S.A.; Brett, C.M.; Cladis, F.; Davis, P.J. Outcomes for extremely premature infants. *Anesth. Analg.* **2015**, *120*, 1337–1351. [CrossRef] [PubMed]
2. Hornik, C.P.; Fort, P.; Clark, R.H.; Watt, K.; Benjamin, D.K., Jr.; Smith, P.B.; Manzoni, P.; Jacqz-Aigrain, E.; Kaguelidou, F.; Cohen-Wolkowiez, M. Early and late onset sepsis in very-low-birth-weight infants from a large group of neonatal intensive care units. *Early Hum. Dev.* **2012**, *88* (Suppl. 2), S69–S74. [CrossRef]
3. Mupsilonller, M.J.; Paul, T.; Seeliger, S. Necrotizing enterocolitis in premature infants and newborns. *J. Neonatal Perinat. Med.* **2016**, *9*, 233–242.
4. Nino, D.F.; Sodhi, C.P.; Hackam, D.J. Necrotizing enterocolitis: New insights into pathogenesis and mechanisms. *Nat. Rev. Gastroenterol. Hepatol.* **2016**, *13*, 590–600. [CrossRef] [PubMed]
5. Henry, M.C.; Moss, R.L. Neonatal necrotizing enterocolitis. *Semin. Pediatr. Surg.* **2008**, *17*, 98–109. [CrossRef] [PubMed]
6. Neu, J.; Walker, W.A. Necrotizing enterocolitis. *N. Engl. J. Med.* **2011**, *364*, 255–264. [CrossRef] [PubMed]
7. Schulzke, S.M.; Deshpande, G.C.; Patole, S.K. Neurodevelopmental outcomes of very low-birth-weight infants with necrotizing enterocolitis: A systematic review of observational studies. *Arch. Pediatr. Adolesc. Med.* **2007**, *161*, 583–590. [CrossRef] [PubMed]
8. Stey, A.; Barnert, E.S.; Tseng, C.H.; Keeler, E.; Needleman, J.; Leng, M.; Kelley-Quon, L.I.; Shew, S.B. Outcomes and costs of surgical treatments of necrotizing enterocolitis. *Pediatrics* **2015**, *135*, e1190–e1197. [CrossRef] [PubMed]
9. Food and Agriculture Organization (FAO); World Health Organization (WHO). Guidelines for the Evaluation of Probiotics in Food: Report of a Joint FAO/WHO Working Group on Drafting Guidelines for the Evaluation of Probiotics in Food 2002. Available online: ftp://ftp.fao.org/es/esn/food/wgreport2.pdf (accessed on 1 October 2017).
10. Rao, R.K.; Samak, G. Protection and Restitution of Gut Barrier by Probiotics: Nutritional and Clinical Implications. *Curr. Nutr. Food Sci.* **2013**, *9*, 99–107. [PubMed]
11. Walker, A. Intestinal colonization and programming of the intestinal immune response. *J. Clin. Gastroenterol.* **2014**, *48* (Suppl. 1), S8–S11. [CrossRef] [PubMed]
12. Deshpande, G.; Rao, S.; Patole, S.; Bulsara, M. Updated meta-analysis of probiotics for preventing necrotizing enterocolitis in preterm neonates. *Pediatrics* **2010**, *125*, 921–930. [CrossRef] [PubMed]
13. AlFaleh, K.; Anabrees, J. Probiotics for prevention of necrotizing enterocolitis in preterm infants. *Evid. Based Child. Health* **2014**, *9*, 584–671. [CrossRef] [PubMed]
14. Deshpande, G.; Rao, S.; Patole, S. Probiotics in neonatal intensive care—Back to the future. *Aust. N. Z. J. Obstet. Gynaecol.* **2015**, *55*, 210–217. [CrossRef] [PubMed]
15. Hartel, C.; Pagel, J.; Rupp, J.; Bendiks, M.; Guthmann, F.; Rieger-Fackeldey, E.; Heckmann, M.; Franz, A.; Schiffmann, J.H.; Zimmermann, B.; et al. Prophylactic use of *Lactobacillus acidophilus/Bifidobacterium infantis* probiotics and outcome in very low birth weight infants. *J. Pediatr.* **2014**, *165*, 285–289. [CrossRef] [PubMed]
16. Janvier, A.; Malo, J.; Barrington, K.J. Cohort study of probiotics in a North American neonatal intensive care unit. *J. Pediatr.* **2014**, *164*, 980–985. [CrossRef] [PubMed]
17. Luoto, R.; Isolauri, E.; Lehtonen, L. Safety of *Lactobacillus GG* probiotic in infants with very low birth weight: Twelve years of experience. *Clin. Infect. Dis.* **2010**, *50*, 1327–1328. [CrossRef] [PubMed]
18. Patole, S.K.; Rao, S.C.; Keil, A.D.; Nathan, E.A.; Doherty, D.A.; Simmer, K.N. Benefits of *Bifidobacterium breve* M-16V Supplementation in Preterm Neonates—A Retrospective Cohort Study. *PLoS ONE* **2016**, *11*, e0150775. [CrossRef] [PubMed]
19. Olsen, R.; Greisen, G.; Schroder, M.; Brok, J. Prophylactic Probiotics for Preterm Infants: A Systematic Review and Meta-Analysis of Observational Studies. *Neonatology* **2016**, *109*, 105–112. [CrossRef] [PubMed]
20. Kataria, J.; Li, N.; Wynn, J.L.; Neu, J. Probiotic microbes: Do they need to be alive to be beneficial? *Nutr. Rev.* **2009**, *67*, 546–550. [CrossRef] [PubMed]
21. C.D.C. Fatal Gastrointestinal Mucormycosis in an Infant Following Ingestion of Contaminated Dietary Supplement—Connecticut. 2014. Available online: https://www.cdc.gov/fungal/outbreaks/rhizopus-investigation.html (accessed on 1 June 2018).

22. Jacobs, S.E.; Tobin, J.M.; Opie, G.F.; Donath, S.; Tabrizi, S.N.; Pirotta, M.; Morley, C.J.; Garland, S.M. Probiotic effects on late-onset sepsis in very preterm infants: A randomized controlled trial. *Pediatrics* **2013**, *132*, 1055–1062. [CrossRef] [PubMed]
23. Boyle, R.J.; Robins-Browne, R.M.; Tang, M.L. Probiotic use in clinical practice: What are the risks? *Am. J. Clin. Nutr.* **2006**, *83*, 1256–1264. [CrossRef] [PubMed]
24. Dani, C.; Coviello, C.C.; Corsini, I.I.; Arena, F.; Antonelli, A.; Rossolini, G.M. *Lactobacillus* Sepsis and Probiotic Therapy in Newborns: Two New Cases and Literature Review. *AJP Rep.* **2016**, *6*, e25–e29. [PubMed]
25. Jenke, A.; Ruf, E.M.; Hoppe, T.; Heldmann, M.; Wirth, S. *Bifidobacterium* septicaemia in an extremely low-birthweight infant under probiotic therapy. *Arch. Dis. Child. Fetal Neonatal Ed.* **2012**, *97*, F217–F218. [CrossRef] [PubMed]
26. Ohishi, A.; Takahashi, S.; Ito, Y.; Ohishi, Y.; Tsukamoto, K.; Nanba, Y.; Ito, N.; Kakiuchi, S.; Saitoh, A.; Morotomi, M.; et al. *Bifidobacterium* septicemia associated with postoperative probiotic therapy in a neonate with omphalocele. *J. Pediatr.* **2010**, *156*, 679–681. [CrossRef] [PubMed]
27. Broughton, R.A.; Gruber, W.C.; Haffar, A.A.; Baker, C.J. Neonatal meningitis due to *Lactobacillus*. *Pediatr. Infect. Dis.* **1983**, *2*, 382–384. [CrossRef] [PubMed]
28. Reddy, V.S.; Patole, S.K.; Rao, S. Role of probiotics in short bowel syndrome in infants and children—A systematic review. *Nutrients* **2013**, *5*, 679–699. [CrossRef] [PubMed]
29. Thompson, C.; McCarter, Y.S.; Krause, P.J.; Herson, V.C. *Lactobacillus acidophilus* sepsis in a neonate. *J. Perinatol.* **2001**, *21*, 258–260. [CrossRef] [PubMed]
30. Kopp, M.V.; Hennemuth, I.; Heinzmann, A.; Urbanek, R. Randomized, double-blind, placebo-controlled trial of probiotics for primary prevention: No clinical effects of *Lactobacillus GG* supplementation. *Pediatrics* **2008**, *121*, e850–e856. [CrossRef] [PubMed]
31. Mater, D.D.; Langella, P.; Corthier, G.; Flores, M.J. A probiotic *Lactobacillus* strain can acquire vancomycin resistance during digestive transit in mice. *J. Mol. Microbiol. Biotechnol.* **2008**, *14*, 123–127. [CrossRef] [PubMed]
32. Rosander, A.; Connolly, E.; Roos, S. Removal of antibiotic resistance gene carrying plasmids from *Lactobacillus reuteri* ATCC 55730 and characterization of the resulting daughter strain, *L. reuteri* DSM 17938. *Appl. Environ. Microbiol.* **2008**, *74*, 6032–6040. [CrossRef] [PubMed]
33. Zheng, M.; Zhang, R.; Tian, X.; Zhou, X.; Pan, X.; Wong, A. Assessing the risk of probiotic dietary supplements in the context of antibiotic resistance. *Front. Microbiol.* **2017**, *8*, 908. [CrossRef] [PubMed]
34. Adams, C.A. The probiotic paradox: Live and dead cells are biological response modifiers. *Nutr. Res. Rev.* **2010**, *23*, 37–46. [CrossRef] [PubMed]
35. Lahtinen, S. Probiotic viability-does it matter? *Microb. Ecol. Health Dis.* **2012**, *23*, 18567. [CrossRef] [PubMed]
36. Nighswonger, B.D.; Brashears, M.M.; Gilliland, S.E. Viability of *Lactobacillus acidophilus* and *Lactobacillus casei* in fermented milk products during refrigerated storage. *J. Dairy Sci.* **1996**, *79*, 212–219. [CrossRef]
37. Taverniti, V.; Guglielmetti, S. The immunomodulatory properties of probiotic microorganisms beyond their viability (ghost probiotics: Proposal of paraprobiotic concept). *Genes Nutr.* **2011**, *6*, 261–274. [CrossRef] [PubMed]
38. Zorzela, L.; Ardestani, S.K.; McFarland, L.V.; Vohra, S. Is there a role for modified probiotics as beneficial microbes: A systematic review of the literature. *Benef. Microbes* **2017**, *8*, 739–754. [CrossRef] [PubMed]
39. Li, N.; Russell, W.M.; Douglas-escobar, M.; Hauser, N.; Lopez, M.; Neu, J. Live and heat-killed *Lactobacillus rhamnosus* GG: Effects on proinflammatory and anti-inflammatory cytokines/chemokines in gastrostomy-fed infant rats. *Pediatr. Res.* **2009**, *66*, 203–207. [CrossRef] [PubMed]
40. Bloise, E.; Torricelli, M.; Novembri, R.; Borges, L.E.; Carrarelli, P.; Reis, F.M.; Petraglia, F. Heat-killed *Lactobacillus rhamnosus* GG modulates urocortin and cytokine release in primary trophoblast cells. *Placenta* **2010**, *31*, 867–872. [CrossRef] [PubMed]
41. Lopez, M.; Li, N.; Kataria, J.; Russell, M.; Neu, J. Live and ultraviolet-inactivated *Lactobacillus rhamnosus* GG decrease flagellin-induced interleukin-8 production in Caco-2 cells. *J. Nutr.* **2008**, *138*, 2264–2268. [CrossRef] [PubMed]
42. Zhang, L.; Li, N.; Caicedo, R.; Neu, J. Alive and dead *Lactobacillus rhamnosus* GG decrease tumor necrosis factor-alpha-induced interleukin-8 production in Caco-2 cells. *J. Nutr.* **2005**, *135*, 1752–1756. [CrossRef] [PubMed]

43. Guglielmetti, S.; Tamagnini, I.; Mora, D.; Minuzzo, M.; Scarafoni, A.; Arioli, S.; Hellman, J.; Karp, M.; Parini, C. Implication of an outer surface lipoprotein in adhesion of *Bifidobacterium bifidum* to Caco-2 cells. *Appl. Environ. Microbiol.* **2008**, *74*, 4695–4702. [CrossRef] [PubMed]
44. Sakai, Y.; Tsukahara, T.; Bukawa, W.; Matsubara, N.; Ushida, K. Cell preparation of *Enterococcus faecalis* strain EC-12 prevents vancomycin-resistant enterococci colonization in the cecum of newly hatched chicks. *Poult. Sci.* **2006**, *85*, 273–277. [CrossRef] [PubMed]
45. Ouwehand, A.C.; Tölkkö, S.; Kulmala, J.; Salminen, S.; Salminen, E. Adhesion of inactivated probiotic strains to intestinal mucus. *Lett. Appl. Microbiol.* **2000**, *31*, 82–86. [CrossRef] [PubMed]
46. Habil, N.; Abate, W.; Beal, J.; Foey, A.D. Heat-killed probiotic bacteria differentially regulate colonic epithelial cell production of human β-defensin-2: Dependence on inflammatory cytokines. *Benef. Microbes* **2014**, *5*, 483–495. [CrossRef] [PubMed]
47. Imaoka, A.; Shima, T.; Kato, K.; Mizuno, S.; Uehara, T.; Matsumoto, S.; Setoyama, H.; Hara, T.; Umesaki, Y. Anti-inflammatory activity of probiotic *Bifidobacterium*: Enhancement of IL-10 production in peripheral blood mononuclear cells from ulcerative colitis patients and inhibition of IL-8 secretion in HT-29 cells. *World J. Gastroenterol.* **2008**, *14*, 2511–2516. [CrossRef] [PubMed]
48. Donkor, O.N.; Ravikumar, M.; Proudfoot, O.; Day, S.L.; Apostolopoulos, V.; Paukovics, G.; Vasiljevic, T.; Nutt, S.L.; Gill, H. Cytokine profile and induction of T helper type 17 and regulatory T cells by human peripheral mononuclear cells after microbial exposure. *Clin. Exp. Immunol.* **2012**, *167*, 282–295. [CrossRef] [PubMed]
49. Szajewska, H.; Guarino, A.; Hojsak, I.; Indrio, F.; Kolacek, S.; Shamir, R.; Vandenplas, Y.; Weizman, Z. European Society for Pediatric Gastroenterology, Hepatology, and Nutrition. Use of probiotics for management of acute gastroenteritis: A position paper by the ESPGHAN Working Group for Probiotics and Prebiotics. *J. Pediatr. Gastroenterol. Nutr.* **2014**, *58*, 531–539. [CrossRef] [PubMed]
50. Sugahara, H.; Yao, R.; Odamaki, T.; Xiao, J.Z. Differences between live and heat-killed *Bifidobacteria* in the regulation of immune function and the intestinal environment. *Benef. Microbes* **2017**, *8*, 463–472. [CrossRef] [PubMed]
51. Schwendicke, F.; Horb, K.; Kneist, S.; Dörfer, C.; Paris, S. Effects of heat-inactivated *Bifidobacterium BB12* on cariogenicity of *Streptococcus mutans* in vitro. *Arch. Oral Biol.* **2014**, *59*, 1384–1390. [CrossRef] [PubMed]
52. Hayes, C.L.; Natividad, J.M.; Jury, J.; Martin, R.; Langella, P.; Verdu, E.F. Efficacy of *Bifidobacterium breve* NCC2950 against DSS-induced colitis is dependent on bacterial preparation and timing of administration. *Benef. Microbes* **2014**, *5*, 79–88. [CrossRef] [PubMed]
53. Natividad, J.M.; Hayes, C.L.; Motta, J.P.; Jury, J.; Galipeau, H.J.; Philip, V.; Garcia-Rodenas, C.L.; Kiyama, H.; Bercik, P.; Verdu, E.F. Differential induction of antimicrobial REGIII by the intestinal microbiota and *Bifidobacterium breve* NCC2950. *Appl. Environ. Microbiol.* **2013**, *79*, 7745–7754. [CrossRef] [PubMed]
54. Nakamura, Y.; Terahara, M.; Iwamoto, T.; Yamada, K.; Asano, M.; Kakuta, S.; Iwakura, Y.; Totsuka, M. Upregulation of Polymeric Immunoglobulin Receptor Expression by the Heat-Inactivated Potential Probiotic *Bifidobacterium bifidum* OLB6378 in a Mouse Intestinal Explant Model. *Scand. J. Immunol.* **2012**, *75*, 176–183. [CrossRef] [PubMed]
55. Athalye-Jape, G.; Rao, S.; Simmer, K.; Patole, S. *Bifidobacterium breve* M-16V as a Probiotic for Preterm Infants: A Strain-Specific Systematic Review. *J. Parenter. Enter. Nutr.* **2017**, *42*, 677–688. [CrossRef] [PubMed]
56. Hikaru, U.; Koichi, S.; Yayoi, S.; Hiromichi, S.; Hiraoki, S.; Yoshikazu, O.; Seigo, S.; Satoru, N.; Toshiaki, S.; Yuichiro, Y. *Bifidobacteria* prevents preterm infants from infection and sepsis. *Int. J. Probiotics Prebiotics* **2010**, *5*, 33–36.
57. Fujii, T.; Ohtsuka, Y.; Lee, T.; Kudo, T.; Shoji, H.; Sato, H.; Nagata, S.; Shimizu, T.; Yamashiro, Y. *Bifidobacterium breve* enhances transforming growth factor beta1 signaling by regulating Smad7 expression in preterm infants. *J. Pediatr. Gastroenterol. Nutr.* **2006**, *43*, 83–88. [CrossRef] [PubMed]
58. Hood, S.K.; Zottola, E.A. Effect of low pH on the ability of *Lactobacillus acidophilus* to survive and adhere to human intestinal cells. *J. Food Sci.* **1988**, *53*, 1514–1516. [CrossRef]
59. Tuomola, E.M.; Ouwehand, A.C.; Salminen, S.J. Chemical, physical and enzymatic pre-treatments of probiotic lactobacilli alter their adhesion to human intestinal mucus glycoproteins. *Int. J. Food Microbiol.* **2000**, *60*, 75–81. [CrossRef]
60. Maldonado Galdeano, C.; Perdigon, G. Role of viability of probiotic strains in their persistence in the gut and in mucosal immune stimulation. *J. Appl. Microbiol.* **2004**, *97*, 673–681. [CrossRef] [PubMed]

61. Chauviere, G.; Coconnier, M.H.; Kerneis, S.; Darfeuille-Michaud, A.; Joly, B.; Servin, A.L. Competitive exclusion of diarrheagenic *Escherichia coli* (ETEC) from human enterocyte-like Caco-2 cells by heat-killed *Lactobacillus*. *FEMS Microbiol. Lett.* **1992**, *70*, 213–217. [CrossRef]
62. Montalto, M.; Maggiano, N.; Ricci, R.; Curigliano, V.; Santoro, L.; Di Nicuolo, F.; Vecchio, F.M.; Gasbarrini, A.; Gasbarrini, G. *Lactobacillus acidophilus* protects tight Sajunctions from aspirin damage in HT-29 cells. *Digestion* **2004**, *69*, 225–228. [CrossRef] [PubMed]
63. Yan, F.; Polk, D.B. Probiotic bacterium prevents cytokine-induced apoptosis in intestinal epithelial cells. *J. Biol. Chem.* **2002**, *277*, 50959–50965. [CrossRef] [PubMed]
64. Solis Pereyra, B.; Lemonnier, D. Induction of human cytokines by bacteria used in dairy foods. *Nutr. Res.* **1993**, *13*, 1127–1140. [CrossRef]
65. Matsuguchi, T.; Takagi, A.; Matsuzaki, T.; Nagaoka, M.; Ishikawa, K.; Yokokura, T.; Yoshikai, Y. Lipoteichoic acids from *Lactobacillus* strains elicit strong tumor necrosis factor alpha-inducing activities in macrophages through Toll-like receptor 2. *Clin. Diagn. Lab. Immunol.* **2003**, *10*, 259–266. [CrossRef] [PubMed]
66. Rachmilewitz, D.; Karmeli, F.; Takabayashi, K.; Hayashi, T.; LeiderTrejo, L.; Lee, J.; Leoni, L.M.; Raz, E. Immunostimulatory DNA ameliorates experimental and spontaneous murine colitis. *Gastroenterology* **2002**, *122*, 1428–1441. [CrossRef] [PubMed]
67. Takahashi, N.; Kitazawa, H.; Iwabuchi, N.; Xiao, J.Z.; Miyaji, K.; Iwatsuki, K.; Saito, T. Immunostimulatory oligodeoxynucleotide from *Bifidobacterium longum* suppresses Th2 immune responses in a murine model. *Clin. Exp. Immunol.* **2006**, *145*, 130–138. [CrossRef] [PubMed]
68. Konstantinov, S.R.; Smidt, H.; de Vos, W.M.; Bruijns, S.C.; Singh, S.K.; Valence, F.; Molle, D.; Lortal, S.; Altermann, E.; Klaenhammer, T.R.; et al. S layer protein A of *Lactobacillus* acidophilus NCFM regulates immature dendritic cell and T cell functions. *Proc. Natl. Acad. Sci. USA* **2008**, *105*. [CrossRef] [PubMed]
69. Kotani, Y.; Shinkai, S.; Okamatsu, H.; Toba, M.; Ogawa, K.; Yoshida, H.; Fukaya, T.; Fujiwara, Y.; Chaves, P.H.; Kakumoto, K.; et al. Oral intake of *Lactobacillus pentosus* strain b240 accelerates salivary immunoglobulin A secretion in the elderly: A randomized, placebo-controlled, double-blind trial. *Immun. Ageing* **2010**, *7*, 11. [CrossRef] [PubMed]
70. Hirose, Y.; Murosaki, S.; Yamamoto, Y.; Yoshikai, Y.; Tsuru, T. Daily intake of heat-killed *Lactobacillus plantarum* L-137 augments acquired immunity in healthy adults. *J. Nutr.* **2006**, *136*, 3069–3073. [CrossRef] [PubMed]
71. Van Baarlen, P.; Troost, F.J.; van Hemert, S.; van der, M.C.; de Vos, W.M.; de Groot, P.J.; Hooiveld, G.J.; Brummer, R.J.; Kleerebezem, M. Differential NF-kappaB pathways induction by *Lactobacillus plantarum* in the duodenum of healthy humans correlating with immune tolerance. *Proc. Natl. Acad. Sci. USA* **2009**, *106*. [CrossRef] [PubMed]
72. Haller, D.; Blum, S.; Bode, C.; Hammes, W.P.; Schiffrin, E.J. Activation of human peripheral blood mononuclear cells by nonpathogenic bacteria in vitro: Evidence of NK cells as primary targets. *Infect. Immun.* **2000**, *68*, 752–759. [CrossRef] [PubMed]
73. Korhonen, R.; Korpela, R.; Saxelin, M.; Maki, M.; Kankaanranta, H.; Moilanen, E. Induction of nitric oxide synthesis by probiotic *Lactobacillus rhamnosus* GG in J774 macrophages and human T84 intestinal epithelial cells. *Inflammation* **2001**, *25*, 223–232. [CrossRef] [PubMed]
74. Perdigon, G.; de Macias, M.E.; Alvarez, S.; Oliver, G.; de Ruiz Holgado, A.A. Effect of perorally administered lactobacilli on macrophage activation in mice. *Infect. Immun.* **1986**, *53*, 404–410. [PubMed]
75. Gill, H.S.; Rutherfurd, K.J. Viability and dose-response studies on the effects of the immunoenhancing lactic acid bacterium *Lactobacillus rhamnosus* in mice. *Br. J. Nutr.* **2001**, *86*, 285–289. [CrossRef] [PubMed]
76. De Simone, C.; Vesely, R.; Negri, R.; Bianchi Salvadori, B.; Zanzoglu, S.; Cilli, A.; Lucci, L. Enhancement of immune response of murine Peyer's patches by a diet supplemented with yogurt. *Immunopharmacol. Immunotoxicol.* **1987**, *9*, 87–100. [CrossRef] [PubMed]
77. Perdigon, G.; Alvarez, S.; Rachid, M.; Aguero, G.; Gobbato, N. Immune system stimulation by probiotics. *J. Dairy Sci.* **1995**, *78*, 1597–1606. [CrossRef]
78. Ibnou-Zekri, N.; Blum, S.; Schiffrin, E.J.; von der Weid, T. Divergent patterns of colonization and immune response elicited from two intestinal *Lactobacillus* strains that display similar properties in vitro. *Infect. Immun.* **2003**, *71*, 428–436. [CrossRef] [PubMed]

79. Mohamadzadeh, M.; Olson, S.; Kalina, W.V.; Ruthel, G.; Demmin, G.L.; Warfield, K.L.; Bavari, S.; Klaenhammer, T.R. Lactobacilli activate human dendritic cells that skew T cells toward T helper 1 polarization. *Proc. Natl. Acad. Sci. USA* **2005**, *102*, 288–305. [CrossRef] [PubMed]
80. Lahtinen, S.J.; Gueimonde, M.; Ouwehand, A.C.; Reinikainen, J.P.; Salminen, S.J. Probiotic bacteria may become dormant during storage. *Appl. Environ. Microbiol.* **2005**, *71*, 1662–1663. [CrossRef] [PubMed]

5

A Metagenomic and in Silico Functional Prediction of Gut Microbiota Profiles may Concur in Discovering New Cystic Fibrosis Patient-Targeted Probiotics

Pamela Vernocchi [1,†], Federica Del Chierico [1,†], Andrea Quagliariello [1], Danilo Ercolini [2], Vincenzina Lucidi [3] and Lorenza Putignani [1,4,*]

1 Unit of Human Microbiome, Bambino Gesù Children's Hospital, IRCCS, Viale San Paolo 15, 00146 Rome, Italy; pamela.vernocchi@opbg.net (P.V.); federica.delchierico@opbg.net (F.D.C.); andrea.quagliariello@opbg.net (A.Q.)
2 Department of Agricultural Sciences, Division of Microbiology, University of Naples Federico II, Via Università 100, Portici, 80055 Napoli, Italy; danilo.ercolini@unina.it
3 Cystic Fibrosis Unit, Bambino Gesù Children's Hospital, IRCCS, Piazza Sant' Onofrio 4, Rome 00165, Italy; vincenzina.lucidi@opbg.net
4 Unit of Parasitology Bambino Gesù Children's Hospital, IRCCS, Piazza Sant' Onofrio 4, Rome 00165, Italy
* Correspondence: lorenza.putignani@opbg.net
† These authors contributed equally to this work.

Abstract: Cystic fibrosis (CF) is a life-limiting hereditary disorder that results in aberrant mucosa in the lungs and digestive tract, chronic respiratory infections, chronic inflammation, and the need for repeated antibiotic treatments. Probiotics have been demonstrated to improve the quality of life of CF patients. We investigated the distribution of gut microbiota (GM) bacteria to identify new potential probiotics for CF patients on the basis of GM patterns. Fecal samples of 28 CF patients and 31 healthy controls (HC) were collected and analyzed by 16S rRNA-based pyrosequencing analysis of GM, to produce CF-HC paired maps of the distribution of operational taxonomic units (OTUs), and by Phylogenetic Investigation of Communities by Reconstruction of Unobserved States (PICRUSt) for Kyoto Encyclopedia of Genes and Genomes (KEGG) biomarker prediction. The maps were scanned to highlight the distribution of bacteria commonly claimed as probiotics, such as bifidobacteria and lactobacilli, and of butyrate-producing colon bacteria, such as *Eubacterium* spp. and *Faecalibacterium prausnitzii*. The analyses highlighted 24 OTUs eligible as putative probiotics. Eleven and nine species were prevalently associated with the GM of CF and HC subjects, respectively. Their KEGG prediction provided differential CF and HC pathways, indeed associated with health-promoting biochemical activities in the latter case. GM profiling and KEGG biomarkers concurred in the evaluation of nine bacterial species as novel putative probiotics that could be investigated for the nutritional management of CF patients.

Keywords: cystic fibrosis; gut microbiota profiling; KEGG prediction-tailored probiotic design

---

1. Introduction

Cystic fibrosis (CF) is an autosomal recessive condition occurring among people with European origins, which is caused by mutations in the cystic fibrosis transmembrane conductance regulator (CFTR) gene. The CFTR mutation leads to the failure or the absence of functional CFTR proteins at the apical membrane of epithelial cells in several body systems [1]. The CFTR protein, in addition to functioning as a chloride channel, can also affect bicarbonate transport. Protein mutations cause the formation of viscous and dehydrated mucus followed by the establishment of aberrant mucosa in the lungs and digestive tract. This condition increases the risk of recurrent and chronic pulmonary infection and inflammation, pancreatic insufficiency (PI), CF-related liver disease, and diabetes [2].

The recurrent destructive airway infections, determined by the progressive inflammatory lung diseases, represent the principal cause of mortality, morbidity, and altered quality of life in CF patients, resulting in respiratory failure in 90% of patients with CF [3].

To reduce pulmonary exacerbation, patients are subjected to an antibiotic therapy which leads to the modification of the gut microbiota (GM) [4]. The CFTR mutations also lead to the alteration of intestinal permeability, determining an impaired composition and function of the intestinal barrier. The production of immune mediators is altered alongside with mucosal inflammation, triggering an increase in the concentrations of fecal calprotectin and rectal nitric oxide [5]. The mutations can also affect the body's endocrine, neural, and immune systems [6]. This clinical status also leads to a compromised nutritional status associated with the severity of CF disease, which unfortunately affects the quality of life and life expectancy [7].

The maintenance of an optimal nutritional status may ameliorate the quality of life of CF patients, especially during rehabilitation programs and therapies targeting the respiratory infections [8]. GM modulation induced by nutritional intervention may have implications in the management of CF-related malnutrition and comorbidities, since diet is perhaps the most modifiable factor that shapes microbiota profiles [9].

The diet-driven functional evolution of the GM has been thoroughly discussed in mammalian species, starting at neonatal age [10,11]. The maintenance of microbiota eubiosis seems to contribute to the prevention and clarification of complex disease phenotypes [12]. In particular, the administration of probiotics also contributes to GM eubiosis maintenance and restoration in CF patients [13].

Probiotics are defined as "live microorganisms that, when administered in adequate amounts, confer a health benefit on the host" [14]. They colonize the intestine and affect either microbiota composition or function, acting on the host epithelial and immunological responses [15], reducing intestinal inflammation, and hence improving the intestinal functions at clinical and biochemical levels [16–18] even when they were altered by an antibiotic therapy [17]. Probiotics have been used with positive outcomes in childhood gastroenteritis, atopic diseases, and *Helicobacter pylori* infection [19]. Specifically, the administration of *Lactobacillus* GG can decrease the incidence of exacerbations and reduce the intestinal inflammation in CF patients, as reported by Bruzzese [20]. Potential mechanisms of action for probiotics in CF include their influence on gut motility and intestinal barrier function and the inhibition of pathogenic bacteria colonization [2].

There is evidence that probiotic administration in these patients reduces pulmonary exacerbation rate and hospital admission [21]. Clinical trials on probiotic administration in CF patients are on the rise [17,22], but there is no evidence of an optimal patient-tailored probiotics regimen to be administered for this chronic disease.

The aim of this study was to evaluate the distribution of *Bifidobacterium* spp., *Lactobacillus* spp., *Eubacterium* spp., and *Faecalibacterium prausntizii* in the GM of CF and healthy subjects. We focused on species commonly claimed as targets for the design of novel probiotics [23]. According to a targeted metagenomics analysis and functional prediction of related Kyoto Encyclopedia of Genes and Genomes (KEGG) pathways, we propose potential probiotics species for CF management.

2. Material and Methods

2.1. Patients

This study was conducted on 28 consecutive CF patients aged 1 to 6 years (average age 3.5 years, SD $\pm$ 1.69; 11 males and 17 females), recruited at the Cystic Fibrosis Unit of the Bambino Gesù Children's Hospital (OPBG, Rome, Italy) over one year (2012). The diagnosis of CF was made on the basis of the results of a pathological sweat test (chloride > 60 mmol/L, reference value), as described by Gibson and Cooke [24], or by the presence of two CF-causing mutations in the CFTR gene [25].

The study protocol was approved by the OPBG Ethics Research Committee (protocol No. 534/RA), and was conducted in accordance with the Declaration of Helsinki (as revised in Seoul, Korea, October 2008). A signed informed consent was obtained from the parents of the enrolled subjects. The patients were age-matched with 31 healthy controls (HC) screened by means of a survey of the OPBG Human Microbiome Unit on pediatric gut microbiota programming.

Inclusion criteria for HC were: absence of any inflammatory, infectious, and chronic diseases at the time of the microbiota analysis and no antibiotic and pre-probiotic intake in the previous two months.

For CF patients, the inclusion criteria consisted of being recruited under clinical stability (i.e., absence of infectious exacerbation of pulmonary symptoms) and no pre-probiotic intake in the previous two weeks.

2.2. Anamnestic and Laboratory Features

Age, gender, and body mass index (BMI) (for patients over 2 years of age) or Z-score (Weight/Length (W/L) of patients under 2 years of age) were collected for both CF patients and HC, whereas sweat chloride test values, pancreatic status (PS), and antibiotic data for chronic regimen were collected only for CF patients (Table 1).

Table 1. Cystic fibrosis (CF) Patients and healthy controls (HC) features.

Subjects	Males	Mean Age	Mean W/L or BMI Z-Score *	Pancreatic Insufficiency: Yes/Not	Mean Value of Sweat Test	Chronic Use of Antibiotic: Yes/No	Disease Severity: Mild/Severe
CF	11/28 (39%)	3.5	±0.9	22/6 79/21 (%)	93	12/16 43/57 (%)	4/24 14/86 (%)
HC	20/31 (64.5%)	3.06	±0.51	nda **	nda	nda	nda

* BMI/Z-Score: body mass index (BMI) (for patients over 2 years of age) or Z-score (Weight/Length (W/L) (for patients under 2 years of age); ** nda: no data associated.

2.3. DNA Extraction and Next Generation Sequencing (NGS) Analysis

Fecal samples (59) were collected from each subject during clinical examination and stored until metagenomics analysis. The genomic DNA was isolated using the QIAamp DNA Stool Mini Kit (Qiagen, Hilden, Germany). The V1–V3 region (520 bp) of the 16S ribosomal RNA locus was amplified for pyrosequencing analysis using a 454-Junior Genome Sequencer (Roche 454 Life Sciences, Branford, CT, USA) according to Del Chierico et al. [26]. The nucleotide barcodes, added in forward primers, were composed of 8 unique nucleotides (Roche 454 Life Sciences). The polymerase chain reactions were performed using Hi-Fi Polymerase Chain Reaction (PCR) Taq polymerase (FastStart™ High Fidelity PCR System, dNTPack, Roche Diagnostics, Mannheim, Germany), guaranteeing high specificity, sensitivity, and accuracy during PCR amplification.

2.4. Statistical Analysis

Reads were analyzed with Qiime 1.8 (Quantitative Insights Into Microbial Ecology, http://qiime.org/1.4.0/) using the default pipeline [27]. After demultiplexing, reads with an average quality score lower than 25, shorter than 300 bp, and with an ambiguous base calling were excluded from the analysis to guarantee a higher level of accuracy in terms of detection of the operational taxonomic units (OTUs). Sequences that passed the quality filter were denoised [28], and singletons were excluded. The denoised sequences *were chimera-checked by identify_chimeric_seqs.py*.

To characterize the taxonomic structure of the samples, the sequences were organized into OTUs by clustering at a threshold of 97% pairwise identity and by classifying the representative sequences using the Greengenes 13_8 database [29]. The representative sequences were submitted to PyNAST for sequence alignment [30] and to UCLUST for sequence clustering [31].

The OTU Kruskal–Wallis tests were performed by QIIME software (http://qiime.org/1.4.0/) using "group_significance.py" script [32]. The Kruskal-Wallis test was performed on OTU distribution with False Discovery Rate (FDR) correction (p-value ≤ 0.1). To gain more insight into the metagenomics-based function of the microbiome of the CF patients and HC, the Phylogenetic Investigation of Communities by Reconstruction of Unobserved States (PICRUSt) v1.1.0 tool was used [33], and the resulting function prediction was analyzed using the HUMAnN2 v0.99 program to get KEGG pathways (http://huttenhower.sph.harvard.edu/humann2) [34]. To find possible OTUs and KEGG biomarkers associated with CF and HC, a linear discriminant effect size (LEfSe) analysis was performed [35] with the α value of the statistical test equal to 0.05 and the logarithmic Linear Discriminant Analysis (LDA) score threshold equal to 2.0.

3. Results

3.1. Putative Probiotic Distribution in the GM Profiles

By targeted metagenomics, a total of 316,000 reads was obtained with an average of 5356 reads/sample and an average length of 487 bp. Genus-level comparisons were performed on 24 OTUs belonging to *Bifidobacterium* spp., *Lactobacillus* spp., *Eubacterium* spp., and *F. prausnitzii* chosen from a total dataset of 165 OTUs, considering their putative probiotic role.

The profiling of targeted metagenomic sequencing pointed out a distribution of 11 bacterial species prevalently associated with the GM of the CF patients (Figure 1, Panel A), and 9 species prevalently associated with the GM of the HC (Figure 1, Panel B) (Table 2). The Kruskal–Wallis test identified a statistically significant difference for *F. prausnitzii* distribution between CF patients and HC, highlighting a higher relative abundance in HC.

On the contrary, the remaining 4 OTUs, namely, *Lactobacillus brevis*, *L. delbrueckii*, *L. helveticus*, and *Eubacterium cylindroides* were comparably distributed in the GM profiles of the CF patients and HC (Figure 1, Panel C).

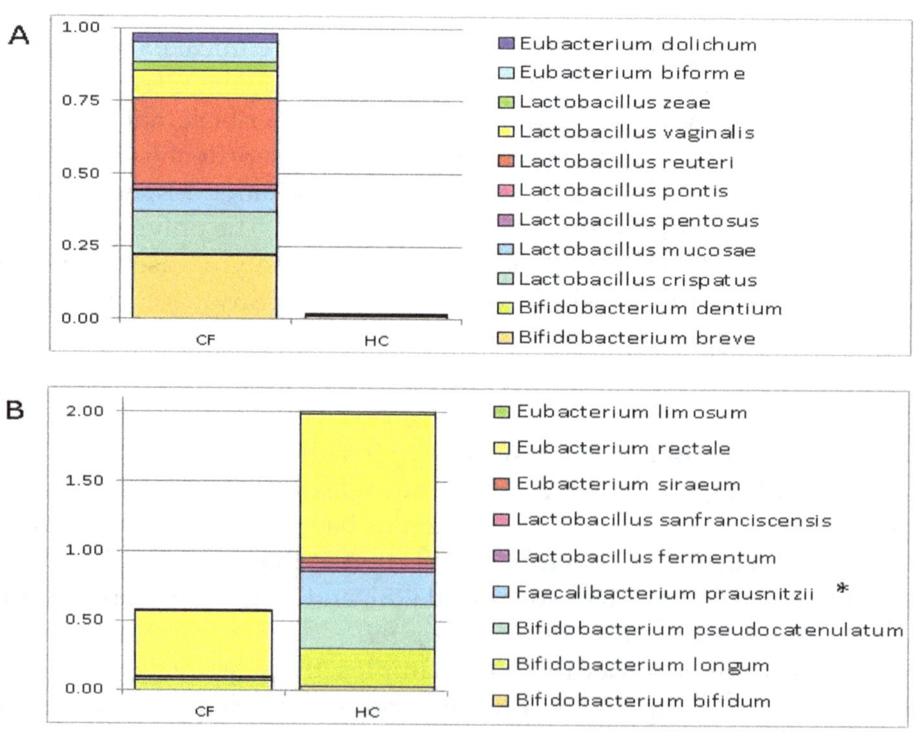

Figure 1. *Cont.*

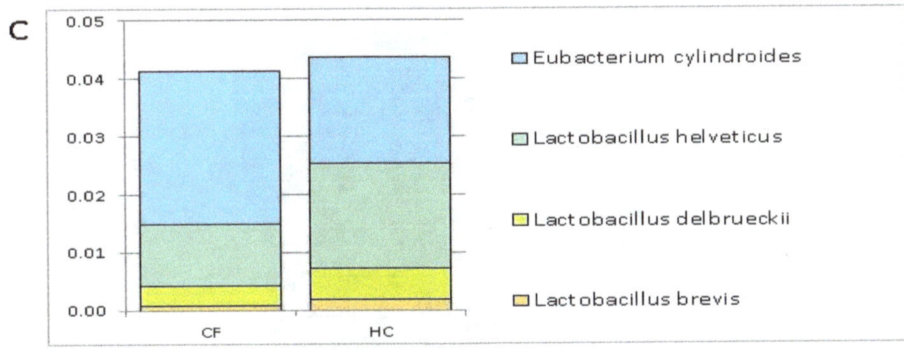

Figure 1. Histograms of the relative abundance of 24 selected operational taxonomic units (OTUs) in the gut microbiota (GM) patterns of cystic fibrosis (CF) patients and healthy controls (HC). These OTUs were chosen for their putative probiotic role. The histograms show the relative abundance of the searched putative probiotic bacteria scanned through the GM patterns of the CF patients and HC. (**Panel A**): 9 OTUs prevalently distributed in the GM profile of the CF subjects (relative abundance > 0.001); (**Panel B**): 11 OTUs prevalently distributed in the GM profile of the HC (relative abundance > 0.02). *Fecalibacterium prausnitzii* shows a statistically significant value False Discovery Rate (FDR) adjusted p value ≤ 0.1); (**Panel C**): 4 OTUs comparably distributed in the GM profiles of the CF patients and HC.

Table 2. List of 20 bacteria prevalently associated with the GM profile of HC and CF patients. These OTUs were chosen for their putative probiotic role.

Bacteria	Group of Subjects
Bifidobacterium bifidum	HC
Bifidobacterium longum	
Bifidobacterium pseudocatenulatum	
Faecalibacterium prausnitzii	
Lactobacillus fermentum	
Lactobacillus sanfranciscensis	
Eubacterium siraeum	
Eubacterium rectale	
Eubacterium limosum	
Bifidobacterium breve	CF
Bifidobacterium dentium	
Lactobacillus crispatus	
Lactobacillus mucosae	
Lactobacillus pentosus	
Lactobacillus pontis	
Lactobacillus reuteri	
Lactobacillus vaginalis	
Lactobacillus zeae	
Eubacterium biforme	
Eubacterium dolichum	

3.2. Metabolic Pathways of Probiotics

To better define the metabolic role of the detected putative probiotic species, a supervised comparison of CF patients' and HC's KEGGs was inferred by LEfSe on the 24 OTU matrix.

The predicted microbial function highlighted differences in metabolic pathways associated with the 24 selected OTUs (Figure 2). In particular, 24 pathways resulted associated with CF and 39 with HC (Table 3).

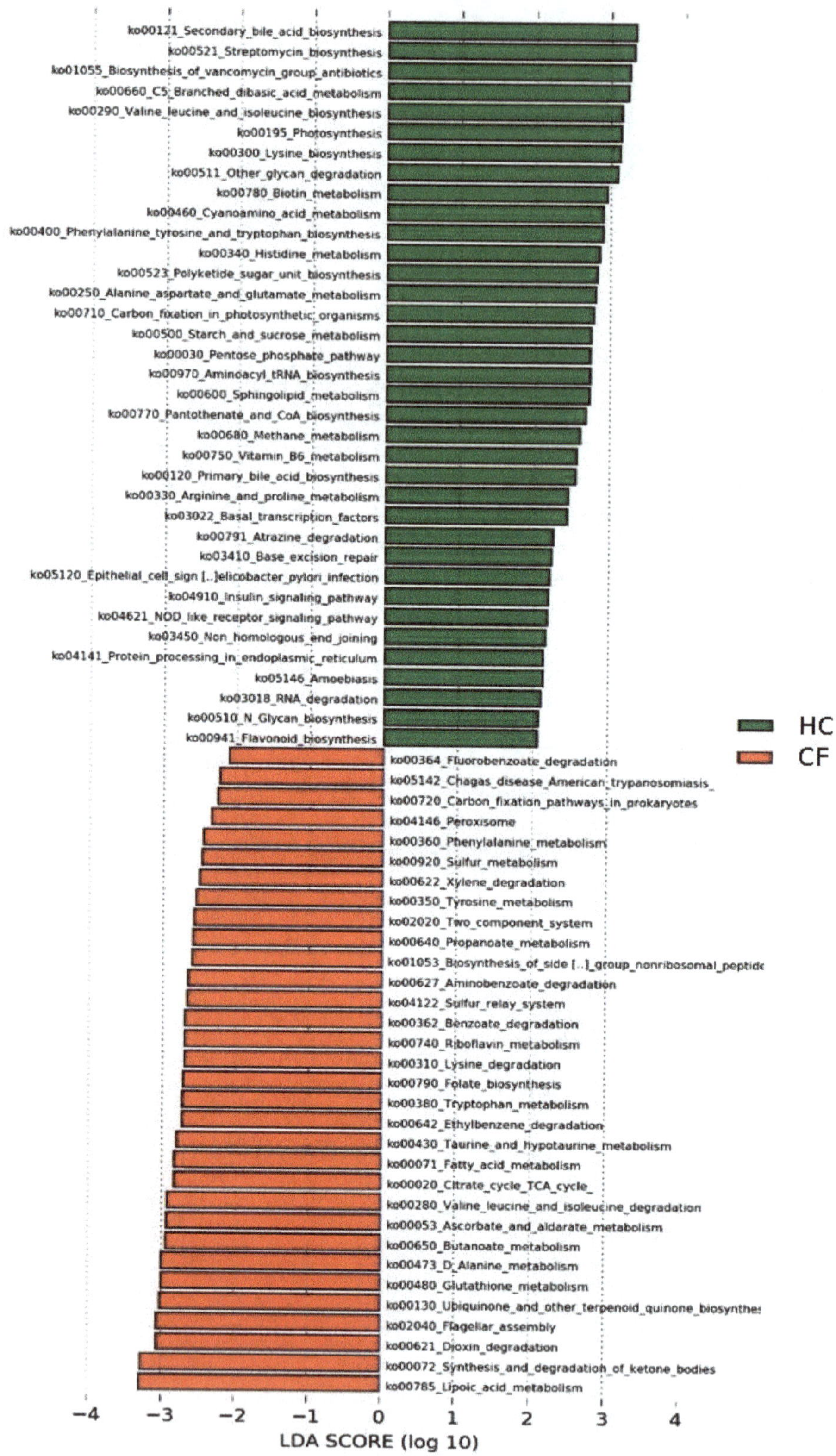

Figure 2. Kyoto Encyclopedia of Genes and Genomes (KEGG) biomarkers inferred from the whole set of 24 OTUs of putative probiotic bacteria scanned through the GM patterns of CF patients and HC subjects. A linear discriminant effect size (LeFse) analysis was performed ($\alpha = 0.05$, logarithmic Linear Discriminant Analysis (LDA) score threshold = 2.0).

Table 3. Kyoto Encyclopedia of Genes and Genomes (KEGG) pathways associated with HC and CF subjects.

KEGG Pathways	Class *	Subclass	Group
Carbon fixation in photosynthetic organisms	1	Energy metabolism	HC
Alanine aspartate and glutamate metabolism		Amino acid metabolism	
Arginine and proline metabolism			
Histidine metabolism			
Lysine biosynthesis			
Phenylalanine tyrosine and tryptophan biosynthesis			
Valine leucine and isoleucine biosynthesis			
Flavonoid biosynthesis		Biosynthesis of other secondary metabolites	
Streptomycin biosynthesis			
C5 Branched dibasic acid metabolism		Carbohydrate metabolism	
Pentose phosphate pathway			
Propanoate metabolism			
Starch and sucrose metabolism			
Methane metabolism		Energy metabolism	
Photosynthesis			
N Glycan biosynthesis		Glycan biosynthesis and metabolism	
Other glycan degradation			
Primary bile acid biosynthesis		Lipid metabolism	
Secondary bile acid biosynthesis			
Sphingolipid metabolism			
Biotin metabolism		Metabolism of cofactors and vitamins	
Pantothenate and CoA biosynthesis			
Riboflavin metabolism			
Vitamin B6 metabolism			
Cyanoamino acid metabolism		Metabolism of other amino acids	
D Alanine metabolism			
Biosynthesis of vancomycin group antibiotics		Metabolism of terpenoids and polyketides	
Polyketide sugar unit biosynthesis			
Atrazine degradation		Xenobiotics biodegradation and metabolism	
Protein processing in endoplasmic reticulum	2	Folding, sorting and degradation	
RNA degradation			
Base excision repair		Replication and repair	
Non homologous end joining			
Basal transcription factors		Transcription	
Aminoacyl tRNA biosynthesis		Translation	

KEGG Pathways	Class	Subclass	Group
Lysine degradation	1	Amino acid metabolism	CF
Phenylalanine metabolism			
Tryptophan metabolism			
Tyrosine metabolism			
Valine leucine and isoleucine degradation			
Ascorbate and aldarate metabolism		Carbohydrate metabolism	
Butanoate metabolism			
Citrate cycle TCA cycle			
Carbon fixation pathways in prokaryotes		Energy metabolism	
Sulfur metabolism			
Fatty acid metabolism		Lipid metabolism	
Synthesis and degradation of ketone bodies			
Folate biosynthesis		Metabolism of cofactors and vitamins	
Lipoic acid metabolism			
Ubiquinone and other terpenoid quinone biosynthesis			
Glutathione metabolism		Metabolism of other amino acids	
Taurine and hypotaurine metabolism			
Biosynthesis of siderophore group nonribosomal peptides		Metabolism of terpenoids and polyketides	
Aminobenzoate degradation		Xenobiotics biodegradation and metabolism	
Benzoate degradation			
Dioxin degradation			
Ethylbenzene degradation			
Fluorobenzoate degradation			
Xylene degradation			
Sulfur relay system	2	Folding, sorting and degradation	
Two component system	3	Signal transduction	

Table 3. Cont.

KEGG Pathways	Class *	Subclass	Group	KEGG Pathways	Class	Subclass	Group
Insulin signaling pathway	5	Endocrine system		Flagellar assembly	4	Cell motility	
Nucleotide oligomerization domain (NOD) like receptor signaling pathway		Immune system		Peroxisome		Transport and catabolism	
Amoebiasis	6	Infectious diseases		Chagas disease American trypanosomiasis	6	Infectious diseases	
Epithelial cell signaling in *Helicobacter pylori* infection							

* Class: 1. Metabolism; 2. Genetic Information Processing; 3. Environmental Information Processing; 4. Cellular Processes; 5. Organismal Systems; 6. Human Diseases.

4. Discussion

4.1. Putative Probiotic Distribution in the GM Profiles

Bifidobacteria and lactobacilli are recognized as beneficial bacteria for their intrinsic probiotic features [23]. *Eubacterium* spp. may aid in the digestion, the absorption, or both of food ingredients and minerals, especially under malnutrition conditions usually occurring in CF because of nutrient absorption defects [36]. More generally, *F. prausntizii* has been recently proposed to provide high butyrate production in the gut [37].

Among the bacteria associated with the CF gut profiles (Table 2), some are actually linked to different pathologic conditions. Indeed, *Bifidobacterium dentium* was detected in the oral cavity in association with dental caries [38], while *Eubacterium dolichum* was associated with frailty in the elderly, a condition that represents the biggest problem associated with population aging [39]. *Lactobacillus mucosae* was detected in the microbiota of short bowel syndrome patients [40]. Other bacterial strains identified for CF patients were associated with metabolic disorders, such as high total cholesterol and low-density lipoprotein levels (*Eubacterium biforme*) [41], obesity (*Lactobacillus reuteri*) [42], and nonalcoholic fatty liver disease (NAFLD) (*L. zeae* and *L. vaginalis*) [24].

Unlike the aforementioned negative roles of the previous reported bacteria in human health, *B. breve* is considered a commensal or even a health-promoting microorganism [43] because it improves symptoms in necrotizing enterocolitis [44] and atopic dermatitis [45], as well as those associated with HIV-induced damages [46]. Moreover, *B. breve* shows antimicrobial activity [47], induces innate immune responses, and has anti-inflammatory effects [48]. Also, *L. pentosus* was reported to ameliorate colitis in the aged rodent by inhibiting the activation of nuclear factor (NF)-κB, activator protein 1 (AP1), and mitogen-activated protein kinases (MAPKs) [49].

No role in the human GM or putative effects as probiotics have been reported for *L. crispatus* and *L. pontis*.

The GM in the HC group seemed to be enriched in species involved in gut integrity and mobility, digestion of specific dietary compounds, and immune system modulation

Indeed, in the research of Kanauchi and co-workers [50], *E. limosum* was presented as an important probiotic candidate for its short-chain fatty acid (SCFA) production, role in maintaining and enhancing mucosal integrity, and anti-inflammatory properties in the intestinal mucosa [50]. Moreover, Bruzzese et al. found that both *E. rectale* and *F. prausnitzii* were reduced in the GM of CF children compared to HC, confirming our results [51].

Eubacterium siraeum is able to degrade wheat bran, contributing to the beneficial effects of cereal fiber in human health through their impact on the GM [52].

L. sanfranciscensis is generally considered the most important lactic acid bacterium in the fermentation of rye and wheat sourdoughs [53]. The strain *L. sanfranciscensis* LBH1068, tested in an induced chronic colitis mouse model, improved mouse health by reducing weight loss, decreasing gut permeability, and modulating cytokine production [54].

In addition, *L. fermentum* demonstrated intestinal anti-inflammatory effects in the model of sodium dextran sulfate-induced colitis in mice. Among the mechanisms proposed, *L. fermentum* restored GM composition and modulated the altered immune response by preserving intestinal barrier integrity, decreasing pro-inflammatory cytokine production, and modulating the expression of Th1-, Th17- and T_{reg}-related cytokines [55].

The study of Moya-Pérez and colleagues demonstrated that *B. pseudocatenulatum* modulated immune cell infiltration and inflammation in the gut in obesity [56].

A reduction in bifidobacteria in CF, especially *B. longum*, was already reported by Duytschaever et al. [57]. High richness of bifidobacteria species was positively correlated with the maturation of the mucosal immune system [58]. *B. longum* was found to be an inhibitor of rotavirus, the predominant cause of sporadic diarrhea in infants [59]. A recent study has demonstrated that acetate produced by *B. longum* acts as an essential cosubstrate for butyrate production and for *E. rectale* growth [60].

B. bifidum and *B. longum* possess numerous pathways involved in the catabolism of human milk oligosaccharides (HMO) and may also consume carbohydrates released by other bacteria [61]. *B. bifidum* and *B. longum* were described as being more abundant in healthy subjects compared to NAFLD patients, suggesting a protective and beneficial role also in obesity and NAFLD [62].

Finally, each of these microbial species, especially those lacking in patients' GM (Table 2, HC-related species), could be considered suitable for the design of CF patient-tailored probiotics.

4.2. Metabolic Pathways of Probiotics

To evaluate the microbial metabolic and functional KEGG pathways of the chosen putative probiotic species, a supervised comparison of CF patients' and HC's KEGGs was performed by LEfSe (Table 3). Pathways associated with fatty acid biosynthesis, metabolism, and synthesis and degradation of ketone bodies were significantly associated with CF patients, as already described by Fouhy et al. [63]. This increase in fat metabolism probably occurs as a result of a combination of factors, including a reduced intestinal absorption and an altered GM in CF patients. Reduced fat absorption is one reason why most CF patients are traditionally prescribed a high-fat diet to ensure adequate weight maintenance. Moreover, it is possible that the altered GM might contribute to the increase in fat metabolism [63].

On the contrary, primary and secondary bile acid biosynthesis pathways were associated with the GM of HC. It is known that CF patients have a variety of intestinal abnormalities in bile acid metabolism at the intestinal level, including increased fecal bile acid losses, reduced bile acid pool size, and duodenal bile acid concentration [64]. These abnormalities appear to be associated with exocrine pancreatic insufficiency and steatorrhoea. Indeed, improvement of bile abnormalities with amelioration in fat malabsorption was reported after pancreatic enzyme therapy [64].

Pathways involved in xenobiotic metabolism have been significantly observed in the GM pattern of CF patients, including benzoate, fluorobenzoate, dioxin, xylene, aminobenzoate, and ethylbenzene degradation pathways. Bacterial pathways involved in xenobiotic metabolism were also observed by Fouhy et al. in CF patients [63]. The increase in bacteria capable of degrading xenobiotic compounds is probably due to the higher exposure to antibiotics and pharmacological treatments, recurrent in CF patients [65]. An enhanced ability of CF patients' GM to metabolize proteins was highlighted by the increase in amino acid catabolism (e.g., valine, leucine, isoleucine, and lysine degradation) prediction. Indeed, the increase in protein catabolism in CF individuals has been well documented, probably due to the breakdown of both cellular and connective tissue proteins, which is related to the degree of impaired lung function and to the systemic inflammatory response [66]. Moreover, also valine, leucine, isoleucine, lysine, phenylalanine, tyrosine, and tryptophan biosynthesis pathways were linked to putative probiotics in HC. Our results nicely agree with the findings of a study carried out by Palmer et al., in which 11 genes involved in branched-chain and aromatic amino acid catabolism were highly upregulated in CF patients' sputum, while genes involved in the biosynthesis of these amino acids were repressed [67].

Moreover, the flagellar assembly pathway was associated with putative probiotics in CF. Bacterial flagellin is classified as a potent mediator of virulence of Gram-negative bacteria. Recurrent infections caused by Gram-negative strains could be linked to this inferred pathway [68].

Finally, the prediction of lipoic acid metabolism and folate biosynthesis pathways were associated with CF patterns. Consistently, Quinn and colleagues reported the abundance of lipoic acid metabolism in the lung of CF patients [65]. Lipoic acid is an antioxidant and a potent quencher of reactive oxygen species (ROS) [69], and it is used as a metabolic cofactor by Proteobacteria, Gram-positive bacteria, and *Pseudomonas aeruginosa* [69,70]. Quinn reported also high abundance of folate synthesis in CF patients [65]. Sulfonamides, such as sulfamethoxazole and trimethoprim, are antibiotics commonly used to treat CF infections that target microbial enzymes required for folate biosynthesis [71].

Prolonged exposure to sulfonamides may select microbes with multiple copies of these genes to overcome the drug's effect on folate synthesis [72].

5. Conclusions

In conclusion, patients with CF usually have an abnormal intestinal microbiota and dysregulated immune mediators resulting from a massive exposure to antibiotics. Probiotics as immunomodulatory and anti-inflammatory substances are considered to improve both the clinical and the biochemical intestinal and pulmonary function in CF patients. The results reported in this study may point out new putative probiotic species on the basis of the GM differential profiles and predicted metabolic pathways of CF patients compared to HC.

On the basis of our data, we speculate that some putative probiotic species, such as *B. longum*, *E. rectale*, *E. limosum*, *E. siraeum*, *L. sanfranciscensis*, *L. fermentum*, *B. pseudocatenulatum*, *B. bifidum*, and *F. prausnitzii* and their produced metabolites may have a protective role against CF disorders. Nevertheless, further in vitro studies and clinical trials should focus on these probiotics to assess whether the administration of selected strains, alone or in combination, may improve the quality of life and the clinical management of CF patients.

Acknowledgments: This work was supported by the Ministry of Health, Ricerca Corrente RC 201702P003961 assigned to L.P., Children's Hospital Bambino Gesù, IRCCS. The authors thank the experts from BioMed Proofreading LLC for their English revision.

Author Contributions: P.V., F.D.C., L.P. conceived and wrote the manuscript. A.Q. performed metagenomic data analysis. D.E. revised the manuscript. V.L. carried out patient recruitment and clinical management.

References

1. Garcia, M.A.S.; Yang, N.; Quinton, P.M. Normal mouse intestinal mucus release requires cystic fibrosis transmembrane regulator-dependent bicarbonate secretion. *J. Clin. Investig.* **2009**, *119*, 2613–2622. [CrossRef] [PubMed]
2. Li, L.; Somerset, S. The clinical significance of the gut microbiota in cystic fibrosis and the potential for dietary therapies. *Clin. Nutr. Edinb. Scotl.* **2014**, *33*, 571–580. [CrossRef]
3. Jafari, S.-A.; Mehdizadeh-Hakkak, A.; Kianifar, H.-R.; Hebrani, P.; Ahanchian, H.; Abbasnejad, E. Effects of probiotics on quality of life in children with cystic fibrosis; a randomized controlled trial. *Iran. J. Pediatr.* **2013**, *23*, 669–674.
4. Claeys, S.; Van Hoecke, H.; Holtappels, G.; Gevaert, P.; De Belder, T.; Verhasselt, B.; Van Cauwenberge, P.; Bachert, C. Nasal polyps in patients with and without cystic fibrosis: A differentiation by innate markers and inflammatory mediators. *Clin. Exp. Allergy* **2005**, *35*, 467–472. [CrossRef] [PubMed]
5. Infante, P.D.; Redecillas, F.S.; Torrent, V.A.; Segarra, C.O.; Maldonado, S.M.; Gartner, T.L.; Hidalgo, A.E. Improvement of intestinal function in cystic fibrosis patients using probiotics. *An. Pediatr.* **2008**, *69*, 501–505.
6. Wells, J.M.; Rossi, O.; Meijerink, M.; van Baarlen, P. Epithelial crosstalk at the microbiota-mucosal interface. *Proc. Natl. Acad. Sci. USA* **2011**, *108* (Suppl. 1), 4607–4614. [CrossRef]
7. Dray, X.; Kanaan, R.; Bienvenu, T.; Desmazes-Dufeu, N.; Dusser, D.; Marteau, P.; Hubert, D. Malnutrition in adults with cystic fibrosis. *Eur. J. Clin. Nutr.* **2005**, *59*, 152–154. [CrossRef] [PubMed]
8. Cohen-Cymberknoh, M.; Shoseyov, D.; Kerem, E. Managing cystic fibrosis: Strategies that increase life expectancy and improve quality of life. *Am. J. Respir. Crit. Care Med.* **2011**, *183*, 1463–1471. [CrossRef]
9. Wu, G.D.; Chen, J.; Hoffmann, C.; Bittinger, K.; Chen, Y.-Y.; Keilbaugh, S.A.; Bewtra, M.; Knights, D.; Walters, W.A.; Knight, R.; et al. Linking long-term dietary patterns with gut microbial enterotypes. *Science* **2011**, *334*, 105–108. [CrossRef]
10. Muegge, B.D.; Kuczynski, J.; Knights, D.; Clemente, J.C.; González, A.; Fontana, L.; Henrissat, B.; Knight, R.; Gordon, J.I. Diet drives convergence in gut microbiome functions across mammalian phylogeny and within humans. *Science* **2011**, *332*, 970–974. [CrossRef]

11. Del Chierico, F.; Vernocchi, P.; Petrucca, A.; Paci, P.; Fuentes, S.; Praticò, G.; Capuani, G.; Masotti, A.; Reddel, S.; Russo, A.; et al. Phylogenetic and Metabolic Tracking of Gut Microbiota during Perinatal Development. *PLoS ONE* **2015**, *10*, e0137347. [CrossRef]
12. Putignani, L.; Dallapiccola, B. Foodomics as part of the host-microbiota-exposome interplay. *J. Proteom.* **2016**, *147*, 3–20. [CrossRef] [PubMed]
13. Anderson, J.L.; Miles, C.; Tierney, A.C. Effect of probiotics on respiratory, gastrointestinal and nutritional outcomes in patients with cystic fibrosis: A systematic review. *J. Cyst. Fibros.* **2017**, *16*, 186–197. [CrossRef] [PubMed]
14. Food and Agriculture Organisation of the United Nations and WHO Working Group. *Guidelines for the Evaluation of Probiotics in Food*; FAO/WHO: Geneva, Switzerland, 2002.
15. Rogers, G.B.; Carroll, M.P.; Hoffman, L.R.; Walker, A.W.; Fine, D.A.; Bruce, K.D. Comparing the microbiota of the cystic fibrosis lung and human gut. *Gut Microbes* **2010**, *1*, 85–93. [CrossRef] [PubMed]
16. Whelan, K.; Quigley, E.M.M. Probiotics in the management of irritable bowel syndrome and inflammatory bowel disease. *Curr. Opin. Gastroenterol.* **2013**, *29*, 184–189. [CrossRef] [PubMed]
17. Gollwitzer, E.S.; Marsland, B.J. Microbiota abnormalities in inflammatory airway diseases—Potential for therapy. *Pharmacol. Ther.* **2014**, *141*, 32–39. [CrossRef] [PubMed]
18. Vernocchi, P.; Del Chierico, F.; Fiocchi, A.G.; El Hachem, M.; Dallapiccola, B.; Rossi, P.; Putignani, L. Understanding probiotics' role in allergic children: The clue of gut microbiota profiling. *Curr. Opin. Allergy Clin. Immunol.* **2015**, *15*, 495–503. [CrossRef] [PubMed]
19. Ahmad, K.; Fatemeh, F.; Mehri, N.; Maryam, S. Probiotics for the treatment of pediatric helicobacter pylori infection: A randomized double blind clinical trial. *Iran. J. Pediatr.* **2013**, *23*, 79–84. [PubMed]
20. Bruzzese, E.; Raia, V.; Gaudiello, G.; Polito, G.; Buccigrossi, V.; Formicola, V.; Guarino, A. Intestinal inflammation is a frequent feature of cystic fibrosis and is reduced by probiotic administration. *Aliment. Pharmacol. Ther.* **2004**, *20*, 813–819. [CrossRef] [PubMed]
21. Weiss, B.; Bujanover, Y.; Yahav, Y.; Vilozni, D.; Fireman, E.; Efrati, O. Probiotic supplementation affects pulmonary exacerbations in patients with cystic fibrosis: A pilot study. *Pediatr. Pulmonol.* **2010**, *45*, 536–540. [CrossRef] [PubMed]
22. Nagalingam, N.A.; Cope, E.K.; Lynch, S.V. Probiotic strategies for treatment of respiratory diseases. *Trends Microbiol.* **2013**, *21*, 485–492. [CrossRef] [PubMed]
23. Rivière, A.; Selak, M.; Lantin, D.; Leroy, F.; De Vuyst, L. Bifidobacteria and Butyrate-Producing Colon Bacteria: Importance and Strategies for Their Stimulation in the Human Gut. *Front. Microbiol.* **2016**, *7*, 979. [CrossRef] [PubMed]
24. Gibson, L.E.; Cooke, R.E. A test for concentration of electrolytes in sweat in cystic fibrosis of the pancreas utilizing pilocarpine by iontophoresis. *Pediatrics* **1959**, *23*, 545–549. [PubMed]
25. Farrell, P.M. The prevalence of cystic fibrosis in the European Union. *J. Cyst. Fibros.* **2008**, *7*, 450–453. [CrossRef] [PubMed]
26. Del Chierico, F.; Nobili, V.; Vernocchi, P.; Russo, A.; Stefanis, C.D.; Gnani, D.; Furlanello, C.; Zandonà, A.; Paci, P.; Capuani, G.; et al. Gut microbiota profiling of pediatric nonalcoholic fatty liver disease and obese patients unveiled by an integrated meta-omics-based approach. *Hepatology* **2017**, *65*, 451–464. [CrossRef] [PubMed]
27. Caporaso, J.G.; Kuczynski, J.; Stombaugh, J.; Bittinger, K.; Bushman, F.D.; Costello, E.K.; Fierer, N.; Peña, A.G.; Goodrich, J.K.; Gordon, J.I.; et al. QIIME allows analysis of high-throughput community sequencing data. *Nat. Methods* **2010**, *7*, 335–336. [CrossRef] [PubMed]
28. Reeder, J.; Knight, R. Rapidly denoising pyrosequencing amplicon reads by exploiting rank-abundance distributions. *Nat. Methods* **2010**, *7*, 668–669. [CrossRef] [PubMed]
29. Rognes, T.; Flouri, T.; Nichols, B.; Quince, C.; Mahé, F. VSEARCH: A versatile open source tool for metagenomics. *PeerJ* **2016**, *4*, e2584. [CrossRef] [PubMed]
30. Caporaso, J.G.; Bittinger, K.; Bushman, F.D.; DeSantis, T.Z.; Andersen, G.L.; Knight, R. PyNAST: A flexible tool for aligning sequences to a template alignment. *Bioinformatics* **2010**, *26*, 266–267. [CrossRef]
31. Edgar, R.C. Search and clustering orders of magnitude faster than BLAST. *Bioinformatics* **2010**, *26*, 2460–2461. [CrossRef]

32. Navas-Molina, J.A.; Peralta-Sánchez, J.M.; González, A.; McMurdie, P.J.; Vázquez-Baeza, Y.; Xu, Z.; Ursell, L.K.; Lauber, C.; Zhou, H.; Song, S.J.; et al. Advancing our understanding of the human microbiome using QIIME. *Methods Enzymol.* **2013**, *531*, 371–444. [CrossRef] [PubMed]
33. Langille, M.G.I.; Zaneveld, J.; Caporaso, J.G.; McDonald, D.; Knights, D.; Reyes, J.A.; Clemente, J.C.; Burkepile, D.E.; Vega Thurber, R.L.; Knight, R.; et al. Predictive functional profiling of microbial communities using 16S rRNA marker gene sequences. *Nat. Biotechnol.* **2013**, *31*, 814–821. [CrossRef] [PubMed]
34. Abubucker, S.; Segata, N.; Goll, J.; Schubert, A.M.; Izard, J.; Cantarel, B.L.; Rodriguez-Mueller, B.; Zucker, J.; Thiagarajan, M.; Henrissat, B.; et al. Metabolic reconstruction for metagenomic data and its application to the human microbiome. *PLoS Comput. Biol.* **2012**, *8*, e1002358. [CrossRef] [PubMed]
35. Segata, N.; Izard, J.; Waldron, L.; Gevers, D.; Miropolsky, L.; Garrett, W.S.; Huttenhower, C. Metagenomic biomarker discovery and explanation. *Genome Biol.* **2011**, *12*, R60. [CrossRef] [PubMed]
36. Gibson, G.R.; Roberfroid, M.B. Dietary modulation of the human colonic microbiota: Introducing the concept of prebiotics. *J. Nutr.* **1995**, *125*, 1401–1412. [PubMed]
37. Louis, P.; Flint, H.J. Diversity, metabolism and microbial ecology of butyrate-producing bacteria from the human large intestine. *FEMS Microbiol. Lett.* **2009**, *294*, 1–8. [CrossRef] [PubMed]
38. Aas, J.A.; Griffen, A.L.; Dardis, S.R.; Lee, A.M.; Olsen, I.; Dewhirst, F.E.; Leys, E.J.; Paster, B.J. Bacteria of dental caries in primary and permanent teeth in children and young adults. *J. Clin. Microbiol.* **2008**, *46*, 1407–1417. [CrossRef] [PubMed]
39. Jackson, M.A.; Jackson, M.; Jeffery, I.B.; Beaumont, M.; Bell, J.T.; Clark, A.G.; Ley, R.E.; O'Toole, P.W.; Spector, T.D.; Steves, C.J. Signatures of early frailty in the gut microbiota. *Genome Med.* **2016**, *8*, 8. [CrossRef] [PubMed]
40. Joly, F.; Mayeur, C.; Bruneau, A.; Noordine, M.-L.; Meylheuc, T.; Langella, P.; Messing, B.; Duée, P.-H.; Cherbuy, C.; Thomas, M. Drastic changes in fecal and mucosa-associated microbiota in adult patients with short bowel syndrome. *Biochimie* **2010**, *92*, 753–761. [CrossRef] [PubMed]
41. Lahti, L.; Salonen, A.; Kekkonen, R.A.; Salojärvi, J.; Jalanka-Tuovinen, J.; Palva, A.; Orešič, M.; de Vos, W.M. Associations between the human intestinal microbiota, *Lactobacillus rhamnosus* GG and serum lipids indicated by integrated analysis of high-throughput profiling data. *PeerJ* **2013**, *1*, e32. [CrossRef] [PubMed]
42. Million, M.; Maraninchi, M.; Henry, M.; Armougom, F.; Richet, H.; Carrieri, P.; Valero, R.; Raccah, D.; Vialettes, B.; Raoult, D. Obesity-associated gut microbiota is enriched in *Lactobacillus reuteri* and depleted in *Bifidobacterium animalis* and *Methanobrevibacter smithii*. *Int. J. Obes.* **2012**, *36*, 817–825. [CrossRef] [PubMed]
43. Sarkar, A.; Mandal, S. Bifidobacteria—Insight into clinical outcomes and mechanisms of its probiotic action. *Microbiol. Res.* **2016**, *192*, 159–171. [CrossRef] [PubMed]
44. Braga, T.D.; da Silva, G.A.P.; de Lira, P.I.C.; de Carvalho Lima, M. Efficacy of *Bifidobacterium breve* and *Lactobacillus casei* oral supplementation on necrotizing enterocolitis in very-low-birth-weight preterm infants: A double-blind, randomized, controlled trial. *Am. J. Clin. Nutr.* **2011**, *93*, 81–86. [CrossRef] [PubMed]
45. Enomoto, N.; Takei, Y.; Yamashina, S.; Ikejima, K.; Kitamura, T.; Sato, N. Anti-inflammatory strategies in alcoholic steatohepatitis. *J. Gastroenterol. Hepatol.* **2007**, *22* (Suppl. 1), S59–S61. [CrossRef]
46. D'Ettorre, G.; Ceccarelli, G.; Giustini, N.; Serafino, S.; Calantone, N.; De Girolamo, G.; Bianchi, L.; Bellelli, V.; Ascoli-Bartoli, T.; Marcellini, S.; et al. Probiotics Reduce Inflammation in Antiretroviral Treated, HIV-Infected Individuals: Results of the "Probio-HIV" Clinical Trial. *PLoS ONE* **2015**, *10*, e0137200. [CrossRef]
47. Tejero-Sariñena, S.; Barlow, J.; Costabile, A.; Gibson, G.R.; Rowland, I. In vitro evaluation of the antimicrobial activity of a range of probiotics against pathogens: Evidence for the effects of organic acids. *Anaerobe* **2012**, *18*, 530–538. [CrossRef] [PubMed]
48. Bermudez-Brito, M.; Muñoz-Quezada, S.; Gomez-Llorente, C.; Matencio, E.; Bernal, M.J.; Romero, F.; Gil, A. Cell-free culture supernatant of *Bifidobacterium breve* CNCM I-4035 decreases pro-inflammatory cytokines in human dendritic cells challenged with *Salmonella typhi* through TLR activation. *PLoS ONE* **2013**, *8*, e59370. [CrossRef]
49. Jeong, J.-J.; Kim, K.-A.; Jang, S.-E.; Woo, J.-Y.; Han, M.J.; Kim, D.-H. Orally administrated *Lactobacillus pentosus* var. plantarum C29 ameliorates age-dependent colitis by inhibiting the nuclear factor-kappa B signaling pathway via the regulation of lipopolysaccharide production by gut microbiota. *PLoS ONE* **2015**, *10*, e0116533. [CrossRef]

50. Kanauchi, O.; Fukuda, M.; Matsumoto, Y.; Ishii, S.; Ozawa, T.; Shimizu, M.; Mitsuyama, K.; Andoh, A. Eubacterium limosum ameliorates experimental colitis and metabolite of microbe attenuates colonic inflammatory action with increase of mucosal integrity. *World J. Gastroenterol.* **2006**, *12*, 1071–1077. [CrossRef] [PubMed]

51. Bruzzese, E.; Callegari, M.L.; Raia, V.; Viscovo, S.; Scotto, R.; Ferrari, S.; Morelli, L.; Buccigrossi, V.; Lo Vecchio, A.; Ruberto, E.; et al. Disrupted intestinal microbiota and intestinal inflammation in children with cystic fibrosis and its restoration with Lactobacillus GG: A randomised clinical trial. *PLoS ONE* **2014**, *9*, e87796. [CrossRef]

52. Duncan, S.H.; Belenguer, A.; Holtrop, G.; Johnstone, A.M.; Flint, H.J.; Lobley, G.E. Reduced dietary intake of carbohydrates by obese subjects results in decreased concentrations of butyrate and butyrate-producing bacteria in feces. *Appl. Environ. Microbiol.* **2007**, *73*, 1073–1078. [CrossRef]

53. De Angelis, M.; Di Cagno, R.; Gallo, G.; Curci, M.; Siragusa, S.; Crecchio, C.; Parente, E.; Gobbetti, M. Molecular and functional characterization of Lactobacillus sanfranciscensis strains isolated from sourdoughs. *Int. J. Food Microbiol.* **2007**, *114*, 69–82. [CrossRef] [PubMed]

54. Torres-Maravilla, E.; Lenoir, M.; Mayorga-Reyes, L.; Allain, T.; Sokol, H.; Langella, P.; Sánchez-Pardo, M.E.; Bermúdez-Humarán, L.G. Identification of novel anti-inflammatory probiotic strains isolated from pulque. *Appl. Microbiol. Biotechnol.* **2016**, *100*, 385–396. [CrossRef]

55. Rodríguez-Nogales, A.; Algieri, F.; Garrido-Mesa, J.; Vezza, T.; Utrilla, M.P.; Chueca, N.; Garcia, F.; Olivares, M.; Rodríguez-Cabezas, M.E.; Gálvez, J. Differential intestinal anti-inflammatory effects of *Lactobacillus fermentum* and *Lactobacillus salivarius* in DSS mouse colitis: Impact on microRNAs expression and microbiota composition. *Mol. Nutr. Food Res.* **2017**. [CrossRef]

56. Moya-Pérez, A.; Neef, A.; Sanz, Y. *Bifidobacterium pseudocatenulatum* CECT 7765 Reduces Obesity-Associated Inflammation by Restoring the Lymphocyte-Macrophage Balance and Gut Microbiota Structure in High-Fat Diet-Fed Mice. *PLoS ONE* **2015**, *10*, e0126976. [CrossRef]

57. Duytschaever, G.; Huys, G.; Bekaert, M.; Boulanger, L.; De Boeck, K.; Vandamme, P. Dysbiosis of bifidobacteria and *Clostridium cluster* XIVa in the cystic fibrosis fecal microbiota. *J. Cyst. Fibros.* **2013**, *12*, 206–215. [CrossRef] [PubMed]

58. Sjögren, Y.M.; Tomicic, S.; Lundberg, A.; Böttcher, M.F.; Björkstén, B.; Sverremark-Ekström, E.; Jenmalm, M.C. Influence of early gut microbiota on the maturation of childhood mucosal and systemic immune responses. *Clin. Exp. Allergy* **2009**, *39*, 1842–1851. [CrossRef]

59. Chenoll, E.; Rivero, M.; Codoñer, F.M.; Martinez-Blanch, J.F.; Ramón, D.; Genovés, S.; Moreno Muñoz, J.A. Complete Genome Sequence of *Bifidobacterium longum* subsp. *infantis* Strain CECT 7210, a Probiotic Strain Active against Rotavirus Infections. *Genome Announc.* **2015**, *3*. [CrossRef]

60. Rivière, A.; Gagnon, M.; Weckx, S.; Roy, D.; De Vuyst, L. Mutual Cross-Feeding Interactions between *Bifidobacterium longum* subsp. *longum* NCC2705 and *Eubacterium rectale* ATCC 33656 Explain the Bifidogenic and Butyrogenic Effects of Arabinoxylan Oligosaccharides. *Appl. Environ. Microbiol.* **2015**, *81*, 7767–7781. [CrossRef]

61. Egan, M.; Motherway, M.O.; Kilcoyne, M.; Kane, M.; Joshi, L.; Ventura, M.; van Sinderen, D. Cross-feeding by *Bifidobacterium breve* UCC2003 during co-cultivation with *Bifidobacterium bifidum* PRL2010 in a mucin-based medium. *BMC Microbiol.* **2014**, *14*, 282. [CrossRef]

62. Nobili, V.; Putignani, L.; Mosca, A.; Chierico, F.D.; Vernocchi, P.; Alisi, A.; Stronati, L.; Cucchiara, S.; Toscano, M.; Drago, L. Bifidobacteria and lactobacilli in the gut microbiome of children with non-alcoholic fatty liver disease: Which strains act as health players? *Arch. Med. Sci.* **2016**. [CrossRef]

63. Fouhy, F.; Ronan, N.J.; O'Sullivan, O.; McCarthy, Y.; Walsh, A.M.; Murphy, D.M.; Daly, M.; Flanagan, E.T.; Fleming, C.; McCarthy, M.; et al. A pilot study demonstrating the altered gut microbiota functionality in stable adults with Cystic Fibrosis. *Sci. Rep.* **2017**, *7*, 6685. [CrossRef] [PubMed]

64. Weizman, Z.; Durie, P.R.; Kopelman, H.R.; Vesely, S.M.; Forstner, G.G. Bile acid secretion in cystic fibrosis: Evidence for a defect unrelated to fat malabsorption. *Gut* **1986**, *27*, 1043–1048. [CrossRef] [PubMed]

65. Quinn, R.A.; Lim, Y.W.; Maughan, H.; Conrad, D.; Rohwer, F.; Whiteson, K.L. Biogeochemical forces shape the composition and physiology of polymicrobial communities in the cystic fibrosis lung. *mBio* **2014**, *5*, e00956-13. [CrossRef] [PubMed]

66. Ionescu, A.A.; Nixon, L.S.; Luzio, S.; Lewis-Jenkins, V.; Evans, W.D.; Stone, M.D.; Owens, D.R.; Routledge, P.A.; Shale, D.J. Pulmonary function, body composition, and protein catabolism in adults with cystic fibrosis. *Am. J. Respir. Crit. Care Med.* **2002**, *165*, 495–500. [CrossRef] [PubMed]
67. Palmer, K.L.; Mashburn, L.M.; Singh, P.K.; Whiteley, M. Cystic fibrosis sputum supports growth and cues key aspects of *Pseudomonas aeruginosa* physiology. *J. Bacteriol.* **2005**, *187*, 5267–5277. [CrossRef]
68. Bacci, G.; Mengoni, A.; Fiscarelli, E.; Segata, N.; Taccetti, G.; Dolce, D.; Paganin, P.; Morelli, P.; Tuccio, V.; De Alessandri, A.; et al. A Different Microbiome Gene Repertoire in the Airways of Cystic Fibrosis Patients with Severe Lung Disease. *Int. J. Mol. Sci.* **2017**, *18*, 1654. [CrossRef] [PubMed]
69. Spalding, M.D.; Prigge, S.T. Lipoic acid metabolism in microbial pathogens. *Microbiol. Mol. Biol. Rev. MMBR* **2010**, *74*, 200–228. [CrossRef] [PubMed]
70. Price-Whelan, A.; Dietrich, L.E.P.; Newman, D.K. Pyocyanin alters redox homeostasis and carbon flux through central metabolic pathways in *Pseudomonas aeruginosa* PA14. *J. Bacteriol.* **2007**, *189*, 6372–6381. [CrossRef] [PubMed]
71. Duytschaever, G.; Huys, G.; Bekaert, M.; Boulanger, L.; De Boeck, K.; Vandamme, P. Cross-sectional and longitudinal comparisons of the predominant fecal microbiota compositions of a group of pediatric patients with cystic fibrosis and their healthy siblings. *Appl. Environ. Microbiol.* **2011**, *77*, 8015–8024. [CrossRef] [PubMed]
72. Lim, Y.W.; Evangelista, J.S.; Schmieder, R.; Bailey, B.; Haynes, M.; Furlan, M.; Maughan, H.; Edwards, R.; Rohwer, F.; Conrad, D. Clinical insights from metagenomic analysis of sputum samples from patients with cystic fibrosis. *J. Clin. Microbiol.* **2014**, *52*, 425–437. [CrossRef] [PubMed]

6

A New Proposal for the Pathogenic Mechanism of Non-Coeliac/Non-Allergic Gluten/Wheat Sensitivity: Piecing Together the Puzzle of Recent Scientific Evidence

Valentina Leccioli [1,*], Mara Oliveri [1], Marcello Romeo [2], Massimiliano Berretta [3] and Paola Rossi [1,*]

1 Department of Biology and Biotechnology "L. Spallanzani", University of Pavia, via Ferrata 1, 27100 Pavia, Italy; mara.oliveri@libero.it
2 C.E.R.H.M. Center for Experimental Research for Human Microbiome Ludes H.E.I., Pietro Stiges Palace, Strait Street, 1436 Valletta, Malta; drmarcelloromeo@gmail.com
3 Department of Medical Oncology, CRO-Aviano, National Cancer Institute, Via Franco Gallini 2, 33081 Aviano, Italy; mberretta@cro.it
* Correspondence: leccioli.valentina@libero.it (V.L.); paola.rossi@unipv.it (P.R.)

Abstract: Non-coeliac/non-allergic gluten/wheat sensitivity (NCG/WS) is a gluten-related disorder, the pathogenesis of which remains unclear. Recently, the involvement of an increased intestinal permeability has been recognized in the onset of this clinical condition. However, mechanisms through which it takes place are still unclear. In this review, we attempt to uncover these mechanisms by providing, for the first time, an integrated vision of recent scientific literature, resulting in a new hypothesis about the pathogenic mechanisms involved in NCG/WS. According to this, the root cause of NCG/WS is a particular dysbiotic profile characterized by decreased butyrate-producing-*Firmicutes* and/or *Bifidobacteria*, leading to low levels of intestinal butyrate. Beyond a critical threshold of the latter, a chain reaction of events and vicious circles occurs, involving other protagonists such as microbial lipopolysaccharide (LPS), intestinal alkaline phosphatase (IAP) and wheat α-amylase trypsin inhibitors (ATIs). NCG/WS is likely to be a multi-factor-onset disorder, probably transient and preventable, related to quality and balance of the diet, and not to the presence of gluten in itself. If future studies confirm our proposal, this would have important implications both for the definition of the disease, as well as for the prevention and therapeutic-nutritional management of individuals with NCG/WS.

Keywords: non-coeliac gluten/wheat sensitivity; pathogenic mechanism; butyrate; amylase trypsin inhibitors; lipopolysaccharide; intestinal alkaline phosphatase; microbiota

---

1. Introduction

Non-coeliac/non-allergic gluten/wheat sensitivity (NCG/WS) is a clinical condition described for the first time in 1978 by Ellis and Linaker [1], and then in 1980 by Cooper et al. [2], who reported cases of patients presenting gluten-responsive clinical picture in absence of coeliac disease (CD). However, it was only in 2012 that NCG/WS has been considered to be within the gluten-related disorder (GRD) spectrum, together with CD and wheat allergy (WA) [3]. In 2012, a consensus on new nomenclature and classification of gluten-related disorders has been published [3], after the first of three International Expert Meetings on GRD, all leading to related publications [3–5] that outlined NCG/WS main clinical and diagnostic features. While CD is a chronic small intestinal, autoimmune enteropathy triggered by gluten and related prolamines in genetically predisposed individuals, and WA is an adverse immunologic reaction to wheat proteins, NCG/WS is "a condition in which symptoms are triggered by gluten ingestion, in the absence of celiac-specific antibodies and of classical celiac villous atrophy, with variable Human Leukocyte Antigen (HLA) status and variable presence of first generation anti-gliadin antibodies (AGA)" [3,4]. HLA-DQ2 and -DQ8 are the genetic markers most strongly associated with CD, being positive in approximately 95% of coeliac patients. HLA haplotypes are found positive in about 50% of NCG/WS patients, only slightly higher than 30% of the general population [4].

The recent renewed interest of scientific community in NCG/WS is due to an increasing number of patients, not affected by CD or WA, referring intestinal and extra-intestinal symptoms after gluten/wheat ingestion; despite the initial skepticism on its very existence as a discrete entity, NCG/WS has been recognized as an independent disorder of clinical, social, and economic relevance. However, there are still questions about its separation from CD [3–9]. This immune-mediated disorder [10] affects individuals for whom CD and WA have been ruled out according to the respective current diagnostic criteria [5,11]. It is characterized by heterogeneous and not specific gastrointestinal (GI) symptoms, including abdominal pain, bloating, bowel habit abnormalities (diarrhea, alternating bowel and constipation), and extra-intestinal symptoms, including chronic tiredness, headache, 'foggy mind', joint and muscle pain, limb numbness, eczema or skin rash, depression, anemia, of variable severity, occurring within hours or a few days after the ingestion of gluten-containing foods; symptoms improve or rapidly disappear with the exclusion of the latter and recur following their reintroduction [3–5,11].

In the last few years, several studies have suggested that both innate and adaptive immunity are involved [9,10,12], but there still remains an absence of confirmed and validated specific biomarkers. Therefore, according to the Salerno Experts, a diagnosis of NCG/WS should be made after a positive double-blind placebo-controlled gluten challenge with crossover (DBPCC) [5,11]. However, this procedure has been shown to be an "imperfect gold standard" [13,14], and in daily clinical practice, the diagnosis remains based on the evaluation of symptoms, the exclusion of CD and WA and improvement in symptoms after elimination of gluten/wheat from the diet (the latter of which is often influenced by placebo effects) [9,15]. Diagnostic difficulty, the lack of correct and scientific diagnostic work-up by some clinicians, and the considerable attention have given by the media to this "young" disorder, have contributed to the spread of the "self-diagnostic" phenomenon and the devotion of many people to gluten-free diets (GDF), which are often self-administered [4,9,12,16,17]. In fact, as for CD and WA, a GFD is the only possible treatment for NCG/WS, to date, but the severity and duration of this diet are not yet well defined, because of the uncertainty about the pathogenesis and triggers, the lack of specific biomarkers, and the strong inter-individual differences among patients [11]. All these factors also hamper the performance of accurate research because of the resulting heterogenous criteria for the selection of patients for the studies, and the following poorly comparable data [12]. Although risk factors for this disorder have not yet been identified, NCG/WS seems to be more common in females and in young/middle age adults [12]. Because of the "self-diagnostic" phenomenon and the absence of biomarkers, the overall prevalence of NCG/WS remains vague and possibly ranging from 0.6% to 6% [4,9]; the prevalence in children is still unknown [12].

There are increasing doubts among the scientific community regarding whether gluten is the trigger of NCG/WS; these doubts are supported by several studies [13,18–24]. It has been suggested that other molecules could determine the onset of NCG/WS [25]; possible candidates are fermentable oligo-, di-, monosaccharides and polyols (FODMAPs) [18], wheat amylase trypsin inhibitors (ATIs) [19–21], wheat germ agglutinin (WGA) [26,27] and exorphins [28].

Regarding the pathogenic mechanism of NCG/WS, a recent study conducted by Uhde et al. [29] clarified some aspects of this condition [10]. This study also suggested that some biomarkers (fatty acid-binding protein 2 or FABP2, soluble CD14 or sCD14, lipopolysaccharide (LPS)-binding protein or LBP, endotoxin-core antibodies or EndoCAb IgM, anti-flagellin IgM and IgG) could be useful as possible diagnostic tools, although they are yet to be confirmed and validated. Uhde demonstrated the presence of enterocyte injury and translocation of microbial components from the intestinal lumen to the blood circulation, resulting in activation of the systemic innate and adaptive immune response [29]. This study confirmed the already verified [30,31] existence of an increased intestinal permeability in individuals with NCG/WS, and provided evidence for a possible pathogenic role of the intestinal microbiota [12]. One of the main questions that remains to be answered is what induces the increased intestinal permeability, allowing microbial and food-borne antigens to cross into the lamina propria, and how does this occur [12].

Starting from the best of our current knowledge, in the present paper we connect some recent scientific evidence, which were never been expressly linked together till now, and propose a new hypothesis on the pathogenic mechanism of NCG/WS, by reconstructing the possible "chain reaction" involved in the onset of this disease. Finally, we provide some starting points for further research that, if confirmed by future studies, could imply important changes both to the substantial definition of the disease and to the therapeutic-nutritional management of individuals with NCG/WS.

2. Scientific Background

2.1. Diagnostic Difficulties

Because a clear pathogenic mechanism and specific, confirmed and validated biomarkers are yet to be identified, the evaluation of symptoms remains fundamental for diagnosis of NCG/WS [9,10,12]. Unfortunately, the symptoms are also shared by CD [3,14], irritable bowel syndrome (IBS) [4,5,14] and non-immunoglobulin E (IgE)-mediated food allergies [4,14,32–34], and, as for CD, symptoms must be considered a poor indicator and predictor of the disease [29,35,36].

The current diagnostic criteria for NCG/WS [5,11] are insufficient for a certain identification of sensitive individuals, both for clinical practice [9,13] and, in our opinion, for research. They are based on the exclusion of CD and WA, and on the clinical responsiveness of individuals to a GFD and gluten rechallenge [5,11]. However, CD and WA cannot always be adequately excluded [14]. According to a recent systematic review [8], up to 20% of NCG/WS patients in literature were eventually reclassified as coeliac patients, after re-evaluation after gluten challenge, or advanced diagnostic investigations, such as characterization of $\gamma\delta$ intraepithelial lymphocytes (IELs), immunohistological detection of anti-tTG2 IgA, duodenal aspirate or biopsy culture, and HLA-DQ2-gliadin tetramer test [9,13]. This subgroup of NCG/WS patients was characterized by lymphocytic enteritis (LE, representing Marsh 1 lesion level), negative serology for CD (anti-endomysial-EmA- and anti-tissue transglutaminase 2-tTG2-IgA), and positive genetics for CD (HLA-DQ2/DQ8 haplotype) [9,13]. Furthermore, according to the current diagnostic criteria, non-IgE-mediated WA can fall within the NCG/WS spectrum [4,32–34]. Non-IgE-mediated food allergies have different systemic and GI symptoms, similar to NCG/WS in terms of quality and time of onset. Without any biomarker, aside from an increased number of eosinophils in normal intestinal mucosa, they can be diagnosed by a positive response to an elimination diet followed by a DBPCC [14,32,34].

With regard to the DBPCC proposed to confirm the diagnosis of NCG/WS [5], besides being cumbersome, time consuming and costly, it is subject to important precebo, placebo, and nocebo effects and presents with a series of parameters that still need standardization and validation [9,13,14]; moreover, Molina-Infante and Carroccio show that more than 80% of recruited patients undergoing a DBPCC cannot reach a formal diagnosis of NCG/WS, 40% have a nocebo response and only 16% show gluten-specific symptoms, reaching 30% when the challenge is performed with wheat [13]. These findings highlight why DBPCC remains an "imperfect gold standard" for NCG/WS, and raise doubts about the role of gluten in the actual triggering of the disease, as suggested by many other studies [13,18–24].

The shared intestinal manifestations also make it hard to distinguish NCG/WS from IBS [14], a chronic functional GI disorder diagnosed exclusively on the basis of non-specific clinical characteristics [37–39]. Many researchers suggest that NCG/WS may be a subgroup of IBS, rather than an independent clinical entity. This hypothesis is supported by the fact that the clinical picture in NCG/WS is almost always dominated by some GI symptoms, among those previously mentioned, most of which are also present in IBS, and that FODMAPs, rather than gluten, are responsible for them [6,18,25,39–43]. FODMAPs are present in grains and related products (especially those gluten-related), legumes, fruit, vegetables, milk and honey [9,44,45], and could in fact induce distension of the intestine because they are osmotically active molecules and fermentative substrates [25,40,46]. However, FODMAPs are known to inhibit rather than cause inflammation, by inducing beneficial changes in the intestinal microbiota and generation of short-chain fatty acids (SCFAs) [42,46–48]. It is unlikely that FODMAPs are the sole responsible for symptoms reported by NCG/WS subjects [42,49]: many individuals in clinical remission with a GFD do continue to ingest FODMAPs from legumes [18], containing quantities of these carbohydrates that are comparable to those of gluten-containing grains [44,45]. In our opinion, rather than triggers, FODMAPs should be considered as possible additional elements of disturbance that, in this specific case, could exacerbate symptoms associated with the gut lumen which is already compromised, due to other causes. Moreover, it is possible that individuals with NCG/WS could also have, at the same time, a lack of one or more enzymes for the digestion of FODMAPs or other nutrients; this would also explain cases of people defining themselves NCG/WS because of an association between the appearance of typical manifestations and the ingestion of gluten-containing foods, but then continuing to report persistent symptoms despite adhesion to a GFD [41]. In this regard, Balakireva [50] claims that both conditions could coexist independently, without necessarily sharing a common pathophysiological basis.

2.2. ATIs as a Trigger of NCG/WS?

Recently, the scientific community has focused on the possible role of ATIs in GRDs [19–21,51–53]. Wheat α-amylase trypsin inhibitors belong to the family of water soluble albumins [21,53], which, together with globulins, represent 10–20% of total wheat proteins [19]; in the endosperm of plant seeds, they support the natural defense against parasites and insects and may regulate starch metabolism during seed development and germination. They are a family of compact protease-resistant proteins with strong disulfide bonds and high secondary structural homology, that copurify specifically with ω-gliadins. ATIs can be grouped into three subfamilies of approximately 50–60, 24–30 and 12–15 kDa [19,21].

Studies on immune stimulating activity of ATIs have been conducted in human and murine macrophages, monocytes and dendritic cells (DCs), in cultures of coeliac intestinal biopsies as well as in vivo in mice [19,21]. These studies have demonstrated that ATIs (in particular CM3 and 0.19 types, of about 15 KDa) are strong activators of dendritic cells (DCs), macrophages and monocytes [19,21]. On these cells they engage the TLR4-MD2-CD14 complex, thereby activating both the classical (nuclear factor kappa B or NF-kB) and the non-classical (interferon responsive factor 3 or IRF-3) pathway. It results in an up-regulation of maturation markers and the early release of innate proinflammatory cytokines, IL-1β, IL-6, TNFα, and then later, IL-8 and MCP-1 [19,21]. Contrary to wild type mice, studies have shown that TLR4- or TLR4-signalling-deficient mice do not show intestinal and systemic innate immune activation after oral challenge with ATIs [20,21]. Furthermore, the in vitro and in vivo experiments performed by Junker [21] found that gliadins or gliadin peptides, such as p31–43 or p31–49, are not innate immunity stimulators. Zevallos [19] reported that in mice fed with an ATI/gluten-free diet for four weeks, a single gavage of about 12 mg/mouse of commercial gluten (containing 0.2 mg ATIs) increased parameters of innate inflammation along the whole intestine; this did not happen in mice challenged with the same dose of gluten that was 70% de-enriched of ATIs by prior extraction. This appears to indicate that pure dietary gluten itself has no relevant immune stimulating activity in normal mice, in contrast to what has been suggested in ex vivo settings [19].

Intestinal myeloid cells probably sense ATIs through DCs body extensions into the gut lumen while probing it for the presence of antigens and/or through an active transport of intact ATIs across the intestinal epithelial layer, as occurs with gliadin peptides [20,54,55]. A direct interaction between ATIs and TLRs may also occur on the surface of enterocyte membrane, leading to the development of intestinal inflammation [56].

Schuppan [20] suggests that ATIs could have an adaptive adjuvant effect on pre-existing intestinal inflammation, in addition to promoting an innate immune response. A healthy adult person with a daily consumption of 150–250 g of wheat flour, therefore exposed to about 0.5–1 g of ATIs, would have a modest or moderate innate intestinal immune activation without development of symptoms, thanks to immune tolerance mechanisms [20,21]. According to Schuppan [20], individuals with NCG/WS could be those with pre-existing or chronic inflammatory diseases in whom the sensing/uptake of ATIs is increased, probably as a consequence of the disruption of intestinal homeostasis and barrier integrity. Thus, even modest activation of innate immunity could exacerbate inflammatory conditions already present, by indirectly promoting an adaptive response through the strengthening of pre-existing antigenic exposition of antigen presenting cells (APC) to T cells. According to Schuppan, such adaptive responses would occur in the gut, as well as in nearby or more remote lymph nodes or lymphatic organs, resulting in the typical NCG/WS extra-intestinal inflammation [20]. Zevallos [19] observed such adjuvant effect of nutritional ATIs in mice with pre-existing dextran sodium sulfate (DSS)-induced small intestinal or colonic inflammation. However, as suggested by Zevallos [19], further preclinical and clinical studies in human are warranted to assess the effect of an ATIs-free diet on intestinal and extra-intestinal inflammatory diseases.

In light of these findings, the recently proposed "FODMAPs hypothesis" concerning NCG/WS would be hardly sustainable, as discussed by Zevallos [19]. As previously mentioned, FODMAPs cannot induce the inflammatory responses occurring in NCG/WS patients, but rather could contribute to "mechanically" worsen their symptoms. In general, scientific evidence seems to better support the role of ATIs as a trigger of NCG/WS, which seems likely to be an immune-mediated disorder [10].

2.3. *Microbial Lipopolysaccharide, Intestinal Alkaline Phosphatase and Intestinal Permeability*

TLR4 activation by ATIs resembles that induced by LPS, the strongest TLR4 agonist. In fact, TLR4 activation by ATIs is CD14-dependent and engages MyD88-mediated downstream signaling (leading to activation of NF-kB and transcriptional upregulation of proinflammatory cytokines and chemokines such as IL-8, TNFα and MCP-1), or TRIF-mediated signaling (resulting in secretion of type I interferons and RANTES) [21].

LPS is the major cell wall component of Gram negative bacteria, consisting of a hydrophobic portion (lipid A) and a hydrophilic portion (an oligosaccharidic core plus an antigenic polysaccharide called O-antigen); it is released from bacterial cell wall by shedding or bacterial lysis [57]. As opposed to ATIs, ingested and luminal LPS is usually completely inactivated by gastric acids and intestinal alkaline phosphatase (IAP) [19–21].

The latter is an important brush-border enzyme involved in preventing intestinal inflammation and preserving the gut microbiota homeostasis. Mainly produced by the proximal small intestine epithelial cells, it is secreted both luminally and basolaterally and inactivates, by dephosphorylation, the microbial components normally present at high concentrations in the gut lumen [58–61]. In particular, IAP may play a pivotal role in the maintenance of intestinal barrier integrity by detoxification of LPS [62]. IAP is downregulated in settings where gut barrier dysfunctions are critical in the development of diseases, such as inflammatory bowel disease (IBD): low levels of IAP have been found in inflamed colonic biopsies of patients with Crohn's disease and ulcerative colitis (UC) [63,64]. Expression levels and activity of duodenal IAP were found to be particularly low, and related to the disrupted intestinal barrier integrity, in severe cases of CD in young patients [62,65]. IAP knock-out (KO) mice show higher LPS influx to the systemic circulation [66]. Exogenous IAP supplementation prevents the development of colitis in both human and mice [67,68], and prevents LPS-induced barrier dysfunctions in vitro [58].

In this regard, in healthy individuals with intact intestinal barriers, plasma concentrations of LPS range from undetectable levels up to 0.2 ng/mL; a variety of physiological factors can result in permeability alterations that lead to plasma LPS levels ranging about 1–2 ng/mL, while patients with intestinal permeability disorders such as necrotizing enterocolitis (NEC) and IBD can reach levels between 2 and 10 ng/mL [69–78]. Guo et al. [57] found that relatively low but physiologically and clinically relevant levels of LPS in the interstitial fluid of enterocytes can lead to a reversible, time-dependent increase in paracellular permeability in vitro (filter-grown Caco-2 monolayers) and in an in vivo (mouse intestinal perfusion) intestinal epithelial model system, without inducing cell death [57]. This occurs through a TLR4-MD2-CD14-mediated intracellular mechanism, engaged by LPS linked to LBP, and involves a TLR4-dependent up-regulation of CD14 membrane expression [57]. A variety of physiological factors such as prolonged physical exertion, high-fat diet, physiological stresses, or intestinal permeability disorders can readily achieve these concentrations of LPS in the interstitial fluid of enterocytes [57]. The consequent paracellular permeability variation occurs within four or five days [57], and can be dynamically regulated by altering both the expression levels and localization of tight junction proteins (TJPs) [58]. Inflammatory pathways, such as LPS-induced NF-kB activation and the consequent production of cytokines, result in disrupted levels and localization of TJPs [79,80]. This, in turn, can increase the passage of intestinal contents to the gut mucosa and to the systemic circulation [57,58]. As circulating LPS is an important determinant of the inflammatory response and multi organ failure, it could therefore play an important role in further deterioration and prolongation of intestinal TJ barrier defects in intestinal permeability disorders and inflammatory gut diseases [57].

Regarding intestinal permeability, the early belief that it was reduced in NCG/WS [81] has been definitively rejected [9]. Several studies have shown that an increased one is present even in non-coeliac patients, in particular in NCG/WS [30,31], IBS [31,82], and generic "non-coeliac" patients with persistent dyspeptic complaints [83]. Barbaro [31] proposed that zonulin could play a role in the pathophysiology of NCG/WS because of increased zonulin serum levels and a correlation with symptoms found in NCG/WS patients, suggesting disassembly of TJs. Hollon [30] analyzed intestinal permability of duodenal biopsy explants in four study groups (coeliacs with active disease (ACD), coeliacs in remission, non-coeliac gluten sensitives and non-coeliac dyspeptic controls) through the measurement of transepithelial electrical resistance (TEER). This study found an increase in permeability in all groups after pepsin-trypsin digested gliadin (PT-gliadin) exposure, compared to the media alone, with a greater increase in individuals with ACD and with NCG/WS. Finally, the findings by Uhde [29] about damage to enterocytes and translocation of microbial components from the lumen to the intestinal mucosa and blood circulation, further support the presence of increased gut permeability in NCG/WS. Uhde [29] also found an association between improvement in symptoms after GFD and normalization of biomarkers levels, although the magnitude of the latter did not correlate significantly with that of the symptoms scores. The damage to enterocytes was deduced by serological levels of FABP2 [29], a cytosolic protein specific to intestinal epithelial cells, rapidly released into systemic circulation after cellular damage, reflecting changes in the rate of enterocyte turnover [84–87]. In individuals with NCG/WS, elevated levels of circulating FABP2 are comparable to those of individuals with CD, and correlate with systemic innate and adaptive immune responses to microbial antigens. These are respectively evidenced by the significant increase in serological levels of soluble CD14 (sCD14) and LBP, and of antibodies towards LPS (EndoCAb IgM) and flagellin (anti-flagellin IgM and IgG). All these serum levels were significantly increased in NCG/WS patients, compared both to healthy and CD cohorts, except anti-flagellin IgM and IgG which were significantly increased only when compared to healthy controls [29]. It has been reported that LBP and sCD14 bind to circulating LPS and, depending on their relative concentrations, transfer LPS either to the TLR4-MD2-CD14 complex on myeloid cells, resulting in inflammatory stimulation, or to high density lipoproteins (HDL), lowering bioactivity of LPS [88,89]. Plasma lipoproteins, and in particular HDL, play an important role in neutralization of circulating LPS by transporting it to the liver for metabolization and excretion in the bile. In humans, low HDL plasma levels were found in septic patients, while raised ones are associated with a reduction in LPS-induced inflammation [90]. Low HDL levels could favour the transfer of LPS to the TLR4-MD2-CD14 complex, favouring inflammatory processes; by failing or decreasing the passage of LPS to HDL, peripheral inflammatory events would have a "green light". In this regard, it would be interesting to assess HDL levels in individuals with NCG/WS to demonstrate a correlation between presence and intensity of symptoms and their improvement after dyslipidemia correction.

We must highlight that in the mentioned studies on intestinal permeability in NCG/WS patients, issues about different inclusion/exclusion criteria recur, as in most of the studies about this condition, due to the lack of specific confirmed biomarkers.

3. New Hypothesis on the Pathogenic Mechanism of NCG/WS

The intestinal epithelial surface is in constant contact with the enteroma; in diseases such as IBD, NEC and HIV infections there is a correlation between compromised epithelial integrity and immune responses consequent to translocation of microbial components from the intestinal lumen to the blood circulation [88,91]. Human microbiota, mainly composed of species belonging to *Firmicutes* and *Bacteroidetes* phyla, is suggested to play immunological, structural and metabolic functions such as, for example, the preservation of GI barrier integrity through the production of SCFAs [88].

Among these, butyrate is the major source of energy for the colonic mucosa, in turn promoting epithelial cell differentiation and injury repair; it also seems to play an important protective role in colorectal carcinogenesis. Butyrate stimulates the secretion of mucin and epithelial antimicrobial peptides, the synthesis of TJPs, and prevents microbial translocation [92–95]. Recently Yan and Ajuwon [92] found that butyrate significantly and dose-dependently protects intestinal barrier integrity from LPS-induced impairment. This effect was indicated by the restoration of paracellular permeability, measured by TEER and paracellular uptake of fluorescein isothiocyanate-dextran (FITC-dextran), and was carried out through the selective stimulation of TJPs and downregulation of TLR-4 expression.

Butyrate-producing bacteria are a functional group within the human gut microbial population [96]. Most of these bacteria belong to *Firmicutes* phylum, in particular Clostridial Clusters IV and XIVa (saccharolytic, strictly anaerobic Gram positive bacteria). Numerically, two of the most important groups appear to be *Faecalibacterium prausnitzii* (Clostridial cluster IV), and *Eubacterium rectale*/*Roseburia* spp. (Clostridial cluster XIVa) with a detection rate in faeces of healthy adults of about 2–15% compared to total bacteria [96,97]. Human studies are often limited to faecal samples analysis that, however, do not provide information about microbiota in the mucus layer, where butyrate-producing *Firmicutes* (b-p*F*) mainly reside, according to a validated in vitro gut model (M-SHIME) [98]. In fact, Clostridial cluster XIVa and IV species constitute respectively 59% and 19% of the mucin-adhered *Firmicutes* microbiota (94% of the mucin layer total community), with major representatives in *Roseburia intestinalis* and *Eubacterium rectale*. In contrast, *Proteobacteria* and *Bacteroidetes* prefer the lumenal milieu [98].

Bifidobacteria (Gram positive, anaerobic, saccharolytic bacteria belonging to the phylum *Actinobacteria*) contribute to the maintainance of adequate levels of intestinal butyrate by providing acetate and lactate to b-p*F*, in turn converting them into butyrate (cross-feeding interaction) [96,97,99].

Similarly, even mucins may indirectly serve as a growth substrate for b-p*F*, possibly via cross-feeding with mucin-degrading microbes, such as *A. muciniphila*, which provide partial breakdown products, acetate and lactate [98,100].

Low levels of b-p*F* are found in patients with IBD and their inflamed tissues compared to healthy individuals [96,101]. Low levels of b-p*F* and *Bifidobacteria* are also found in IBS and are associated with increased IBS symptoms [102,103]. Furthermore, the absence of butyrate in colonic tissue is associated with mucosal atrophy and coloncyte apoptosis [104,105].

In light of the above findings and considerations, a particular dysbiotic profile characterized by low levels of b-p*F* and *Bifidobacteria* could not provide an adequate butyrate level for enterocytes, resulting in reduced or absent butyrate trophic and protective effects. This would "starve" enterocytes, would negatively influence TJPs expression and localization, and would also predispose GI epithelial cells to possible cell damage or premature death. In fact, Uhde observed high FAPB2 serum levels in NCG/WS patients [29]. Moreover, as butyrate stimulates mucine secretion [95], a decrease or lack of butyrate could result in mucus layer alterations. Mucus is produced by goblet cells and forms a protective physical barrier covering enterocytes, thus preventing microrganisms and noxious substances from reaching epithelial surface [106]; so mucus layer impairment could further enhance the direct contact between enterocytes and microbial and food-borne antigens, and would create unfavorable conditions for b-p*F*, thereby creating a vicious circle. For example, recent in vivo and in vitro studies have revealed that IBD, in which the mucus layer becomes thinner and more discontinuous, is associated with low levels of mucosal butyrate producers, such as *Roseburia* and *Faecalibacterium*, indicating that a damaged mucus layer may lower the ecological fitness of specific butyrate producers [98].

Such a situation could allow sufficient LPS quantities to arrive in the interstitial fluid, resulting in a further increase in permeability, as explained by Guo [57]. In our opinion, this could constitute the pre-existing condition allowing the onset of NCG/WS. As a consequence, simultaneous paracellular translocation of microbial components and food-borne antigens, such as intact ATIs, could occur. Active ATIs would directly, and in greater quantities, stimulate the maturation of DCs, monocytes and macrophages of the GI tract, leading to activation of the innate immune response in the lamina propria [19–21]. Here, the stimulation of the TLR4-MD2-CD14 complex by ATIs would be additional to that of translocated LPS, amplifying the proinflammatory effect. Further, direct stimulation of the TLR4-MD2-CD14 complex on the surface of epithelial cells may occur to a greater extent because of the impaired mucus layer. Such a mechanism may also be amplified because TLR4 and CD14 expression and membrane co-localization are increased after LPS exposure in vitro and in vivo [57]. This would explain the typical local and rapid-onset intestinal symptoms of NCG/WS after the ingestion of gluten/ATI-containing foods. Uhde found that these translocated molecules could also arrive in the bloodstream and activate both innate and adaptive systemic immunity, as shown by the respective detection of serum LBP and sCD14, and EndoCAb and anti-flagellin antibodies. Translocated circulating antigens could bind to TLRs on other cells to trigger inflammatory responses in other parts of the body, explaining the extra-intestinal manifestations of NCG/WS [29].

Luminal LPS is usually completely inactivated by IAP: the latter, although exclusively secreted by brush border epithelial cells of the proximal small intestine, preserves its activity along the entire GI tract [107,108]. Several in vitro and in vivo studies in mice and rats have shown that IAP prevents adhesion of both pathogenic and commensal bacteria to the intestinal epithelial cells [109], prevents their translocation [107,110,111], inactivates possibly translocated pathogen-associated molecular patterns (PAMPs), and inhibits PAMP-induced NF-kB-mediated inflammatory responses [60,108]. IAP also stimulates gene expression of TJPs, such as ZO-1, ZO-2 and occludin, and their correct cellular localization, thus playing a direct role in intestinal barrier functionality [58]. However, we must highlight that butyrate is an inducer of IAP expression, and increases its activity [93,107,112,113]. Therefore, it is likely that a dysbiosis characterized by low levels of b-p*F* and/or *Bifidobacteria* could indirectly cause a decrease in IAP levels and activity, resulting in an insufficient detoxification of luminal microbial components, including LPS. The latter would have a greater green light for translocation across the previously described compromised NCG/WS GI barrier. In support of this hypothesis, also Goldberg [107] asserts that IAP silencing could result in impairment of the host's ability to protect itself from luminal LPS exposure. Moreover, butyrate-induced IAP gene expression is inhibited by cytokines such as IL-1β and TNFα, and according to Malo [114], "cytokine-mediated IAP gene silencing may have important implications for gut epithelial function in the setting of intestinal inflammatory conditions". Interestingly, IL-1β and TNFα are two of the cytokines produced after ATI stimulation [19], so that the GI inflammation, triggered by translocated antigens, could contribute to further silencing IAP, resulting in another vicious cycle.

In Junker's in vivo experiments in mice to characterize the inflammatory activity of ATIs, orally ingested LPS was not found to cause increased transcription of cytokines, and thus, inflammation [21]. Junker, and later Schuppan and Zevallos, properly described this finding to be attributed to LPS inactivation by gastric acids and IAP activity [19–21]. In a paper on NCG/WS, Schuppan [20] defined ATIs as "the only relevant luminal TLR4 activator in the gastrointestinal tract". In light of what discussed above, it could be that not only ATIs, but also luminal LPS from the resident microbiota, are involved in immune response activation in NCG/WS, thus accumulating their stimulating effects.

In NCG/WS individuals AGA are detected in a variable trend: AGA IgG are found in about half of patients [81,115], finding that created great discussion about their possible utility as a diagnostic tool for this disease [49,115–118], while AGA IgA are rarely detected [29,115]. Interestingly, in the study by Uhde [29] IgM responses to gliadin and microbial components (LPS and flagellin) were also investigated and found enhanced, in clear contrast with CD and healthy cohorts. Uhde suggests that acute microbial translocation from the gut would be expected to enhance the secretion of IgM antibodies in the periphery via a TLR9-dependent activation of B cells, independent of direct contact with respective antigens or T-cell involvement. IgM B cells would be further stimulated by direct interaction with specific antigens, such as translocated gliadins and microbial components, thus contributing to the observed IgM antibody responses [29]. However, according to our hypothesis, the triggers of NCG/WS are ATIs and microbial components, LPS in particular; we think that the host immune response would be mainly addressed against these ones, that should be further investigated in this regard. Even if our hypothesis is confirmed by future studies, further research will be necessary to understand pathophysiological and immunological events, and most of aspects of NCG/WS, such as variability in antibody reactivity among patients.

Contrary to CD patients, individuals with NCG/WS do not present villous atrophy or mucosal architecture abnormalities at duodenal level. For this reason, regarding NCG/WS, several authors have recently suggested possible elective damage sites aside from the duodenum [11,29,119]. Di Liberto et al. [119] suggested that in sensitive patients the immunological response could be greater in the colon rather than in the duodenal mucosa, because NCG/WS is generally characterized by GI symptoms also present in IBS, which is very often characterized by colonic mucosal inflammation [40,120,121]. In fact, Di Liberto observed innate lymphoid cell infiltrates (ILC1) in the rectal mucosa of individuals with NCG/WS, where a greater expression of proinflammatory cytokines such as IFNγ was also detected [119]. Uhde suggested the jejunum as an alternative damage location because it is the primary expression site of FABP2 [29]. On the basis of our proposal, we believe that the whole intestine could be involved in NCG/WS, maybe with an increasing trend in the colon. This hypothesis is based on several factors: first, the stimulating activity of ATIs progressively increases along the intestinal tract and is more marked in the colon rather than in the small intestine [19]; second, the colon contains the most "dense" and metabolically active microbiota within the adult GI tract, however the Clostridial cluster XIVa spp. is also present in the small intestine [97]. Regardless, it could be that epithelial changes associated with NCG/WS do not lead to overt remodelling of the mucosa, and therefore, they could require confocal laser endomicroscopy (CLE) for visualization [10,29].

In summary, the "culture medium" for the rooting of NCG/WS appears to be a pre-existing dysbiosis characterized by low levels of b-p*F* and/or *Bifidobacteria*, leading to a decrease in butyrate. Beyond a critical threshold of the latter, the gut would no longer be capable of dealing with different inflammatory stimuli, these being, an exogenous one from the diet (ATIs) and an endogenous one from the resident microbiota (LPS and other microbial components); as a consequence, it would begin a chain reaction as illustrated in Figure 1. In line with this, although no consensus has been agreed upon, Bennet [122] declared that in IBS patients there is a temporary decreased stability of the gut microbiota, leading to a dysbiosis generically defined as a weak tendency for a reduction in the beneficial bacteria of the gut countered with an increase in pathogenic species. Furthermore, Bennet highlighted the beneficial effects of butyrate and suggested that, although inconsistent, reduced levels of butyrate-producing *Eubacterium, Faecalibacterium* and *Roseburia* spp. could potentially be an ancillary cause of IBS symptoms in some patients [122]. Chassard [103] suggests that low levels of butyrate found in a subgroup of IBS patients could be due to the lowering of some butyrate-producing bacteria and may reduce the potential health benefit of this metabolite, including anti-inflammatory effects and the colonic defence barrier. All of this could be important in our perspective, considering that, to date, NCG/WS patients may be still diagnosed as suffering from IBS. Finally, with regard to NCG/WS, Volta [9] suggests that microbial dysbiosis driven by aberrant changes in the normal composition of the gut microbiota may contribute to intestinal barrier defects and inflammatory responses.

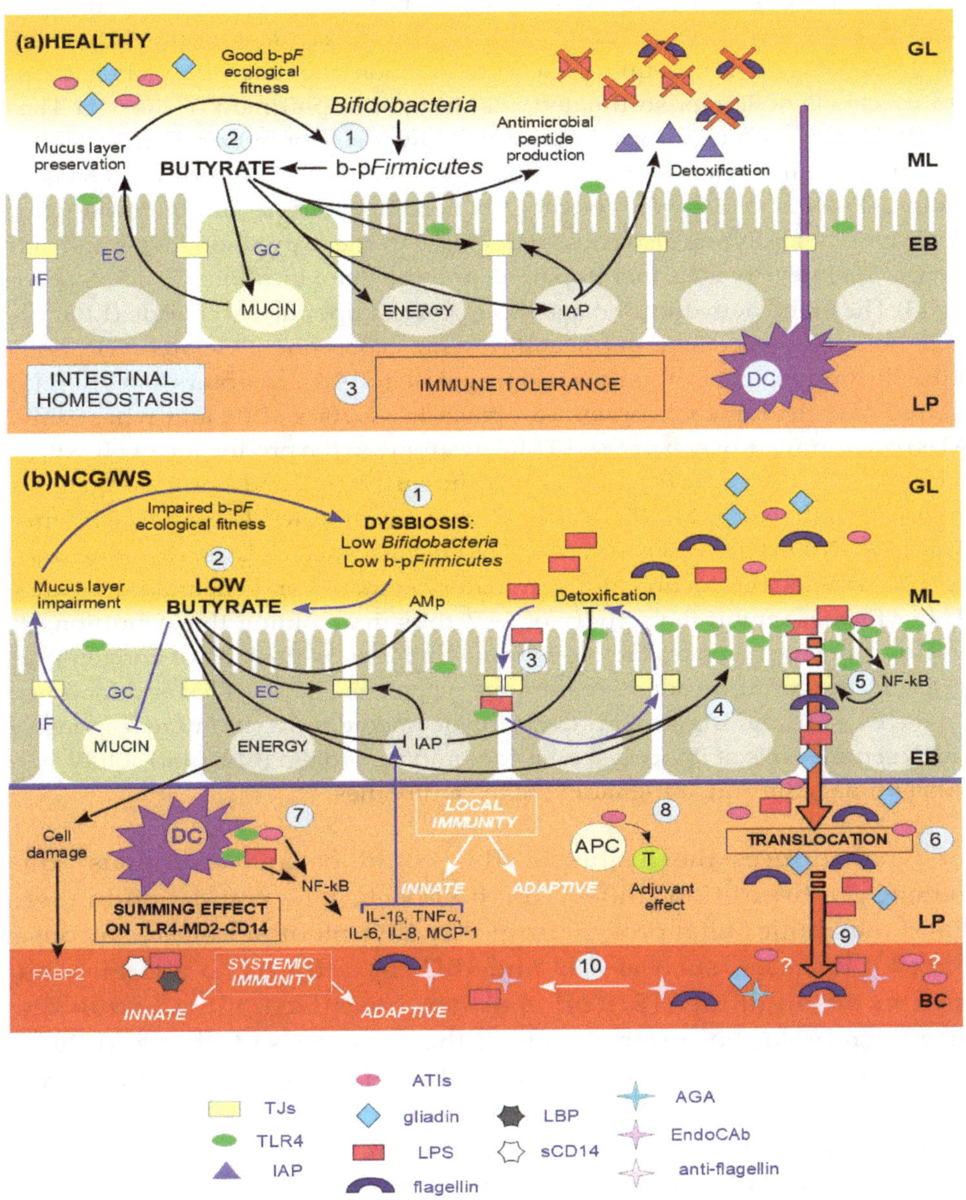

Figure 1. Schematic drawing that shows what happens in a healthy gut versus a non-coeliac gluten/wheat sensitivity gut according to our hypothesis. **NCG/WS** = non-coeliac gluten/wheat sensitivity; **EC** = enterocyte; **GC** = goblet cell; **IF** = interstitial fluid; **GL** = gut lumen; **ML** = mucus layer; **EB** = epithelial barrier; **LP** = lamina propria; **BC** = blood circulation; numbers in light blue balloons indicate the various steps in the chain reaction; → indicates stimulation; ⊣ indicates inhibition. (**a**) HEALTHY: 1. Butyrate-producing *Firmicutes* (b-p*F*) provide adequate levels of butyrate

in the ML and *Bifidobacteria* support the production of butyrate thanks to cross-feeding interactions with b-p*F*; 2. Butyrate in the ML, close to ECs, plays different trophic and protective functions: it stimulates GCs in the production of mucins, resulting in the preservation of the ML, and thus in a good b-p*F* ecological fitness. Butyrate constitutes the major energy supply for ECs; it favours the preservation of tight junctions (TJs) integrity by stimulating the expression and membrane co-localization of tight junction proteins (TJPs). Butyrate stimulates the production of antimicrobial peptides (AMp), and the expression and activity of intestinal alkaline phosphatase (IAP), thereby favouring the detoxification of microbial components; 3. All these functions together prevent that the content of the GL directly contacts and/or translocates across the EB, and, together with dendritic cells (DCs) which probe the GL for the presence of antigens, allow gut homeostasis and immune tolerance. (**b**) NCG/WS: (1) A dysbiosis characterized by low levels of b-p*F* and/or *Bifidobacteria* results in not sufficient levels of butyrate in the ML; (2) As a consequence, a chain reaction of events and vicious circles occur: the production of mucins is no longer stimulated, resulting in impairment of the ML. The consequent lowering of b-p*F* ecological fitness further promotes low levels of butyrate. ECs, without adequate energy source, run into inefficiency and cell damage, resulting in high serum levels of fatty acids binding protein 2 (FABP2). Moreover, TJs integrity is compromised, and the production of AMp is decreased. Low levels of butyrate also cause a decrease in the expression levels and activity of IAP; as a consequence, TJs integrity is further impaired, and the detoxification of microbial components is not sufficient; (3) The failed detoxification enables microbial lipopolysaccharide (LPS) to penetrate in the IF, where it increases paracellular permeability, with a consequent vicious cycle; (4) Furthermore, both LPS in the IF and low levels of butyrate upregulate toll-like receptors 4 (TLR4); (5) Because of the compromised ML, the lumenal content can reach EC surface. LPS and wheat amylase trypsin inhibitors (ATIs) can stimulate overexpressed TLR4, resulting in the production of NF-kB, and then later, inflammatory cytokines, which further damage TJs integrity; (6) Food-borne antigens and microbial components can cross the leaky EB; (7) In the LP, both translocated LPS and ATIs stimulate, at the same time, the TLR4-MD2-CD14 complex on myeloid cells, such as DCs, resulting in a local innate immune response with the production of inflammatory cyokines and chemokines. Among the latter, IL-1β and TNFα further inhibit the activity of IAP, thus maintaining this condition; (8) Moreover, ATIs have an adjuvant effect on possible pre-existing antigenic exposition of antigen-presenting cells (APC) to T-cells (T), triggering an adaptive immune response; (9) Microbial and food-borne antigens translocate in the BC (10), and trigger a systemic innate and adaptive immune response, respectively resulting in high serum levels of lipopolysaccharide-binding protein (LBP) and soluble CD14 (sCD14), and EndoCAb, anti-flagellin and anti-gliadin (AGA) antibodies.

In terms of what induces the dysbiosis, this could be an "erroneous" diet and lifestyle, and/or an epigenetic predisposition. In fact, the first bacterial colonization in utero can modulate immunological and metabolic "fetal programming", with potential long-term consequences on the risk of developing GI diseases, such as CD and IBD, in addition to allergies, autoimmune and metabolic diseases in the adult life [123,124]. Further, breastfeeding and adult diet are known to strongly influence microbiota. For example, given the scarceness of fiber and the excess of animal fats and proteins, "Western-like diets" are associated with an increase in the secretion of bile salts, resulting in the selection of bile-resistant and sulfate-reducer bacteria with proteolytic and putrefactive action. This is in contrast with a healthy saccharolytic microbiota, promoted, for example, by the "Mediterranean diet", which allows the preservation of adequate leves of SCFAs and butyrate in particular. Moreover, the richness of Western diets, particularly with regard to trans and satured fats, could result in a greater translocation of LPS and greater inflammation [94,123–129].

4. Implications of the New Hypothesis

Based on the previously described literature and evaluations, it could be considered that NCG/WS is a potentially transient and preventable condition, strongly related to diet quality and balance, rather than to the presence or absence of gluten-containing foods. Without the suggested dysbiotic conditions, the extent of gliadin exposure effects would remain limited to those described in healthy subjects by Hollon [30]. This hypothesis could also be supported by the current lack, to the best of our knowledge, of both a specific and proven genetic background [12,14], and clear and defined evidence of hypersensitivity to gliadin [23,115] in NCG/WS patients.

Regardless, a GFD is currently the cornerstone of treatment for NCG/WS [11]. Undertaking a GFD, if self-administered, means exposure to a series of nutritional risks, and the possibility of obesity and related comorbidities, or in the least excessive weight gain. Moreover, a GFD is usually not economical and is very difficult to follow because of cross-contaminations and/or the presence of small amounts of gluten in food and drugs. In general a GFD appears to be unbalanced and inadequate in terms of both macro- and micronutrients, so it is fundamental that people start a GFD only if, and for the time, strictly necessary [11,50,130–135]. Also according to the current NASPGHAN guidelines on GRDs [11], given the uncertainty about the pathogenesis and triggers of NCG/WS, it is not clear if a GFD is actually the optimal treatment for this disease, although it could lead to improved symptoms in self-reported or diagnosed sensitives; it is also not clear how strict and how prolonged this diet should be, and how its efficacy should be monitored independently from the clinical response, given the strong inter-individual differences and the lack of clear guidelines for a standardized follow-up [8,11].

The validation of a co-causal role of specific alterations of the intestinal microbiota in this disorder would be fundamental to the management of NCG/WS patients at a nutritional level. As such, sensitive individuals would no longer need to follow a prolonged, if not permanent, restrictive diet based on the exclusion of gluten. All the more so that this restriction has been shown to affect microbiota richness and composition by reducing beneficial bacteria such as *F. prausnitzii* and *B. longum* [43,136]. On the contrary, by directing the dietetic choice of these patients towards a targeted "prebiotic" type, we could aim to restore a state of eubiosis thanks to the food's ability to shape the microbiota [126,137,138].

According to what is hypothesized here, targeted probiotic intake could be another fundamental aspect of the treatment of individuals with NCG/WS. In line with this, we might speculate if the weak correlation between magnitude of change in analyzed biomarkers and magnitude of change in symptom score after GFD in the study by Uhde [29] could be explained simply by the absence of an associated probiotic therapy.

One of the chief contributions of our microbiota is its partecipation in food digestion, mainly through a saccharolytic or a proteolytic catabolic pathway [125,139]. With the first one, saccharolytic bacteria, such as *Bifidobacteria* and *Lactobacilli*, hydrolize complex polysaccharides in monomeric sugars, then converted in SCFAs (mainly acetate, propionate, and butyrate). The latter seem to to have a positive role in regulating some physiological processes [94], well summarized in a review by Macfarlane G.T. and Macfarlane S. [139]. For example, SCFAs are known to affect lipid, cholesterol and glucose metabolism in various tissues, and to control the release of satiety hormones; recently, they have also been suggested to play a critical role in the regulation of the gut-microbiota-brain cross talk [94]. Furthermore, SCFAs have been shown to promote intestinal barrier integrity, affect epithelial cell transport and metabolism, epithelial cell growth and differentiation, and elicit direct transcriptional responses in immune cells [125,139]. Both carbohydrate and protein fermentation result in SCFAs production, although in quantitative terms, protein is a minor contributor [139]. Furthermore, besides SCFAs, the proteolytic pathway yields a variety of end-products including co-metabolites such as CO_2, H_2, H_2S, ammonia, amines, thiols, phenols, and indoles, many of which are potentially toxic and are believed to promote the onset of "Western diseases", such as colon cancer and chronic systemic disorders [125,139]. Saccharolytic bacteria contribute to protect the host from toxic products associated with putrefaction, by requiring them for incorporation into cellular proteins [139]. For these reasons, although the composition of microbiota is a highly personalized peculiarity influenced by several factors such as diet, drugs and lifestyle, it seems that a healthy and balanced microbiota should be mainly saccharolytic with a prevalence of *Bifidobacteria* and *Lactobacilli* [125]. Among SCFAs, butyrate seems to be the most interesting one, thanks to its many important physiological properties [139], some of which have been previously mentioned. Among butyrate-producing bacteria that colonize the human gut, *F. prausnitzii*, *Roseburia* spp., and *E. hallii* belong to the so called *"emerging probiotics"* [100,140]. Of particular interest, *F. prausnitzii* has well characterized immunomodulatory properties in vitro and in vivo [100]: it is able to abolish the NF-kB pathway in intestinal epithelial cells, and prevents colitis in animal models [141]. Currently, *emerging probiotics* culturing and functional characterization difficulties do not allow well-designed pre-clinical and intervention studies yet [140]. For this reason, we have to wait for developing new probiotic products aimed to directly restore butyrate-producing bacteria levels in NCG/WS subjects.

Fortunately, the contribution of cross-feeding interactions between *Bifidobacteria* and butyrate-producing *Firmicutes* is remarkable in the stimulation of butyrate production [99] and thus we believe it could be a strategy in the "attack phase" of NCG/WS treatment. For this purpose, *Bifidobacteria* such as *B. bifidum*, *B. longum* and *B. adolescentis*, the colonic dominant species of the genus, could be useful [97,99]: besides their role in butyrate production, they promote other important anti-inflammatory effects [142–147]. For example, some strains of *B. bifidum* have been shown to promote strong anti-inflammatory effects through the inhibition of LPS-induced NF-kB-activation in a strain and dose-dependent manner [142]; some strains of *B. longum* ssp. *longum* and *B. longum* ssp. *infantis*, as well as *B. adolescentis* and *B. animalis* have been shown to induce significant levels of IL-10 in different human cell cultures and in human colonic lamina propria [144]; IL-10 is a regulatory cytokine with an important role in the maintenance of intestinal homeostasis [148,149], and it is absent in gut explants from NCG/WS patients, according to Hollon [30]. *B. longum* ssp. *longum* CCM 7952, is able to increase expression of zonulin-1 and occludin in the intestinal epithelium, preserving TJs and epithelial barrier function [144], thus potentially contributing to a reduction in inflammatory stimuli in the intestinal mucosa of patients with NCG/WS. Finally, *Bifidobacteria*, alone or together with particular *Lactobacilli* and *Streptococci* strains in specific multispecies probiotic mixtures, have been shown to be effective in the prevention and/or treatment of DSS-induced colitis [144,146,150], IBS symptoms [151] and GI inflammatory diseases, such as UC in mice and humans [143,146,147,152,153]. In particular, *Bifidobacterium bifidum* BGN 4 seems to reduce the production of pro-inflammatory cytokines, thanks to the chiro-inositol present in its cell membrane [154]. According to a recent study [155], the administration of a specific probiotic blend containing *Bifidobacterium bifidum* BGN 4, *Lactobacillus salivarius* and *Lactobacillus acidophilus* (Acronelle®, Bromatech srl, Milan, Italy) decreases inflammation in patients with IBD, in combination with mesalazine treatment.

Other microbes besides *Bifidobacteria* have demonstrated important anti-inflammatory activities that could be useful in the treatment of NCG/WS: *L. rhamnosus* GG, found in the mucus layer environment [98], has been shown to attenuate intestinal barrier dysfunctions and proinflammatory signals [156], and in particular, to restore in vitro gliadin-induced epithelial barrier disruption and related TEER in the presence of polyamines [157]; *Akkermansia muciniphila*, a Gram-negative strictly anaerobic mucin-degrader, contributes to the production of SCFAs and the maintenance of a healthy protective GI barrier by continuously renovating the mucosae cover [100]. The use of probiotic therapy could be strengthened by the association with prebiotics such as resistant starch, inulin, xylans and fructo-oligosaccharides (FOS) which would, directly and indirectly, stimulate butyrate production [94,96–99,126].

Obviously, if our hypothesis is validated in future studies, further research would be necessary to define the best formulation of treatment, including correct dosages and posology.

5. NCG/WS Is a Cancer Risk Factor?

Whether CD is associated with an increased risk of cancer malignancy is still under debate. However, some literature seems to support this hypothesis. A European multi-centre study reported more than a three-fold increased risk of non-Hodgkin's Lymphoma (NHL) in patients with clinically diagnosed CD [158]. Also an increased incidence and/or mortality for NHL have been reported in patients with CD [159]. An increased risk of GI cancers, duodenal ones in particular, was also documented [160]. On the contrary, other studies suggested that CD may be associated with a reduced risk of some cancers, including breast and lung ones [161,162], although the rationale for this relationship remains unknown.

Overall, it has been observed that the correlation between all types of cancer and CD remained significant for more than one year after diagnosis.

As regards possible correlations between malignancies and NCG/WS, to date data are missing [12]. However, Elfestrom et al. [163] in a study including 28.882 CD patients, 12.860 subjects with small intestinal inflammation (Marsh 1–2) and 3.705 patients with latent CD, found that all the three groups had an increased risk for GI cancers in the first year after diagnosis, but not thereafter. Moreover, an Irish population-based retrospective cohort study [164] reported that malignancy and mortality from malignant neoplasms were increased in patients with positive AGA and negative EmA tests. However, only on the basis of those serological results, the authors could not classify patients as having CD or NCG/WS according to recognised diagnostic criteria, so they could not provide reliable information about a real correlation between NCG/WS and cancer risk.

In conclusion, more investigations are necessary in this field to determine if NCG/WS may be correlated with cancer malignancy.

6. Starting Points for Future Research

The data and hypotheses described herein could contribute to the clarification of some controversial aspects of this "young" clinical condition, and could provide some novel avenues for future research. First, it would be interesting to verify the existence of an actual association between the particular dysbiotic profile proposed and NCG/WS. Second, it is of interest to reassess, at the colonic level, the expression of TJPs and TLRs. In this regard, according to a study by Sheth [165] on the effects of LPS on cholangiocytes TJs, LPS disrupts barrier function and increases paracellular permeability in a time- and dose-dependent manner, and also induces a redistribution of TJPs from intercellular junction sites. This study also reported that the LPS-induced disruption of TJs is mediated by TLR4 and LBP [165]. This could raise the question whether, in individuals with NCG/WS, the localization mechanisms of TJPs could be altered, rather than their expression levels. Third, we could speculate that individuals with NCG/WS may have an "overactive" TLR4, attributable to "gain-of-function" mutations. This could also contribute to explain the LPS-induced increase in gut permeability, according to the mechanisms proposed by Guo [57] and Sheth [165], and even more so, may help explain the extent of the immune response caused by the hypothetical combined stimulating effect of ATIs and LPS on the TLR4-MD2-CD14 complex.

Finally, future verification that critical intestinal butyrate levels are pivotal for the onset of NCG/WS could also provide the premise for studies regarding possible associated long-term major complications, such as intestinal lymphoma or gastrointestinal malignancies, as observed in CD. In the current literature there are no such reports, due to a lack of longitudinal data and prospective studies on the natural history of NCG/WS [12]. However, as previously mentioned, butyrate has been suggested to play an important protective role in colorectal carcinogenesis, and has been shown to reduce size and number of tumors in rat models of bowel cancer. Moreover, in vitro, it influences morphology and motility, inhibits proliferation and induces apoptosis in a variety of cancer cells [93,139].

The starting points for future research offered by this paper are described in Table 1.

Table 1. Starting points for research. The listed starting points are suggested for testing our hypothesis on the pathogenic mechanism of non-coeliac gluten/wheat sensitivity (NCG/WS). b-p*F* = butyrate-producing Firmicutes, IAP = intestinal alkaline phosphatase, TJPs = tight junctions proteins, TLR4 = toll-like receptor 4, ATIs = amylase trypsin inhibitors, LPS = lypopolysaccharide, HDL=high density lipoproteins.

Suggested Starting Points For Testing Our Hypothesis On NCG/WS
1. Association between NCG/WS and dysbiosis, in particular focusing on b-p*F* and *Bifidobacteria* levels
2. Association between NCG/WS and an impaired mucus barrier
3. Roles of butyrate and IAP
4. Presence of TJPs co-localization defects and role in the alteration of gut permeability
5. Expression of TJPs and TLR4 at the colonic level
6. Presence of simultaneous stimulation of the TLR4-MD2-CD14 complex by ATIs and LPS
7. Existence of anti-ATIs antibodies
8. Mutations of TLR4 coding gene and related functional studies
9. Association between NCG/WS and HDL levels

7. Conclusions

This review investigates and discusses, for the first time, novel plausible connections among recent scientific evidence, which have never been linked together in an integrated vision. We also propose a new theory on the pathogenic mechanism of NCG/WS, schematized in Figure 1.

NCG/WS may be considered a multi-factor-onset disorder, potentially transient and preventable, to date without a specific genetic pattern. It may have, instead, an epigenetic component, strongly related to quality and balance of the diet, and consequently, to the microbiota. If the hypotheses posed here are confirmed, NCG/WS could be still defined as a gluten-related disease because of the substantial coexistence of gluten and the stimulating activity of ATIs, for which a GFD is essentially ATIs-free [19].

More precisely, NCG/WS could be considered to be an ATIs/low butyrate-producing *Firmicutes*/low *Bifidobacteria*-dysbiosis-induced disorder, which would more appropriately be referred to as "dysbiosis-induced ATIs sensitivity" (DIAS).

In future, once excluded CD and WA in all their forms, the diagnosis of NCG/WS could ideally be determined also thanks to the aid of the immunological and enterocyte damage biomarkers suggested by Uhde, and the analysis of gut microbiota. According to our hypothesis, host immune system may be mainly addressed towards two different inflammatory stimuli, an exogenous one from the diet (ATIs) and an endogenous one from the resident microbiota, LPS in particular. In our opinion, further studies should be focused into this field, including possible existence of anti-ATIs antibodies. However, first of all, more appropriate diagnostic criteria for NCG/WS and standardized inclusion/exclusion criteria are warranted to perform more reliable studies on it. In our opinion, more appropriate diagnostic criteria are warranted for GRDs in general, because even a certain exclusion of CD still does not seem to be guaranteed, as well as exclusion of non-IgE mediated WA, with a consequent possible contamination of NCG/WS sample, thus creating confounding and possibly biased results. In this regard, it is important to underline that HLA haplotypes should not to be considered as suggestive of NCG/WS: according to the systematic review by Molina-Infante [8], not all studies on this disorder could adequately exclude CD and confirm diagnosis of NCG/WS, as well as not all studies performed, clearly defined and fully described genetic tests, and related the latter to histology [14]. Positive HLA-DQ2/DQ8 haplotypes are necessary, but not sufficient, to develop CD, and their absence excludes the latter, but so far, no genetic markers have been identified for NCG/WS [9], and according to Bardella [14], "other haplotypes, not CD-related, should be investigated".

According to our hypothesis, the treatment for NCG/WS would be completely different, and no longer necessarily based only on a restrictive and prolonged GFD, but on a targeted "prebiotic" type of nutrition together with specific probiotic therapy, all to be formulated in the future. In particular, we suggest that such a treatment should be specifically addressed to the direct or indirect restoration of adequate levels of butyrate-producing *Firmicutes*, and consequently of intestinal butyrate. In fact, in our opinion, the decrease of bp-*F* is at the basis of increased intestinal permeability of NCG/WS, via insufficient butyrate levels, according to the supposed chain reaction. However, we do not know at the moment what should be exactly referred to as "adequate levels" of b-p*F* or intestinal butyrate, also considering that a state of eubiosis results from a balance among all species of our microbiota. Because of culturing and functional characterization difficulties, new strategies are warranted to study the functional group of bp-*F*, later allowing pre-clinical and intervention studies necessary to confirm their usefulness in the treatment of this condition. Furthermore, clinical studies on human are necessary also to define if patients would benefit from an ATI-reduced or -free diet, as well as from IAP and/or butyrate supplementation.

We are aware that the objective which we aim at with this paper could seem ambitious, but we think that it is our duty as part of scientific community, to continuously pose questions and formulate related hypothetical plausible theories, even if not yet supported by experimental evidence: such theories could be at the basis of developing new research projects, which could lead to a step forward in the comprehension of critical aspects in a field, even if negative results are obtained. With this paper, in a very humbly way, we would like to make our idea/intuition available to scientific community, to stimulate it in investigating at various levels about aspects not yet taken into account, and that could have a role in the onset of NCG/WS. In our hypothesis we have critically put together recent scientific evidence in NCG/WS, highlighting diagnostic difficulties and absence of standardized procedures. We are aware that our proposed integrated vision opens up more questions than it closes, by taking into account many aspects which were never been expressly linked together till now in regard to NCG/WS, such as ATIs, IAP, LPS, butyrate and microbiota.

Coordinated studies in different areas of research will be necessary to confirm or reject our hypotheses, and to develop a full understanding of the pathogenesis of NCG/WS, that still seems to retain many intriguing secrets to uncover.

Acknowledgments: The authors thank Anna Vallerugo, Scientific English Teacher of CRO-Aviano, Scientific Direction, National Cancer Institute, for editing the English text.

Author Contributions: V.L. collected and reviewed the literature, wrote the manuscript and created figures; M.O., M.R. and P.R. critically analyzed and reviewed the manuscript; M.B. collected and reviewed the literature on oncological issues, and helped in writing the relative section of manuscript; P.R. was also the overall guarantor of this manuscript.

References

1. Ellis, A.; Linaker, B.D. Non-coeliac gluten sensitivity? *Lancet* **1978**, *1*, 1358–1359. [CrossRef]
2. Cooper, B.T.; Holmes, G.K.; Ferguson, R.; Thompson, R.A.; Allan, R.N.; Cooke, W.T. Gluten-sensitive diarrhea without evidence of celiac disease. *Gastroenterology* **1980**, *79*, 801–806. [PubMed]
3. Sapone, A.; Bai, J.C.; Ciacci, C.; Dolinsek, J.; Green, P.H.; Hadjivassiliou, M.; Kaukinen, K.; Rostami, K.; Sanders, D.S.; Schumann, M.; et al. Spectrum of gluten-related disorders: Consensus on new nomenclature and classification. *BMC Med.* **2012**, *10*, 13. [CrossRef] [PubMed]
4. Catassi, C.; Bai, J.C.; Bonaz, B.; Bouma, G.; Calabrò, A.; Carroccio, A.; Castillejo, G.; Ciacci, C.; Cristofori, F.; Dolinsek, J.; et al. Non-celiac Gluten Sensitivity: The New Frontier of Gluten Related Disorders. *Nutrients* **2013**, *5*, 3839–3853. [CrossRef] [PubMed]
5. Catassi, C.; Elli, L.; Bonaz, B.; Bouma, G.; Carroccio, A.; Castillejo, G.; Cellier, C.; Cristofori, F.; de Magistris, L.; Dolinsek, J.; et al. Diagnosis of Non-Celiac Gluten Sensitivity (NCGS): The Salerno Experts' Criteria. *Nutrients* **2015**, *7*, 4966–4977. [CrossRef] [PubMed]
6. Vanga, R.; Leffler, D.A. Gluten sensitivity: Not celiac and not certain. *Gastroenterology* **2013**, *145*, 276–279. [CrossRef] [PubMed]
7. Sapone, A.; Lammers, K.M.; Mazzarella, G.; Mikhailenko, I.; Cartenì, M.; Casolaro, V.; Fasano, A. Differential Mucosal IL-17 Expression in Two Gliadin-Induced Disorders: Gluten Sensitivity and the Autoimmune Enteropathy Celiac Disease. *Int. Arch. Allergy Immunol.* **2010**, *152*, 75–80. [CrossRef] [PubMed]

8. Molina-Infante, J.; Santolaria, S.; Sanders, D.S.; Fernández-Bañares, F. Systematic review: Noncoeliac gluten sensitivity. *Aliment. Pharmacol. Ther.* **2015**, *41*, 807–820. [CrossRef] [PubMed]
9. Volta, U.; Caio, G.; Karunaratne, T.B.; Alaedini, A.; De Giorgio, R. Non-coeliac gluten/wheat sensitivity: Advances in knowledge and relevant questions. *Exp. Rev. Gastroenterol. Hepatol.* **2017**, *11*, 9–18. [CrossRef] [PubMed]
10. Carroccio, A. Searching for the immunological basis of wheat sensitivity. *Nat. Rev. Gastroenterol. Hepatol.* **2016**, *13*, 628–630. [CrossRef] [PubMed]
11. Hill, I.D.; Fasano, A.; Guandalini, S.; Hoffenberg, E.; Levy, J.; Reilly, N.; Verma, R. NASPGHAN Clinical Report on the Diagnosis and Treatment of Gluten-related Disorders. *J. Pediatr. Gastroenterol. Nutr.* **2016**, *63*, 156–165. [CrossRef] [PubMed]
12. Caio, G.; Riegler, G.; Patturelli, M.; Facchiano, A.; DE Magistris, L.; Sapone, A. Pathophysiology of non-celiac gluten sensitivity: Where are we now? *Minerva Gastroenterol. Dietol.* **2017**, *63*, 16–21. [CrossRef] [PubMed]
13. Molina-Infante, J.; Carroccio, A. Suspected non-celiac gluten sensitivity confirmed in few patients after gluten challenge in double-blind, placebo-controlled trials. *Clin. Gastroenterol. Hepatol.* **2017**, *15*, 339–348. [CrossRef] [PubMed]
14. Bardella, M.T.; Elli, L.; Ferretti, F. Non Celiac Gluten Sensitivity. *Curr. Gastroenterol. Rep.* **2016**, *18*, 63. [CrossRef] [PubMed]
15. Elli, L.; Roncoroni, L.; Bardella, M.T. Non-celiac gluten sensitivity: Time for sifting the grain. *World J. Gastroenterol.* **2015**, *21*, 8221–8226. [CrossRef] [PubMed]
16. Di Sabatino, A.; Corazza, G.R. Nonceliac gluten sensitivity: Sense or sensibility? *Ann. Intern. Med.* **2012**, *156*, 309–311. [CrossRef] [PubMed]
17. Elli, L.; Tomba, C.; Branchi, F.; Roncoroni, L.; Lombardo, V.; Bardella, M.T.; Ferretti, F.; Conte, D.; Valiante, F.; Fini, L.; et al. Evidence for the Presence of Non-Celiac Gluten Sensitivity in Patiens with Functional Gastrointestinal Symptoms: Results from a Multicenter Randomized Double-Blind Placebo-Controlled Gluten Challange. *Nutrients* **2016**, *8*, 84. [CrossRef] [PubMed]
18. Biesiekierski, J.R.; Peters, S.L.; Newnham, E.D.; Rosella, O.; Muir, J.G.; Gibson, P.R. No Effects of Gluten in Patients With Self-Reported Non-Celiac Gluten Sensitivity After Dietary Reduction of Fermentable, Poorly Absorbed, Short-Chain Carbohydrates. *Gastroenterology* **2013**, *145*, 320–328. [CrossRef] [PubMed]
19. Zevallos, V.F.; Raker, V.; Tenzer, S.; Jimenez-Calvente, C.; Ashfaq-Khan, M.; Rüssel, N.; Pickert, G.; Schild, H.; Steinbrink, K.; Schuppan, D. Nutritional Wheat Amylase-Trypsin Inhibitors Promote Intestinal Inflammation via Activation of Myeloid Cells. *Gastroenterology* **2017**, *152*, 1100–1113. [CrossRef] [PubMed]
20. Schuppan, D.; Pickert, G.; Ashfaq-Khan, M.; Zevallos, V. Non-celiac wheat sensitivity: Differential diagnosis, triggers and implications. *Best Pract. Res. Clin. Gastroenterol.* **2015**, *29*, 469–476. [CrossRef] [PubMed]
21. Junker, Y.; Zeissig, S.; Kim, S.J.; Barisani, D.; Wieser, H.; Leffler, D.A.; Zevallos, V.; Libermann, T.A.; Dillon, S.; Freitag, T.L.; et al. Wheat amylase trypsin inhibitors drive intestinal inflammation via activation of toll-like receptor 4. *J. Exp. Med.* **2012**, *209*, 2395–2408. [CrossRef] [PubMed]
22. Zanini, B.; Basché, R.; Ferraresi, A.; Ricci, C.; Lanzarotto, F.; Marullo, M.; Villanacci, V.; Hidalgo, A.; Lanzini, A. Randomised clinical study: Gluten challenge induces symptom recurrence in only a minority of patients who meet clinical criteria for non-coeliac gluten sensitivity. *Aliment. Pharmacol. Ther.* **2015**, *42*, 968–976. [CrossRef] [PubMed]
23. Bucci, C.; Zingone, F.; Russo, I.; Morra, I.; Tortora, R.; Pogna, N.; Scalia, G.; Iovino, P.; Ciacci, C. Gliadin Does Not Induce Mucosal Inflammation or Basophil Activation in Patiens With Nonceliac Gluten Sensitivity. *Clin. Gastroenterol. Hepatol.* **2013**, *11*, 1294–1299. [CrossRef] [PubMed]
24. Rosinach, M.; Fernández-Bañares, F.; Carrasco, A.; Ibarra, M.; Temiño, R.; Salas, A.; Esteve, M. Double-Blind Randomized Clinical Trial: Gluten versus Placebo Rechallange in Patiens with Lymphocytic Enteritis and Suspected Celiac Disease. *PLoS ONE* **2016**, *11*, e0157879. [CrossRef] [PubMed]
25. Gibson, P.R.; Muir, J.G.; Newnham, E.D. Other Dietary Confounders: FODMAPs et al. *Dig. Dis.* **2015**, *33*, 269–276. [CrossRef] [PubMed]
26. De Punder, K.; Pruimboom, L. The dietary intake of wheat and other cereal grains and their role in inflammation. *Nutrients* **2013**, *5*, 771–787. [CrossRef] [PubMed]
27. Dalla Pellegrina, C.; Perbellini, O.; Scupoli, M.T.; Tomelleri, C.; Zanetti, C.; Zoccatelli, G.; Fusi, M.; Peruffo, A.; Rizzi, C.; Chignola, R. Effects of wheat germ agglutinin on human gastrointestinal epithelium: Insights from an experimental model of immune/epithelial cell interaction. *Toxicol. Appl. Pharmacol.* **2009**, *237*, 146–153. [CrossRef] [PubMed]

28. Pruimboom, L.; de Punder, K. The opioid effects of gluten exorphins: Asymptomatic celiac disease. *J. Health Popul. Nutr.* **2015**, *33*, 24. [CrossRef] [PubMed]
29. Uhde, M.; Ajamian, M.; Caio, G.; De Giorgio, R.; Indart, A.; Green, P.H.; Verna, E.C.; Volta, U.; Alaedini, A. Intestinal cell damage and systemic immune activation in individuals reporting sensitivity to wheat in the absence of coelic disease. *Gut* **2016**, *65*, 1930–1937. [CrossRef] [PubMed]
30. Hollon, J.; Puppa, E.L.; Greenwald, B.; Goldberg, E.; Guerrerio, A.; Fasano, A. Effect of gliadin on permeability of intestinal biopsy explants from celiac disease patients and patients with non-celiac gluten sensitivity. *Nutrients* **2015**, *7*, 1565–1576. [CrossRef] [PubMed]
31. Barbaro, M.R.; Cremon, C.; Caio, G.; Bellacosa, L.; De Giorgio, R.; Volta, U.; Stanghellini, V.; Barbara, G. Increased zonulin serum levels and correlation with symptoms in non-celiac gluten sensitivity and irritable bowel syndrome with diarrhea. In Proceedings of the UEG Week 2014, Vienna, Austria, 18–22 October 2014.
32. Elli, L.; Villalta, D.; Roncoroni, L.; Barisani, D.; Ferrero, S.; Pellegrini, N.; Bardella, M.T.; Valiante, F.; Tomba, C.; Carroccio, A.; et al. Nomenclature and diagnosis of gluten-related disorders: A position statement by the Italian Association of Hospital Gastroenterologists and Endoscopists (AIGO). *Dig. Liver Dis.* **2017**, *49*, 138–146. [CrossRef] [PubMed]
33. Carroccio, A.; Mansueto, P.; D'Alcamo, A.; Iacono, G. Non-celiac wheat sensitivity as an allergic condition: Personal experience and narrative review. *Am. J. Gastroenterol.* **2013**, *108*, 1845–1852. [CrossRef] [PubMed]
34. Cianferoni, A. Wheat allergy: Diagnosis and management. *J. Asthma Allergy* **2016**, *9*, 13–25. [CrossRef] [PubMed]
35. Katz, K.D.; Rashtak, S.; Lahr, B.D.; Melton, L.J.; Krause, P.K.; Maggi, K.; Talley, N.J.; Murray, J.A. Screening for celiac disease in a North American population: Sequential serology and gastrointestinal symptoms. *Am. J. Gastroenterol.* **2011**, *106*, 1333–1339. [CrossRef] [PubMed]
36. Leffler, D.A.; Dennis, M.; Hyett, B.; Kelly, E.; Schuppan, D.; Kelly, C.P. Etiologies and predictors of diagnosis in nonresponsive celiac disease. *Clin. Gastroenterol. Hepatol.* **2007**, *5*, 445–450. [CrossRef] [PubMed]
37. Drossman, D.A. Functional gastrointestinal disorders: History, pathophysiology, clinical features, and Rome IV. *Gastroenterology* **2016**, *150*, 1262–1279. [CrossRef] [PubMed]
38. Palsson, O.S.; Whitehead, W.E.; van Tilburg, M.A.; Chang, L.; Chey, W.; Crowell, M.D.; Keefer, L.; Lembo, A.J.; Parkman, H.P.; Rao, S.S.; et al. Development and Validation of the Rome IV Diagnostic Questionnaire for Adults. *Gastroenterology* **2016**, *150*, 1481–1491. [CrossRef] [PubMed]
39. Makharia, A.; Catassi, C.; Makharia, G.K. The overlap between irritable bowel syndrome and non-celiac gluten sensitivity: A clinical dilemma. *Nutrients* **2015**, *7*, 10417–10426. [CrossRef] [PubMed]
40. De Giorgio, R.; Volta, U.; Gibson, P.R. Sensitivity to wheat, gluten and FODMAPs in IBS: Facts or fiction? *Gut* **2016**, *65*, 169–178. [CrossRef] [PubMed]
41. Biesiekierski, J.R.; Newnham, E.D.; Shepherd, S.J.; Muir, J.G.; Gibson, P.R. Characterization of adults with a self-diagnosis of nonceliac gluten sensitivity. *Nutr. Clin. Pract.* **2014**, *29*, 504–509. [CrossRef] [PubMed]
42. Fasano, A.; Sapone, A.; Zevallos, V.; Schuppan, D. Nonceliac Gluten Sensitivity. *Gastroenterology* **2015**, *148*, 1195–1204. [CrossRef] [PubMed]
43. Volta, U.; Pinto-Sanchez, M.I.; Boschetti, E.; Caio, G.; De Giorgio, R.; Verdu, E.F. Dietary Triggers in Irritable Bowel Syndrome: Is There a Role for Gluten? *J. Neurogastroenterol. Motil.* **2016**, *22*, 547–557. [CrossRef] [PubMed]
44. Biesiekierski, J.R.; Rosella, O.; Rose, R.; Liels, K.; Barrett, J.S.; Shepherd, S.J.; Gibson, P.R.; Muir, J.G. Quantification of fructans, galacto-oligosaccharides and other short-chain carbohydrates in processed grains and cereals. *J. Hum. Nutr. Diet.* **2011**, *24*, 154–176. [CrossRef] [PubMed]
45. Varney, J.; Barrett, J.; Scarlata, K.; Catsos, P.; Gibson, P.R.; Muir, J.G. FODMAPs: Food composition, defining cutoff values and international application. *J. Gastroenterol. Hepatol.* **2017**, *32*, 53–61. [CrossRef] [PubMed]
46. Tuck, C.J.; Muir, J.G.; Barrett, J.S.; Gibson, P.R. Fermentable oligo-, di-, monosaccharide and polyols: Role in irritable bowel syndrome. *Expert Rev. Gastroenterol. Hepatol.* **2014**, *8*, 819–834. [CrossRef] [PubMed]
47. Halmos, E.P.; Christophersen, C.T.; Bird, A.R.; Shepherd, S.J.; Gibson, P.R.; Muir, J.G. Diets that differ in their FODMAP content alter the colonic luminal microenvironment. *Gut* **2015**, *64*, 93–100. [CrossRef] [PubMed]
48. Puertollano, E.; Kolida, S.; Yaqoob, P. Biological significance of short-chain fatty acid metabolism by the intestinal microbiome. *Curr. Opin. Clin. Nutr. Metab. Care* **2014**, *17*, 139–144. [CrossRef] [PubMed]

49. Catassi, C. Gluten Sensitivity. *Ann. Nutr. Metab.* **2015**, *67*, 16–26. [CrossRef] [PubMed]
50. Balakireva, A.V.; Zamyatnin, A.A. Properties of Gluten Intolerance: Gluten Structure, Evolution, Pathogenicity and Detoxification Capabilities. *Nutrients* **2016**, *8*, 644. [CrossRef] [PubMed]
51. Tilg, H.; Koch, R.; Moschen, A.R. Proinflammatory Wheat Attacks on the Intestine: Alpha-Amylase Trypsin Inhibitors as New Players. *Gastroenterology* **2013**, *144*, 1561–1563. [CrossRef] [PubMed]
52. Schuppan, D.; Gisbert-Schuppan, K. Reply. *Gastroenterology* **2013**, *144*, 1563–1564. [CrossRef]
53. Cuccioloni, M.; Mozzicafreddo, M.; Ali, I.; Bonfili, L.; Cecarini, V.; Eleuteri, A.M.; Angeletti, M. Interaction between wheat alpha-amylase/trypsin bi-functional inhibitor and mammalian digestive enzymes: Kinetic, equilibrium and structural characterization of binding. *Food Chem.* **2016**, *213*, 571–578. [CrossRef] [PubMed]
54. Niess, J.H.; Brand, S.; Gu, X.; Landsman, L.; Jung, S.; McCormick, B.A.; Vyas, J.M.; Boes, M.; Ploegh, H.L.; Fox, J.G.; et al. CX3CR1-mediated dendritic cell access to the intestinal lumen and bacterial clearance. *Science* **2005**, *307*, 254–258. [CrossRef] [PubMed]
55. Matysiak-Budnik, T.; Candalh, C.; Dugave, C.; Namane, A.; Cellier, C.; Cerf-Bensussan, N.; Heyman, M. Alterations of the intestinal transport and processing of gliadin peptides in celiac disease. *Gastroenterology* **2003**, *125*, 696–707. [CrossRef]
56. Gribar, S.C.; Richardson, W.M.; Sodhi, C.P.; Hackam, D.J. No longer an innocent bystander: Epithelial toll-like receptor signaling in the development of mucosal inflammation. *Mol. Med.* **2008**, *14*, 645–659. [CrossRef] [PubMed]
57. Guo, S.; Al-Sadi, R.; Said, H.M.; Ma, T.Y. Lipopolysaccharide Causes an Increase in Intestinal Tight Junction Permeability in Vitro and in Vivo by Inducing Enterocyte Membrane Expression and Localization of TLR-4 and CD14. *Am. J. Pathol.* **2013**, *182*, 375–387. [CrossRef] [PubMed]
58. Liu, W.; Hu, D.; Huo, H.; Zhang, W.; Adiliaghdam, F.; Morrison, S.; Ramirez, J.M.; Gul, S.S.; Hamarneh, S.R.; Hodin, R.A. Intestinal Alkaline Phosphatase Regulates Tight Junction Protein Levels. *J. Am. Coll. Surg.* **2016**, *222*, 1009–1017. [CrossRef] [PubMed]
59. Chen, K.T.; Malo, M.S.; Moss, A.K.; Zeller, S.; Johnson, P.; Ebrahimi, F.; Mostafa, G.; Alam, S.N.; Ramasamy, S.; Warren, H.S.; et al. Identification of specific targets for the gut mucosal defense factor intestinal alkaline phosphatase. *Am. J. Physiol. Gastrointest. Liver Physiol.* **2010**, *299*, G467–G475. [CrossRef] [PubMed]
60. Lallès, J.P. Intestinal alkaline phosphatase: Novel functions and protective effects. *Nutr. Rev.* **2014**, *72*, 82–94. [CrossRef] [PubMed]
61. Bilski, J.; Mazur-Bialy, A.; Wojcik, D.; Zahradnik-Bilska, J.; Brzozowski, B.; Magierowski, M.; Mach, T.; Magierowska, K.; Brzozowski, T. The Role of Intestinal Alkaline Phosphatase in Inflammatory Disorders of Gastrointestinal Tract. *Mediat. Inflamm.* **2017**, *2017*, 9074601. [CrossRef] [PubMed]
62. Molnár, K.; Vannay, A.; Sziksz, E.; Bánki, N.F.; Győrffy, H.; Arató, A.; Dezsőfi, A.; Veres, G. Decreased mucosal expression of intestinal alkaline phosphatase in children with coeliac disease. *Virchows Arch.* **2012**, *460*, 157–161. [CrossRef] [PubMed]
63. Tuin, A.; Poelstra, K.; de Jager-Krikken, A.; Bok, L.; Raaben, W.; Velders, M.P.; Dijkstra, G. Role of alkaline phosphatase in colitis in man and rats. *Gut* **2009**, *58*, 379–387. [CrossRef] [PubMed]
64. Molnár, K.; Vannay, A.; Szebeni, B.; Bánki, N.F.; Sziksz, E.; Cseh, A.; Győrffy, H.; Lakatos, P.L.; Papp, M.; Arató, A.; et al. Intestinal alkaline phosphatase in the colonic mucosa of children with inflammatory bowel disease. *World J. Gastroenterol.* **2012**, *18*, 3254–3259. [CrossRef] [PubMed]
65. Prasad, K.K.; Thapa, B.R.; Nain, C.K.; Sharma, A.K.; Singh, K. Brush border enzyme activities in relation to histological lesion in pediatric celiac disease. *J. Gastroenterol. Hepatol.* **2008**, *23*, e348–e352. [CrossRef] [PubMed]
66. Kaliannan, K.; Hamarneh, S.R.; Economopoulos, K.P.; Nasrin Alam, S.; Moaven, O.; Patel, P.; Malo, N.S.; Ray, M.; Abtahi, S.M.; Muhammad, N.; et al. Intestinal alkaline phosphatase prevents metabolic syndrome in mice. *Proc. Natl. Acad. Sci. USA* **2013**, *110*, 7003–7008. [CrossRef] [PubMed]
67. Ramasamy, S.; Nguyen, D.D.; Eston, M.A.; Alam, S.N.; Moss, A.K.; Ebrahimi, F.; Biswas, B.; Mostafa, G.; Chen, K.T.; Kaliannan, K.; et al. Intestinal alkaline phosphatase has beneficial effects in mouse models of chronic colitis. *Inflamm. Bowel Dis.* **2011**, *17*, 532–542. [CrossRef] [PubMed]
68. Lukas, M.; Drastich, P.; Konecny, M.; Gionchetti, P.; Urban, O.; Cantoni, F.; Bortlik, M.; Duricova, D.; Bulitta, M. Exogenous alkaline phosphatase for the treatment of patients with moderate to severe ulcerative colitis. *Inflamm. Bowel Dis.* **2010**, *16*, 1180–1186. [CrossRef] [PubMed]
69. Hurley, J.C. Endotoxemia: Methods of detection and clinical correlates. *Clin. Microbiol. Rev.* **1995**, *8*, 268–292. [PubMed]

70. Andreasen, A.S.; Krabbe, K.S.; Krogh-Madsen, R.; Taudorf, S.; Pedersen, B.K.; Møller, K. Human endotoxemia as a model of systemic inflammation. *Curr. Med. Chem.* **2008**, *15*, 1697–1705. [CrossRef] [PubMed]
71. Marshall, J.C.; Walker, P.M.; Foster, D.M.; Harris, D.; Ribeiro, M.; Paice, J.; Romaschin, A.D.; Derzko, A.N. Measurement of endotoxin activity in critically ill patients using whole blood neutrophil dependent chemiluminescence. *Crit. Care* **2002**, *6*, 342–348. [CrossRef] [PubMed]
72. Wellmann, W.; Fink, P.C.; Benner, F.; Schmidt, F.W. Endotoxaemia in active Crohn's disease. Treatment with whole gut irrigation and 5-aminosalicylic acid. *Gut* **1986**, *27*, 814–820. [CrossRef] [PubMed]
73. Sharma, R.; Tepas, J.J., 3rd; Hudak, M.L.; Mollitt, D.L.; Wludyka, P.S.; Teng, R.J.; Premachandra, B.R. Neonatal gut barrier and multiple organ failure: Role of endotoxin and proinflammatory cytokines in sepsis and necrotizing enterocolitis. *J. Pediatr. Surg.* **2007**, *42*, 454–461. [CrossRef] [PubMed]
74. Brock-Utne, J.G.; Gaffin, S.L.; Wells, M.T.; Gathiram, P.; Sohar, E.; James, M.F.; Morrell, D.F.; Norman, R.J. Endotoxaemia in exhausted runners after a long-distance race. *S. Afr. Med. J.* **1988**, *73*, 533–536. [PubMed]
75. Amar, J.; Burcelin, R.; Ruidavets, J.B.; Cani, P.D.; Fauvel, J.; Alessi, M.C.; Chamontin, B.; Ferriéres, J. Energy intake is associated with endotoxemia in apparently healthy men. *Am. J. Clin. Nutr.* **2008**, *87*, 1219–1223. [PubMed]
76. Lira, F.S.; Rosa, J.C.; Pimentel, G.D.; Souza, H.A.; Caperuto, E.C.; Carnevali, L.C., Jr.; Seelaender, M.; Damaso, A.R.; Oyama, L.M.; de Mello, M.T.; et al. Endotoxin levels correlate positively with a sedentary lifestyle and negatively with highly trained subjects. *Lipids Health Dis.* **2010**, *9*, 82. [CrossRef] [PubMed]
77. Bosenberg, A.T.; Brock-Utne, J.G.; Gaffin, S.L.; Wells, M.T.; Blake, G.T. Strenuous exercise causes systemic endotoxemia. *J. Appl. Physiol.* **1988**, *65*, 106–108. [PubMed]
78. Liu, H.; Li, W.; Wang, X.; Li, J.; Yu, W. Early gut mucosal dysfunction in patients with acute pancreatitis. *Pancreas* **2008**, *36*, 192–196. [CrossRef] [PubMed]
79. Ma, T.Y.; Iwamoto, G.K.; Hoa, N.T.; Akotia, V.; Pedram, A.; Boivin, M.A.; Said, H.M. TNF-alpha-induced increase in intestinal epithelial tight junction permeability requires NF-kappa B activation. *Am. J. Physiol. Gastrointest. Liver Physiol.* **2004**, *286*, 367–376. [CrossRef] [PubMed]
80. Al-Sadi, R.; Ye, D.; Dokladny, K.; Ma, T.Y. Mechanism of IL-1beta-induced increase in intestinal epithelial tight junction permeability. *J. Immunol.* **2008**, *180*, 5653–5661. [CrossRef] [PubMed]
81. Sapone, A.; Lammers, K.M.; Casolaro, V.; Cammarota, M.; Giuliano, M.T.; De Rosa, M.; Stefanile, R.; Mazzarella, G.; Tolone, C.; Russo, M.I.; et al. Divergence of gut permeability and mucosal immune gene expression in two gluten-associated conditions: Celiac disease and gluten sensitivity. *BMC Med.* **2011**, *9*, 23. [CrossRef] [PubMed]
82. Vazquez-Roque, M.I.; Camilleri, M.; Smyrk, T.; Murray, J.A.; Marietta, E.; O'Neill, J.; Carlson, P.; Lamsam, J.; Janzow, D.; Eckert, D.; et al. A controlled trial of gluten-free diet in patients with irritable bowel syndrome-diarrhea: Effects on bowel frequency and intestinal function. *Gastroenterology* **2013**, *144*, 903–911. [CrossRef] [PubMed]
83. Drago, S.; El Asmar, R.; Di Pierro, M.; Grazia Clemente, M.; Tripathi, A.; Sapone, A.; Thakar, M.; Iacono, G.; Carroccio, A.; D'Agate, C.; et al. Gliadin, zonulin and gut permeability: Effects on celiac and non-celiac intestinal mucosa and intestinal cell lines. *Scand. J. Gastroenterol.* **2006**, *41*, 408–419. [CrossRef] [PubMed]
84. Pelsers, M.M.; Hermens, W.T.; Glatz, J.F. Fatty acid-binding proteins as plasma markers of tissue injury. *Clin. Chim. Acta* **2005**, *352*, 15–35. [CrossRef] [PubMed]
85. Pelsers, M.M.; Namiot, Z.; Kisielewski, W.; Namiot, A.; Januszkiewicz, M.; Hermens, W.T.; Glatz, J.F. Intestinal-type and liver-type fatty acid-binding protein in the intestine. Tissue distribution and clinical utility. *Clin. Biochem.* **2003**, *36*, 529–535. [CrossRef]
86. Sandler, N.G.; Koh, C.; Roque, A.; Eccleston, J.L.; Siegel, R.B.; Demino, M.; Kleiner, D.E.; Deeks, S.G.; Liang, T.J.; Heller, T.; et al. Host response to translocated microbial products predicts outcomes of patients with HBV or HCV infection. *Gastroenterology* **2011**, *141*, 1220–1230. [CrossRef] [PubMed]
87. Levy, E.; Ménard, D.; Delvin, E.; Montoudis, A.; Beaulieu, J.F.; Mailhot, G.; Dubé, N.; Sinnett, D.; Seidman, E.; Bendayan, M. Localization, function and regulation of the two intestinal fatty acid-binding protein types. *Histochem. Cell Biol.* **2009**, *132*, 351–367. [CrossRef] [PubMed]
88. Brenchley, J.M.; Douek, D.C. Microbial translocation across the GI tract. *Annu. Rev. Immunol.* **2012**, *30*, 149–173. [CrossRef] [PubMed]
89. Kitchens, R.L.; Thompson, P.A. Modulatory effects of sCD14 and LBP on LPS-host cell interactions. *J. Endotoxin Res.* **2005** *11*, 225–229. [CrossRef] [PubMed]

90. Sharifov, O.F.; Xu, X.; Gaggar, A.; Grizzle, W.E.; Mishra, V.K.; Honavar, J.; Litovsky, S.H.; Palgunachari, M.N.; White, C.R.; Anantharamaiah, G.M.; et al. Anti-inflammatory mechanisms of apolipoprotein A-I mimetic peptide in acute respiratory distress syndrome secondary to sepsis. *PLoS ONE* **2013**, *8*, e64486. [CrossRef] [PubMed]
91. Estes, J.D.; Harris, L.D.; Klatt, N.R.; Tabb, B.; Pittaluga, S.; Paiardini, M.; Barclay, G.R.; Smedley, J.; Pung, R.; Oliveira, K.M.; et al. Damaged intestinal epithelial integrity linked to microbial translocation in pathogenic simian immunodeficiency virus infections. *PLoS Pathog.* **2010**, *6*, e1001052. [CrossRef] [PubMed]
92. Yan, H.; Ajuwon, K.M. Butyrate modifies intestinal barrier function in IPEC-J2 cells through a selective upregulation of tight junction proteins and activation of the Akt signaling pathway. *PLoS ONE* **2017**, *12*, e0179586. [CrossRef] [PubMed]
93. Orchel, A.; Dzierzewicz, Z.; Parfiniewicz, B.; Weglarz, L.; Wilczok, T. Butyrate-Induced Differentiation of Colon Cancer Cells Is PKC and JNK Dependent. *Dig. Dis. Sci.* **2005**, *50*, 490–498. [CrossRef] [PubMed]
94. Sandhu, K.V.; Sherwin, E.; Schellekens, H.; Stanton, C.; Dinan, T.G.; Cryan, J.F. Feeding the microbiota-gut-brain axis: Diet, microbiome, and neuropsychiatry. *Transl. Res.* **2016**, *179*, 223–244. [CrossRef] [PubMed]
95. Jung, T.H.; Park, J.H.; Jeon, W.M.; Han, K.S. Butyrate modulates bacterial adherence on LS174T human colorectal cells by stimulating mucin secretion and MAPK signaling pathway. *Nutr. Res. Pract.* **2015**, *9*, 343–349. [CrossRef] [PubMed]
96. Louis, P.; Flint, H.J. Diversity, metabolism and microbial ecology of butyrate-producing bacteria from the human large intestine. *FEMS Microbiol. Lett.* **2009**, *294*, 1–8. [CrossRef] [PubMed]
97. Rivière, A.; Selak, M.; Lantin, D.; Leroy, F.; De Vuyst, L. Bifidobacteria and Butyrate-Producing Colon Bacteria: Importance and Strategies for Their Stimulation in the Human Gut. *Front. Microbiol.* **2016**, *7*, 979. [CrossRef] [PubMed]
98. Van den Abbeele, P.; Belzer, C.; Goossens, M.; Kleerebezem, M.; De Vos, W.M.; Thas, O.; De Weirdt, R.; Kerckhof, F.M.; Van de Wiele, T. Butyrate-producing Clostridium cluster XIVa species specifically colonize mucins in an in vitro gut model. *ISME J.* **2013**, *7*, 949–961. [CrossRef] [PubMed]
99. Belenguer, A.; Duncan, S.H.; Calder, A.G.; Holtrop, G.; Louis, P.; Lobley, G.E.; Flint, H.J. Two routes of metabolic cross-feeding between Bifidobacterium adolescentis and butyrate-producing anaerobes from the human gut. *Appl. Environ. Microbiol.* **2006**, *72*, 3593–3599. [CrossRef] [PubMed]
100. Hevia, A.; Delgado, S.; Sánchez, B.; Margolles, A. Molecular Players Involved in the Interaction between Beneficial Bacteria and the Immune System. *Front. Microbiol.* **2015**, *6*, 1285. [CrossRef] [PubMed]
101. Walker, A.W.; Sanderson, J.D.; Churcher, C.; Parkes, G.C.; Hudspith, B.N.; Rayment, N.; Brostoff, J.; Parkhill, J.; Dougan, G.; Petrovska, L. High-throughput clone library analysis of the mucosa-associated microbiota reveals dysbiosis and differences between inflamed and non-inflamed regions of the intestine in inflammatory bowel disease. *BMC Microbiol.* **2010**, *11*, 7. [CrossRef] [PubMed]
102. Rajilić-Stojanović, M.; Biagi, E.; Heilig, H.G.; Kajander, K.; Kekkonen, R.A.; Tims, S.; de Vos, W.M. Global and deep molecular analysis of microbiota signatures in fecal samples from patients with irritable bowel syndrome. *Gastroenterology* **2011**, *141*, 1792–1801. [CrossRef] [PubMed]
103. Chassard, C.; Dapoigny, M.; Scott, K.P.; Crouzet, L.; Del'homme, C.; Marquet, P.; Martin, J.C.; Pickering, G.; Ardid, D.; Eschalier, A.; et al. Functional dysbiosis within the gut microbiota of patients with constipated-irritable bowel syndrome. *Aliment. Pharmacol. Ther.* **2012**, *35*, 828–838. [CrossRef] [PubMed]
104. Kripke, S.A.; Fox, A.D.; Berman, J.M.; Settle, R.G.; Rombeau, J.L. Stimulation of intestinal mucosal growth with intracolonic infusion of short-chain fatty acids. *J. Parent. Enter. Nutr.* **1989**, *13*, 109–116. [CrossRef] [PubMed]
105. Hass, R.; Busche, R.; Luciano, L.; Reale, E.; Engelhardt, W.V. Lack of butyrate is associated with induction of Bax and subsequent apoptosis in the proximal colon of guinea pig. *Gastroenterology* **1997**, *112*, 875–881. [CrossRef] [PubMed]
106. Cornick, S.; Tawiah, A.; Chadee, K. Roles and regulation of the mucus barrier in the gut. *Tissue Barriers* **2015**, *3*, e982426. [CrossRef] [PubMed]
107. Goldberg, R.F.; Austen, W.G.; Zhang, X., Jr.; Munene, G.; Mostafa, G.; Biswas, S.; McCormack, M.; Eberlin, K.R.; Nguyen, J.T.; Tatlidede, H.S.; et al. Intestinal alkaline phosphatase is a gut mucosal defense factor maintained by enteral nutrition. *Proc. Natl. Acad. Sci. USA* **2008**, *105*, 3551–3556. [CrossRef] [PubMed]
108. Lallès, J.P. Microbiota-host interplay at the gut epithelial level, health and nutrition. *J. Anim. Sci. Biotechnol.* **2016**, *7*, 66. [CrossRef] [PubMed]

109. Shifrin, D.A., Jr.; McConnell, R.E.; Nambiar, R.; Higginbotham, J.N.; Coffey, R.J.; Tyska, M.J. Enterocyte microvillus-derived vesicles detoxify bacterial products and regulate epithelial-microbial interactions. *Curr. Biol.* **2012**, *22*, 627–631. [CrossRef] [PubMed]
110. Wang, W.; Chen, S.W.; Zhu, J.; Zuo, S.; Ma, Y.Y.; Chen, Z.Y.; Zhang, J.L.; Chen, G.W.; Liu, Y.C.; Wang, P.Y. Intestinal alkaline phosphatase inhibits the translocation of bacteria of gut-origin in mice with peritonitis: Mechanism of action. *PLoS ONE* **2015**, *10*, e0124835. [CrossRef] [PubMed]
111. Martínez-Moya, P.; Ortega-González, M.; González, R.; Anzola, A.; Ocón, B.; Hernández-Chirlaque, C.; López-Posadas, R.; Suárez, M.D.; Zarzuelo, A.; Martínez-Augustin, O.; et al. Exogenous alkaline phosphatase treatment complements endogenous enzyme protection in colonic inflammation and reduces bacterial translocation in rats. *Pharmacol. Res.* **2012**, *66*, 144–153. [CrossRef] [PubMed]
112. Bol-Schoenmakers, M.; Fiechter, D.; Raaben, W.; Hassing, I.; Bleumink, R.; Kruijswijk, D.; Maijoor, K.; Tersteeg-Zijderveld, M.; Brands, R.; Pieters, R. Intestinal alkaline phosphatase contributes to the reduction of severe intestinal epithelial damage. *Eur. J. Pharmacol.* **2010**, *633*, 71–77. [CrossRef] [PubMed]
113. Melo, A.D.; Silveira, H.; Bortoluzzi, C.; Lara, L.J.; Garbossa, C.A.; Preis, G.; Costa, L.B.; Rostagno, M.H. Intestinal alkaline phosphatase and sodium butyrate may be beneficial in attenuating LPS-induced intestinal inflammation. *Genet. Mol. Res.* **2016**, *15*, 15048875. [CrossRef] [PubMed]
114. Malo, M.S.; Biswas, S.; Abedrapo, M.A.; Yeh, L.; Chen, A.; Hodin, R.A. The pro-inflammatory cytokines, IL-1beta and TNF-alpha, inhibit intestinal alkaline phosphatase gene expression. *DNA Cell Biol.* **2006**, *25*, 684–695. [CrossRef] [PubMed]
115. Volta, U.; Tovoli, F.; Cicola, R.; Parisi, C.; Fabbri, A.; Piscaglia, M.; Fiorini, E.; Caio, G. Serological tests in gluten sensitivity (nonceliac gluten intolerance). *J. Clin. Gastroenterol.* **2012**, *46*, 680–685. [CrossRef] [PubMed]
116. Infantino, M.; Manfredi, M.; Meacci, F.; Grossi, V.; Severino, M.; Benucci, M.; Bellio, E.; Bellio, V.; Nucci, A.; Zolfanelli, F.; et al. Diagnostic accuracy of anti-gliadin antibodies in Non Celiac Gluten Sensitivity (NCGS) patients: A dual statistical approach. *Clin. Chim. Acta* **2015**, *451*, 135–141. [CrossRef] [PubMed]
117. Infantino, M.; Meacci, F.; Grossi, V.; Macchia, D.; Manfredi, M. Anti-gliadin antibodies in non-celiac gluten sensitivity. *Minerva Gastroenterol. Dietol.* **2017**, *63*, 1–4. [CrossRef] [PubMed]
118. Caio, G.; Volta, U.; Tovoli, F.; De Giorgio, R. Effect of gluten free diet on immune response to gliadin in patients with non-celiac gluten sensitivity. *BMC Gastroenterol.* **2014**, *14*, 26. [CrossRef] [PubMed]
119. Di Liberto, D.; Mansueto, P.; D'Alcamo, A.; Lo Pizzo, M.; Lo Presti, E.; Geraci, G.; Fayer, F.; Guggino, G.; Iacono, G.; Dieli, F.; et al. Predominance of type 1 innate lymphoid cells in the rectal mucosa of patients with non-celiac wheat sensitivity: Reversal after a wheat-free diet. *Clin. Transl. Gastroenterol.* **2016**, *7*, e178. [CrossRef] [PubMed]
120. Barbara, G.; Stanghellini, V.; De Giorgio, R.; Cremon, C.; Cottrell, G.S.; Santini, D.; Pasquinelli, G.; Morselli-Labate, A.M.; Grady, E.F.; Bunnett, N.W.; et al. Activated mast cells in proximity to colonic nerves correlate with abdominal pain in irritable bowel syndrome. *Gastroenterology* **2004**, *126*, 693–702. [CrossRef] [PubMed]
121. Barbara, G.; Cremon, C.; Carini, G.; Bellacosa, L.; Zecchi, L.; De Giorgio, R.; Corinaldesi, R.; Stanghellini, V. The immune system in irritable bowel syndrome. *J. Neurogastroenterol. Motil.* **2011**, *17*, 349–359. [CrossRef] [PubMed]
122. Bennet, S.M.; Ohman, L.; Simren, M. Gut microbiota as potential orchestrators of irritable bowel syndrome. *Gut Liver* **2015**, *9*, 318–331. [CrossRef] [PubMed]
123. Stinson, L.F.; Payne, M.S.; Keelan, J.A. Planting the seed: Origins, composition, and postnatal health significance of the fetal gastrointestinal microbiota. *Crit. Rev. Microbiol.* **2017**, *43*, 352–369. [CrossRef] [PubMed]
124. Thum, C.; Cookson, A.L.; Otter, D.E.; McNabb, W.C.; Hodgkinson, A.J.; Dyer, J.; Roy, N.C. Can nutritional modulation of maternal intestinal microbiota influence the development of the infant gastrointestinal tract? *J. Nutr.* **2012**, *142*, 1921–1928. [CrossRef] [PubMed]
125. Montemurno, E.; Cosola, C.; Dalfino, G.; Daidone, G.; De Angelis, M.; Gobbetti, M.; Gesualdo, L. What would you like to eat, Mr CKD Microbiota? A Mediterranean Diet, please! *Kidney Blood Press. Res.* **2014**, *39*, 114–123. [CrossRef] [PubMed]

126. Alou, M.T.; Lagier, J.C.; Raoult, D. Diet influence on the gut microbiota and dysbiosis related to nutritional disorders. *Hum. Microbiome J.* **2016**, *1*, 3–11. [CrossRef]
127. Cani, P.D.; Delzenne, N.M. The role of the gut microbiota in energy metabolism and metabolic disease. *Curr. Pharm. Des.* **2009**, *15*, 1546–1558. [CrossRef] [PubMed]
128. Rocha, D.M.; Caldas, A.P.; Oliveira, L.L.; Bressan, J.; Hermsdorff, H.H. Saturated fatty acids trigger TLR4-mediated inflammatory response. *Atherosclerosis* **2016**, *244*, 211–215. [CrossRef] [PubMed]
129. Rodriguez-Castaño, G.P.; Caro-Quintero, A.; Reyes, A.; Lizcano, F. Advances in Gut Microbiome Research, Opening New Strategies to Cope with a Western Lifestyle. *Front. Genet.* **2016**, *7*, 224. [CrossRef] [PubMed]
130. Vici, G.; Belli, L.; Biondi, M.; Polzonetti, V. Gluten free diet and nutrient deficiencies: A review. *Clin. Nutr.* **2016**, *35*, 1236–1241. [CrossRef] [PubMed]
131. Saturni, L.; Ferretti, G.; Bacchetti, T. The gluten-free diet: Safety and nutritional quality. *Nutrients* **2010**, *2*, 16–34. [CrossRef] [PubMed]
132. Wild, D.; Robins, G.G.; Burley, V.J.; Howdle, P.D. Evidence of high sugar intake, and low fibre and mineral intake, in the gluten-free diet. *Aliment. Pharmacol. Ther.* **2010**, *32*, 573–581. [CrossRef] [PubMed]
133. Shepherd, S.J.; Gibson, P.R. Nutritional inadequacies of the gluten-free diet in both recently-diagnosed and long-term patients with coeliac disease. *J. Hum. Nutr. Diet.* **2013**, *26*, 349–358. [CrossRef] [PubMed]
134. Tortora, R.; Capone, P.; De Stefano, G.; Imperatore, N.; Gerbino, N.; Donetto, S.; Monaco, V.; Caporaso, N.; Rispo, A. Metabolic syndrome in patients with coeliac disease on a gluten-free diet. *Aliment. Pharmacol. Ther.* **2015**, *41*, 352–359. [CrossRef] [PubMed]
135. Lebwohl, B.; Cao, Y.; Zong, G.; Hu, F.B.; Green, P.H.R.; Neugut, A.I.; Rimm, E.B.; Sampson, L.; Dougherty, L.W.; Giovannucci, E.; et al. Long term gluten consumption in adults without celiac disease and risk of coronary heart disease: Prospective cohort study. *BMJ* **2017**, *357*, 1892. [CrossRef] [PubMed]
136. De Palma, G.; Nadal, I.; Collado, M.C.; Sanz, Y. Effects of a gluten-free diet on gut microbiota and immune function in healthy adult human subjects. *Br. J. Nutr.* **2009**, *102*, 1154–1160. [CrossRef] [PubMed]
137. Shanahan, F.; van Sinderen, D.; O'Toole, P.W.; Stanton, C. Feeding the microbiota: Transducer of nutrient signals for the host. *Gut* **2017**, *66*, 1–9. [CrossRef] [PubMed]
138. Donovan, S.M. Introduction to the special focus issue on the impact of diet on gut microbiota composition and function and future opportunities for nutritional modulation of the gut microbiome to improve human health. *Gut Microbes* **2017**, *8*, 75–81. [CrossRef] [PubMed]
139. Macfarlane, G.T.; Macfarlane, S. Bacteria, colonic fermentation, and gastrointestinal health. *J. AOAC Int.* **2012**, *95*, 50–60. [CrossRef] [PubMed]
140. Hill, C.; Guarner, F.; Reid, G.; Gibson, G.R.; Merenstein, D.J.; Pot, B.; Morelli, L.; Canani, R.B.; Flint, H.J.; Salminen, S.; et al. Expert consensus document. The International Scientific Association for Probiotics and Prebiotics consensus statement on the scope and appropriate use of the term probiotic. *Nat. Rev. Gastroenterol. Hepatol.* **2014**, *11*, 506–514. [CrossRef] [PubMed]
141. Quévrain, E.; Maubert, M.A.; Michon, C.; Chain, F.; Marquant, R.; Tailhades, J.; Miquel, S.; Carlier, L.; Bermúdez-Humarán, L.G.; Pigneur, B.; et al. Identification of an anti-inflammatory protein from Faecalibacterium prausnitzii, a commensal bacterium deficient in Crohn's diseas. *Gut* **2016**, *65*, 415–425. [CrossRef] [PubMed]
142. Riedel, C.U.; Foata, F.; Philippe, D.; Adolfsson, O.; Eikmanns, B.J.; Blum, S. Anti-inflammatory effects of bifidobacteria by inhibition of LPS-induced NF-kappaB activation. *World J. Gastroenterol.* **2006**, *12*, 3729–3735. [CrossRef] [PubMed]
143. Furrie, E.; Macfarlane, S.; Kennedy, A.; Cummings, J.H.; Walsh, S.V.; O'Neil, D.A.; Macfarlane, G.T. Synbiotic therapy (*Bifidobacterium longum*/Synergy 1) initiates resolution of inflammation in patients with active ulcerative colitis: A randomised controlled pilot trial. *Gut* **2005**, *54*, 242–249. [CrossRef] [PubMed]
144. Srutkova, D.; Schwarzer, M.; Hudcovic, T.; Zakostelska, Z.; Drab, V.; Spanova, A.; Rittich, B.; Kozakova, H.; Schabussova, I. Bifidobacterium longum CCM 7952 Promotes Epithelial Barrier Function and Prevents Acute DSS-Induced Colitis in Strictly Strain-Specific Manner. *PLoS ONE* **2015**, *10*, e0134050. [CrossRef] [PubMed]
145. Khokhlova, E.V.; Smeianov, V.V.; Efimov, B.A.; Kafarskaia, L.I.; Pavlova, S.I.; Shkoporov, A.N. Anti-inflammatory properties of intestinal Bifidobacterium strains isolated from healthy infants. *Microbiol. Immunol.* **2012**, *56*, 27–39. [CrossRef] [PubMed]

146. Fujiwara, M.; Kaneko, T.; Iwana, H.; Taketomo, N.; Tsunoo, H.; Kanno, J.; Ohkusa, T.; Okayasu, I. Inhibitory effects of Bifidobacterium longum on experimental ulcerative colitis induced in mice by synthetic dextran sulfate sodium. *Digestion* **2003**, *67*, 90–95. [CrossRef] [PubMed]
147. Plaza-Díaz, J.; Ruiz-Ojeda, F.J.; Vilchez-Padial, L.M.; Gil, A. Evidence of the Anti-Inflammatory Effects of Probiotics and Synbiotics in Intestinal Chronic Diseases. *Nutrients* **2017**, *9*, 555. [CrossRef] [PubMed]
148. Moore, K.W.; de Waal Malefyt, R.; Coffman, R.L.; O'Garra, A. Interleukin-10 and the interleukin-10 receptor. *Annu. Rev. Immunol.* **2001**, *19*, 683–765. [CrossRef] [PubMed]
149. Madsen, K.L.; Malfair, D.; Gray, D.; Doyle, J.S.; Jewell, L.D.; Fedorak, R.N. Interleukin-10 gene-deficient mice develop a primary intestinal permeability defect in response to enteric microflora. *Inflamm. Bowel Dis.* **1999**, *5*, 262–270. [CrossRef] [PubMed]
150. Hong, Y.S.; Ahn, Y.T.; Park, J.C.; Lee, J.H.; Lee, H.; Huh, C.S.; Kim, D.H.; Ryu, D.H.; Hwang, G.S. 1H NMR-based metabonomic assessment of probiotic effects in a colitis mouse model. *Arch. Pharm Res.* **2010**, *33*, 1091–1101. [CrossRef] [PubMed]
151. Ki Cha, B.; Mun Jung, S.; Hwan Choi, C.; Song, I.D.; Woong Lee, H.; Joon Kim, H.; Hyuk, J.; Kyung Chang, S.; Kim, K.; Chung, W.S.; et al. The effect of a multispecies probiotic mixture on the symptoms and fecal microbiota in diarrhea-dominant irritable bowel syndrome: A randomized, double-blind, placebo-controlled trial. *J. Clin. Gastroenterol.* **2012**, *46*, 220–227. [CrossRef] [PubMed]
152. Bibiloni, R.; Fedorak, R.N.; Tannock, G.W.; Madsen, K.L.; Gionchetti, P.; Campieri, M.; De Simone, C.; Sartor, R.B. VSL#3 probiotic-mixture induces remission in patients with active ulcerative colitis. *Am. J. Gastroenterol.* **2005**, *100*, 1539–1546. [CrossRef] [PubMed]
153. Miele, E.; Pascarella, F.; Giannetti, E.; Quaglietta, L.; Baldassano, R.N.; Staiano, A. Effect of a probiotic preparation (VSL#3) on induction and maintenance of remission in children with ulcerative colitis. *Am. J. Gastroenterol.* **2009**, *104*, 437–443. [CrossRef] [PubMed]
154. You, H.J.; Oh, D.K.; Ji, G.E. Anticancerogenic effect of a novel chiroinositol-containing polysaccharide from Bifidobacterium bifidum BGN4. *FEMS Microbiol. Lett.* **2004**, *240*, 131–136. [CrossRef] [PubMed]
155. Palumbo, V.D.; Romeo, M.; Marino Gammazza, A.; Carini, F.; Damiani, P.; Damiano, G.; Buscemi, S.; Lo Monte, A.I.; Gerges-Geagea, A.; Jurjus, A.; et al. The long-term effects of probiotics in the therapy of ulcerative colitis: A clinical study. *Biomed. Pap. Med. Fac. Univ. Palacky Olomouc Czechoslov.* **2016**, *160*, 372–377. [CrossRef] [PubMed]
156. Donato, K.A.; Gareau, M.G.; Wang, Y.J.; Sherman, P.M. Lactobacillus rhamnosus GG attenuates interferon-{gamma} and tumour necrosis factor-alpha-induced barrier dysfunction and pro-inflammatory signalling. *Microbiology* **2010**, *156*, 3288–3297. [CrossRef] [PubMed]
157. Orlando, A.; Linsalata, M.; Notarnicola, M.; Tutino, V.; Russo, F. Lactobacillus GG restoration of the gliadin induced epithelial barrier disruption: The role of cellular polyamines. *BMC Microbiol.* **2014**, *14*, 19. [CrossRef] [PubMed]
158. Mearin, M.L.; Catassi, C.; Brousse, N.; Brand, R.; Collin, P.; Fabiani, E.; Schweizer, J.J.; Abuzakouk, M.; Szajewska, H.; Hallert, C. European multi-centre study on coeliac disease and non-Hodgkin lymphoma. *Eur. J. Gastroenterol. Hepatol.* **2006**, *18*, 187–194. [CrossRef] [PubMed]
159. Corrao, G.; Corazza, G.R.; Bagnardi, V.; Brusco, G.; Ciacci, C.; Cottone, M.; Sategna Guidetti, C.; Usai, P.; Cesari, P.; Pelli, M.A. Mortality in patients with coeliac disease and their relatives: A cohort study. *Lancet* **2001**, *358*, 356–361. [CrossRef]
160. Green, P.H.; Fleischauer, A.T.; Bhagat, G.; Goyal, R.; Jabri, B.; Neugut, A.I. Risk of malignancy in patients with celiac disease. *Am. J. Med.* **2003**, *115*, 191–195. [CrossRef]
161. Askling, J.; Linet, M.; Gridley, G.; Halstensen, T.S.; Ekström, K.; Ekbom, A. Cancer incidence in a population-based cohort of individuals hospitalized with celiac disease or dermatitis herpetiformis. *Gastroenterology* **2002**, *123*, 1428–1435. [CrossRef] [PubMed]
162. West, J.; Logan, R.F.; Smith, C.J.; Hubbard, R.B.; Card, T.R. Malignancy and mortality in people with coeliac disease: Population based cohort study. *BMJ* **2004**, *329*, 716–719. [CrossRef] [PubMed]
163. Elfström, P.; Granath, F.; Ye, W.; Ludvigsson, J.F. Low risk of gastrointestinal cancer among patients with celiac disease, inflammation, or latent celiac disease. *Clin. Gastroenterol. Hepatol.* **2012**, *10*, 30–36. [CrossRef] [PubMed]

164. Anderson, L.A.; McMillan, S.A.; Watson, R.G.; Monaghan, P.; Gavin, A.T.; Fox, C.; Murray, L.J. Malignancy and mortality in a population-based cohort of patients with celiac disease or "gluten sensitivity". *World J. Gastroenterol.* **2007**, *13*, 146–151. [CrossRef] [PubMed]
165. Sheth, P.; Delos Santos, N.; Seth, A.; LaRusso, N.F.; Rao, R.K. Lipopolysaccharide disrupts tight junctions in cholangiocyte monolayers by a c-Src-, TLR4-, and LBP-dependent mechanism. *Am. J. Physiol. Gastrointest. Liver Physiol.* **2007**, *293*, 308–318. [CrossRef] [PubMed]

7

Effect of Probiotics on Metabolic Outcomes in Pregnant Women with Gestational Diabetes

Bonnie L. Taylor, Georgia E. Woodfall, Katherine E. Sheedy, Meggan L. O'Riley, Kelsie A. Rainbow, Elsa L. Bramwell and Nicole J. Kellow *

Be Active Sleep & Eat (BASE) Facility, Department of Nutrition, Dietetics & Food, Monash University, Notting Hill, VIC 3168, Australia; bltay9@student.monash.edu (B.L.T.); gewoo1@student.monash.edu (G.E.W.); keshe5@student.monash.edu (K.E.S.); mlori1@student.monash.edu (M.L.O.); karia3@student.monash.edu (K.A.R.); elbra3@student.monash.edu (E.L.B.)

* Correspondence: nicole.kellow@monash.edu

Abstract: The metabolic effects of probiotic administration in women with gestational diabetes mellitus (GDM) is unknown. The objective of this review was to investigate the effect of probiotics on fasting plasma glucose (FPG), insulin resistance (HOMA-IR) and LDL-cholesterol levels in pregnant women diagnosed with GDM. Seven electronic databases were searched for RCTs published in English between 2001 and 2017 investigating the metabolic effects of a 6–8 week dietary probiotic intervention in pregnant women following diagnosis with GDM. Eligible studies were assessed for risk of bias and subjected to qualitative and quantitative synthesis using a random effects model meta-analyses. Four high quality RCTs involving 288 participants were included in the review. Probiotic supplementation was not effective in decreasing FBG (Mean Difference = −0.13; 95% CI −0.32, 0.06, p = 0.18) or LDL-cholesterol (−0.16; 95% CI −0.45, 0.13, p = 0.67) in women with GDM. However, a significant reduction in HOMA-IR was observed following probiotic supplementation (−0.69; 95% CI −1.24, −0.14, p = 0.01). There were no significant differences in gestational weight gain, delivery method or neonatal outcomes between experimental and control groups, and no adverse effects of the probiotics were reported. Probiotic supplementation for 6–8 weeks resulted in a significant reduction in insulin resistance in pregnant women diagnosed with GDM. The use of probiotic supplementation is promising as a potential therapy to assist in the metabolic management of GDM. Further high quality studies of longer duration are required to determine the safety, optimal dose and ideal bacterial composition of probiotics before their routine use can be recommended in this patient group.

Keywords: probiotics; gut microbiota; Gestational Diabetes Mellitus; pregnancy; insulin resistance

---

1. Introduction

The gut microbiota is a collective term used to refer to the microorganisms colonizing the human gastrointestinal tract [1]. It is an important ecosystem consisting of both residential and pathogenic bacteria [2,3]. Residential intestinal microbes coexist in a symbiotic relationship with their host by extracting energy from dietary components which humans lack the enzymes to digest. In return, the microbiota produce bioactive compounds shown to benefit host metabolism. Manipulation of the gut microbiome and its fermentation by-products is emerging as a promising therapeutic treatment strategy for many chronic medical conditions [4]. A variety of factors influence the gut microbiome, including host genetics, illness, antibiotic use, dietary patterns, weight loss and pregnancy [5–8].

Perturbations in the composition of the gut microbiota have been hypothesized to contribute to the pathogenesis of obesity, inflammation and insulin resistance [9].

Throughout pregnancy the gut microbiota undergoes significant changes. From the first (T1) to the third trimester (T3), the species richness of the gut microbiome decreases [8], although this has not been observed in all studies [10]. There is an increase in Proteobacteria and Actinobacteria phyla and a reduction in beneficial bacterial species *Roseburia intestinalis* and *Faecalibacterium prausnitzii* [8,11]. These changes in gut microbial composition cause inflammation and correlate with increases in fat mass, blood glucose, insulin resistance and circulating pro-inflammatory cytokines in the expectant mother [12]. This "diabetic-like" state observed during the later stages of all healthy pregnancies is thought to maximize nutrient provision to the developing fetus [13]. However, increased insulin resistance combined with an inability to secrete the additional insulin required to maintain glucose homeostasis can result in the development of gestational diabetes mellitus (GDM) in the mother and macrosomia in the baby.

GDM is defined as the development of glucose intolerance, with first onset during pregnancy [14]. This condition is associated with adverse maternal and infant health outcomes during gestation, childbirth and postpartum. Maternal comorbidities include pre-eclampsia and increased risk of infection throughout pregnancy [15]. A seven-fold increased risk of the mother developing type 2 diabetes (T2DM) postpartum has also been reported [16]. Infant morbidity includes risk of fetal malformations and diabetic fetopathy which may cause macrosomia and subsequent mechanical complications during labor [17,18]. Additionally, studies suggest that children born to mothers with GDM have an increased risk of diabetes mellitus and metabolic dysfunction later in life [19,20]. In order to reduce the risk of such adverse health outcomes, current best practice GDM management requires modification of the maternal diet with or without pharmacological treatment such as Metformin and/or insulin [21]. Despite its benefits, pharmacotherapy may result in significant side effects including abdominal discomfort, dizziness, diarrhea and hypoglycemia [22]. As research suggests that probiotic interventions may attenuate some of the adverse metabolic effects of type 2 diabetes [23,24], probiotics may also provide an acceptable treatment option in women with GDM.

Probiotics have been defined by the World Health Organization (WHO) as 'live micro-organisms which when administered in adequate amounts confer a health benefit on the host' [25]. Regular consumption of probiotics have been found to beneficially modulate the composition of the gut microbiota [26]. Increases in colonic microbial diversity have been linked to improved glucose homeostasis, attenuation of inflammation, regulation of insulin production, maintenance of the integrity of the gastrointestinal lining, and the harvesting of nutrients from the host diet [7,8,27]. Safe and effective evidence-based interventions are vital for both the prevention and optimal management of GDM. A recent RCT conducted in healthy pregnant women suggest that probiotic supplementation may improve blood glucose control during the third trimester [28] and potentially reduce the risk of developing GDM [29]. To our knowledge, no systematic reviews have investigated the effect of maternal probiotic supplementation on the metabolic health of women with established GDM, highlighting the need for further exploration of this topic. The aim of this review was to determine the effect of 6–8 week probiotic supplementation versus placebo on glucose homeostasis, lipid levels and gestational weight gain in pregnant women diagnosed with GDM.

2. Methods

This review was conducted in accordance with the Preferred Reporting Items for Systematic Reviews and Meta-Analyses: The PRISMA Statement [30]. A systematic computer search of the databases Proquest, Scopus, Embase, Ovid MEDLINE, Web of science, CINAHL, and the Cochrane Database of Systematic Reviews was performed for the period between 1 January 2001 and 1 January 2017. In 2001, the WHO recognized the need for guidelines to evaluate probiotic use and to substantiate health claims. The rationale for excluding papers before 2001 was due to a lack of international guidelines and criteria regulating the use of probiotics prior to this date [31]. The following search terms were used:

(1) (pregnan * OR Gestation * OR Matern * OR Obstetric * OR expectan * OR "gestational diabetes" OR "gestational diabetes mellitus"), (probiotic * OR Lactobacill * OR bacteria * OR ferment * OR microorganism * OR acidophilus OR streptococc *), and (glucose OR "blood glucose" OR insulin OR HbA1c OR "birth weight" OR metabol * OR intervention * OR "pharmaceutical Intervention"); (2) limit 1 to year '2001–2017'; limit 2 to humans; limit 3 exclude males and non-pregnant subjects. Trials were included if they were published in English, utilized an RCT study design, involved human participants diagnosed with GDM by OGTT and if at least one group of participants were randomized to receive a dietary probiotic supplement for a period of 6–8 weeks.

Studies in patients with pre-existing conditions such as type 1 diabetes, type 2 diabetes or gastrointestinal pathologies were considered beyond the scope of this review, and were therefore excluded. Intervention trials involving the administration of fermented foods (which contain unknown quantities of bacteria), prebiotics (which contain no live bacteria) or synbiotics (which contain both pre- and probiotics) were also excluded.

Resultant studies were combined and duplicates removed. All articles were independently screened for eligibility by two authors based on title and abstract. Articles were excluded if they reported a non-RCT study design, subjects were not diagnosed with GDM or there was no probiotic intervention. The reference lists of included studies were hand-searched to identify additional relevant trials. The methodological quality of all included trials was independently assessed by two authors using the Cochrane Risk of Bias tool for Quality Assessment of Randomized Controlled Trials [32]. This tool rates primary research based on the use of sequence generation, allocation concealment, blinding of participants and personnel, blinding of outcome assessors, completeness of outcome data, non-selective outcome reporting, and other measures of bias. Trials were assessed as satisfying each of the quality criteria using "yes", "no", or "unsure", with studies meeting the majority of quality criteria considered to have a low risk of bias, while those assigned "no" or "unsure" for most criteria were designated as moderate or high risk of bias. Discrepancies between authors risk of bias assessments were resolved through collaborative discussion until consensus was reached.

Data was independently extracted from each article by two authors using a data collection form. Data items collected included first author, article title, journal name, year of publication, country in which trial was conducted, number of trial participants: intervention group (n) and control group (n), mean participant age (year), mean participant BMI (kg/m^2), mean gestational age (week), mean length of intervention (week), composition of probiotic supplement (genus, species), number of micro-organisms in probiotic supplement (CFU/g), mean gestational weight gain (kg), mean fasting blood glucose (mmol/L), mean Homeostasis Model Assessment—Insulin Resistance (HOMA-IR) (units), mean LDL-cholesterol (mmol/L), mean number of normal deliveries (n), mean number of caesarian sections (n), mean number of interventions during delivery (n), maternal complications (n), infant complications (n), and infant birth weight (g).

Trials measuring FBG, LDL-cholesterol and insulin resistance (HOMA-IR) in pregnant women with GDM were subjected to a random-effects model meta-analysis using Revman 5.1 (The Cochrane Collaboration, Copenhagen, Denmark, 2014). Treatment effects and 95% CI were calculated using the Mean Difference (MD). Limited numbers of studies investigating comparable outcomes, small sample sizes and heterogeneity among prebiotic supplements and outcome measures limited the majority of data synthesis to a narrative analysis.

3. Results

3.1. Description of Selected Trials

A total of 944 citations were identified at the time of the initial database search based on the predefined inclusion and exclusion criteria. After removal of duplicate publications and exclusion of irrelevant articles, four articles [33–36] reporting on four randomized controlled trials involving 288 participants were ultimately included (Figure 1). Characteristics of the included studies are shown in Table 1. All studies included otherwise healthy pregnant women diagnosed with GDM at 24–30 weeks gestation by oral glucose tolerance test. Participant ages ranged between 18–40 years and pre-pregnancy BMI from 26–32 kg/m^2. All trial participants were randomized to receive either a daily probiotic supplement or a placebo. Probiotic composition varied between studies, but all trials provided *Lactobacillus* spp., and three [34–36] provided *Bifidobacterium* spp. The duration of intervention ranged from 6–8 weeks. A variety of post-intervention outcome measures were reported including fasting plasma glucose, fasting insulin, C-peptide, HOMA-IR, lipid studies, inflammatory markers, pro-inflammatory cytokines, gestational weight gain, requirement for glucose-lowering pharmacotherapy, interventions required during childbirth, infant birthweight, incidence of macrosomia (birthweight > 4 kg), fetal anomalies, admissions to the neonatal intensive care unit, and 5-min Apgar score.

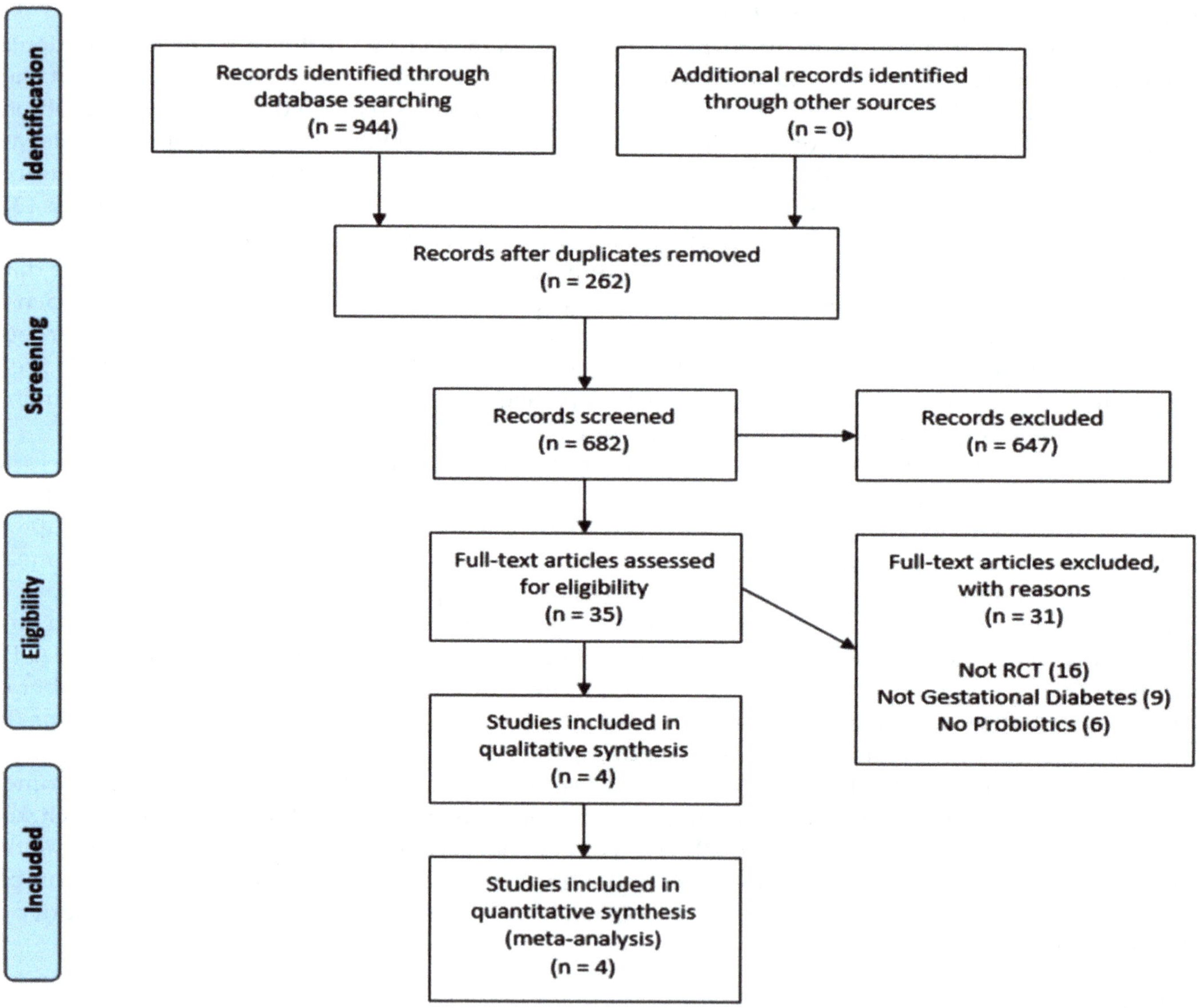

Figure 1. PRISMA flowchart showing the progression of trials through each stage of the selection process.

Table 1. Characteristics of randomised controlled trials included in the review.

Study Author/Year	Participants	Study Design/Blinding	Dietary Probiotic Intervention	Effect of Dietary Probiotic Supplement on Metabolic Outcomes
Karamali et al. (2016) [34]	Iran, *n* 60 pregnant women with GDM in third trimester (age range 18–40 years)	Parallel RCT, double-blinded	Random assignment to 6-week probiotic or placebo capsules. Each probiotic capsule contained *L. acidophilus* (2×10^9 CFU/g), *L. casei* (2×10^9 CFU/g) and *B. bifidum* (2×10^9 CFU/g)	↓ Fasting plasma glucose ↓ HOMA-IR ↔ Total cholesterol ↔ LDL cholesterol ↓ VLDL cholesterol ↓ Triglyceride ↔ gestational weight gain
Dolatkhah et al. (2015) [36]	Iran, *n* 64 pregnant women with GDM (mean age intervention 28.1 years, control 26.5 years; mean BMI intervention 31.4 kg/m^2, control 29.9 kg/m^2)	Parallel RCT, double-blinded	Random assignment to 8-week probiotic capsule with dietary advice or placebo capsule with dietary advice. Each probiotic capsule contained *L. acidophilus* LA-5, *Bifidobacterium* BB-12, S. thermophilus STY-31 and *L. delbrueckii* subsp. Bulgaricus LBY-27 (>4×10^9 CFU/g)	↓ Fasting plasma glucose ↓ HOMA-IR ↓ gestational weight gain
Jafarnejad et al. (2016) [35]	Iran, *n* 82 pregnant women with GDM (mean age intervention 32.4 years control 31.9 years; mean BMI intervention 26.8 kg/m^2, control 27.4 kg/m^2)	Parallel RCT, double-blinded	Random assignment to 8-week probiotic or placebo capsules. Each probiotic capsule contained VSL#3 (*S. thermophilus*, *B. breve*, *B. longum*, *B. infantis*, *L. acidophilus*, *L. plantarum*, *L. paracasei*, *L. delbrueckii* subsp. Bulgaricus, 15×10^9 CFU/g)	↓ Fasting plasma glucose ↔ gestational weight gain ↓ HOMA-IR ↓ Interleukin-6 ↓ Tumor Necrosis Factor-aplha ↓ hs-CRP
Lindsay et al. (2015) [33]	Ireland, *n* 149 women with GDM (mean age intervention 33.5 years control 32.6 years; mean BMI intervention 29.1 kg/m^2, control 29.0 kg/m^2)	Parallel RCT, double-blinded	Random assignment to 6-week probiotic or placebo capsules. Each capsule contained *L. salivarius* UCC118 (1×10^9 CFU/g)	↔ Fasting plasma glucose ↔ HOMA-IR ↔ C-peptide ↓ Total cholesterol ↔ CRP ↔ Triglyceride ↓ LDL cholesterol ↔ HDL cholesterol ↔ gestational weight gain

RCT: Randomised Controlled Trial; GDM: Gestational Diabetes Mellitus; HOMA-IR score: homeostatic model of assessment of insulin resistance; hs-CRP: High sensitivity C-reactive protein; HDL cholesterol: High density lipoprotein; LDL cholesterol: Low density lipoprotein; HbA1c: Glycosylated haemoglobin; *n*: number of participants randomised; ↓ significantly lower than that in the comparison control group after intervention; ↑ significantly higher than that in the comparison control group after intervention; ↔ no significant difference between the probiotic-supplemented and control groups after intervention.

All of the studies included in the present review had a low risk of bias, as assessed using the Cochrane Collaboration Risk of Bias tool (Table 2). Methodological strengths of the trials included double-blinding and randomization of participants to intervention and control groups. Methodological limitations of the trials included small sample sizes and short study duration. Additionally, one of the trials had not been registered on a clinical trials registry prior to commencement, so it could not be determined whether primary outcomes reported were pre-specified before the trial began [35].

Table 2. Risk of bias summary for included studies.

Author/Year	Risk of Bias [a]	Bias Minimisation Items [b]						
		1	2	3	4	5	6	Other
Dolatkhah, 2015 [36]	Low	+	+	+	+	+	?	Funding & sponsorship free from bias, statistical analysis appropriate
Lindsay, 2015 [33]	Low	+	+	+	+	+	?	Funding & sponsorship free from bias
Jafarnejad, 2015 [35]	Low	+	+	+	+	?	?	Funding & sponsorship free from bias
Karamali, 2015 [34]	Low	+	+	+	+	+	?	Funding & sponsorship free from bias

"+" = response of "yes" to use of the bias minimization item; "?" = response of "uncertain" to the use of the bias minimization item; [a] Assessed using the Cochrane Collaboration tool for assessing risk of bias in RCTs (ref); [b] Bias minimization items: 1. Random sequence generation (selection bias); 2. Allocation concealment (selection bias); 3. Blinding of participants and personnel (performance bias); 4. Blinding of outcome assessment (detection bias); 5. Complete outcome data (attrition bias); 6. Non-selective reporting (reporting bias). Trials receiving a + response for most items are likely to have a low risk of bias.

3.2. Fasting Blood Glucose

Four studies investigated the effect of probiotic supplementation on FBG levels in pregnant women with GDM [32–35]. Two [33,35] of the four studies reported statistically significant reductions in FBG levels in the groups receiving probiotics in comparison to the groups receiving the placebo. However, a meta-analysis of all four trials (n = 288) indicated no significant reduction in FBG following probiotic supplementation (Mean Difference = −0.13; 95% CI −0.32, 0.06, $p = 0.18$) (Figure 2). While each of the studies included in the pooled analysis had a low risk of bias and administered probiotic supplements to women with GDM over a similar intervention period, significant interstudy heterogeneity was observed (I^2 = 88%, $p < 0.001$), so the calculated mean difference should be interpreted as an average intervention effect.

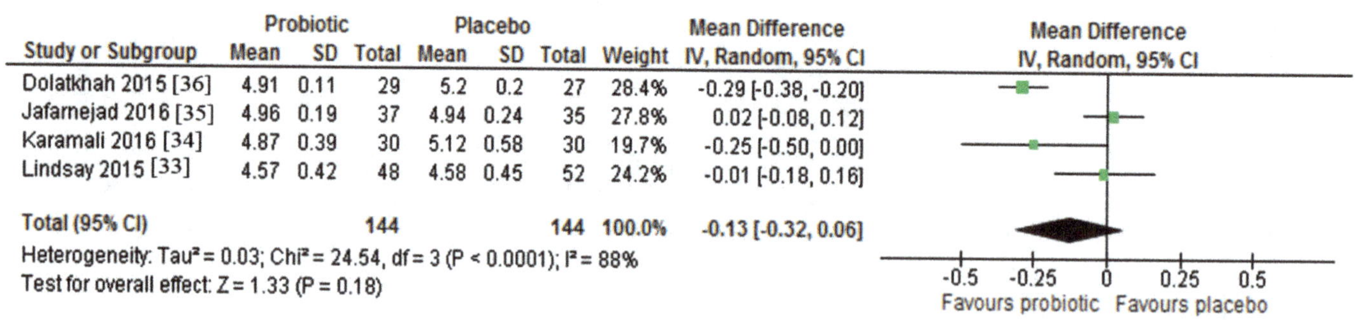

Figure 2. Effect of probiotic supplementation on fasting plasma glucose (mmol/L) in pregnant women with gestational diabetes.

3.3. Insulin Resistance

Four trials estimated insulin resistance in study participants by calculating HOMA-IR from fasting glucose and insulin values [33–36]. While one study found no change in insulin resistance between intervention and control groups following probiotic supplementation [33], three studies reported significant reductions in insulin resistance in the women receiving probiotics [34–36]. After meta-analysis (n = 288), the pooled mean difference in HOMA-IR was −0.69 (95% CI −1.24,

-0.14, $p = 0.01$), indicating a statistically significant effect favoring probiotic supplementation over placebo (Figure 3). Significant evidence of interstudy heterogeneity was observed across studies ($I^2 = 79\%$, $p < 0.01$).

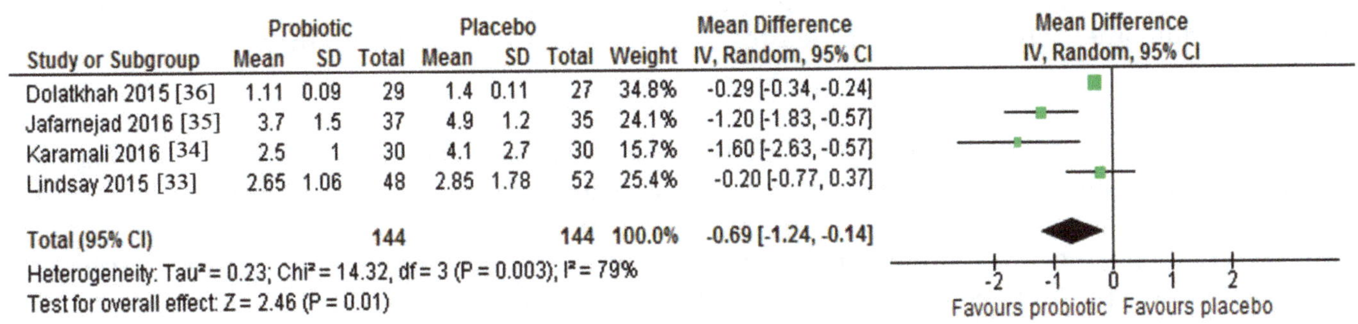

Figure 3. Effect of probiotic supplementation on HOMA-IR in pregnant women with gestational diabetes.

3.4. LDL-Cholesterol

Lindsay et al. [33] found that the usual rise in total cholesterol and LDL-cholesterol usually observed during the late stages of pregnancy was significantly attenuated in the probiotic group (both $p < 0.05$). In contrast, the study by Karamali et al. [34] reported no change in total cholesterol ($p = 0.33$) and LDL-cholesterol ($p = 0.07$) between treatment and control groups, but described significant reductions in VLDL-cholesterol and serum TG in the probiotic group (both < 0.05). When the data from both studies were pooled for meta-analysis ($n = 160$), there was no significant reduction in LDL-cholesterol following probiotic supplementation (MD = -0.16; 95% CI -0.45, 0.13, $p = 0.67$) (Figure 4).

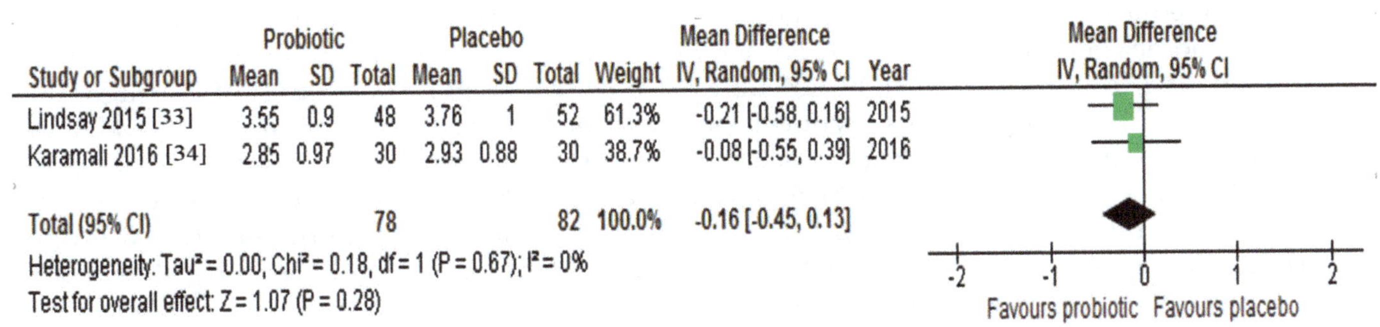

Figure 4. Effect of probiotic supplementation on LDL-cholesterol (mmol/L) in pregnant women with gestational diabetes.

3.5. Gestational Weight Gain

During the final 2 weeks of an 8-week intervention, one study reported that the weight gain of the women in the probiotic group was significantly less than the weight gain of those receiving the placebo (0.74 ± 0.14 kg vs. 1.22 ± 0.11 kg respectively), which remained significant after adjusting for daily energy intake ($p < 0.05$) [36]. However, the remaining three studies found no differences in gestational weight gain between intervention and control groups [33–35]. Two studies also reported no significant differences in infant birthweights between those born to mothers receiving the probiotic and those whose mothers received the placebo [33,34].

3.6. Obstetric Outcomes

No significant differences were found between probiotic and control groups for rates of pregnancy-induced hypertension, requirement for labor induction, commencement of glucose-lowering medications, blood loss at delivery, postpartum hemorrhage, fetal anomalies, admission of the infant to neonatal intensive care [33], and rates of delivery by caesarian section [33,34]. No adverse outcomes related to use of the probiotics were reported in any of the trials.

4. Discussion

Fasting hyperglycemia in women with GDM is associated with increased short and long-term morbidity in the offspring [37]. There is a clear need for safe, low-cost therapies to assist in the prevention and management of GDM. The gut microbial composition is altered during pregnancy, and given that specific micro-organisms in the gastrointestinal tract are able to positively influence host metabolism, probiotic supplements may contribute to the maintenance of bacterial diversity and glucose homeostasis in individuals with metabolic disturbances [38,39]. Research investigating probiotic use during pregnancy and its effect on the outcomes of GDM is an emerging area of interest. This systematic literature review aimed to explore the current evidence regarding the effect of probiotic supplementation on glucose and lipid homeostasis in pregnant women with GDM. Assessment of four randomized controlled trials in this review involving 288 pregnant women with GDM found that a 6–8 week probiotic intervention did not improve FBG or LDL-cholesterol levels. However, probiotic supplementation in women with GDM was associated with significant reductions in insulin resistance which could potentially reduce their requirement for glucose-lowering medication later in their pregnancy.

The mechanisms whereby probiotics alter glucose homeostasis are not completely understood. One proposed method is by the production of short chain fatty acids (SCFAs), generated as a by-product of bacterial fermentation of dietary fibers. SCFAs act as an energy source for intestinal cells and have been found to regulate the production of hormones effecting energy intake and expenditure such as leptin and grehlin [40]. The binding of SCFAs to G protein-coupled receptors GPR41 and GPR43 increases the intestinal expression of Peptide YY and Glucagon-like peptide-1 (GLP-1) hormones which act to reduce appetite by slowing intestinal transit time and increasing insulin sensitivity [11]. Another hypothesized mechanism of SCFA action includes reducing gastrointestinal permeability by upregulating transcription of tight junction proteins, enhancing production of Glucagon-like peptide-2 (GLP-2) which promotes crypt cell proliferation, and reducing inflammation in colonic epithelial cells by increasing PPAR-gamma activation [41]. Maintenance of the integrity of the gut barrier minimizes the concentration of lipopolysaccharide (LPS) in circulation. LPS is a structural component of gram negative bacterial cell walls, which induces an immune-cell response upon absorption into the human bloodstream, stimulating proinflammatory cytokine production and the onset of insulin resistance and hyperglycemia [42]. In support of this mechanism of probiotic action, Jafarnejad et al. [35] demonstrated probiotic-induced reductions in high sensitivity CRP, IL-6 and TNFα in their 8-week trial in women with GDM.

While this review found no significant effect of probiotic supplementation on FBG in women with GDM, a number of studies have reported positive outcomes. A study conducted in 256 pregnant women with normal glucose tolerance found significant reductions in FBG, insulin concentrations and insulin resistance following probiotic supplementation, potentially reducing participants' GDM risk [28]. However, the length of the intervention (18 months) was significantly longer than the trials included in the current meta-analysis, and fasting glucose and insulin levels were measured during pregnancy and up to 12 months postpartum in the study subjects. A Cochrane systematic review exploring the effect of probiotic supplementation during normal pregnancies concluded that although there was a reduction in the incidence of GDM in one trial, there were insufficient studies to perform a quantitative meta-analysis [43]. Further research is therefore required before probiotics can be recommended to pregnant women to reduce their risk of GDM. A meta-analysis of six RCTs demonstrated a significant reduction in FBG in 252 subjects with type 2 diabetes [44], however changes in HbA1c, inflammatory markers, fasting insulin and HOMA-IR were inconclusive, possibly due to the brief duration of the intervention (4–8 weeks). It was also unknown whether trial participants were also receiving pharmacological therapy such as Metformin, which can influence the composition of the gut microbiota. The authors postulated that probiotics may elicit hypoglycemic effects by increasing the level of antioxidative enzymes capable of scavenging reactive oxygen species, thereby reducing oxidative stress levels [44]. Similarly, a systematic review of 12 RCTs explored the effect of probiotics on glucose tolerance in people with type 2 diabetes, concluding that probiotic supplementation significantly reduced FBG [45]. This review included trials which varied substantially in methodological quality, and a number of the probiotic treatments included yoghurts or other foodstuffs containing unknown quantities of uncertain bacterial species. Finally, a systematic review of 17 RCTs reported significant reductions in FBG, fasting insulin and HOMA-IR [46]. Trial participants represented a range of demographics with various forms of metabolic disease including GDM, hypercholesterolemia and T2DM [46], which was likely to have contributed to the large interstudy heterogeneity observed.

The contradictory findings of this review in comparison to other published reviews investigating the effect of probiotics on FBG may be related to the small sample sizes (n = 60–149) and short study durations (6–8 weeks) in the women with GDM. Moreover, the current review included trials involving only participants with GDM, which may be more resistant to the effects of probiotic supplementation than the variety of other forms of glucose intolerance included in the other reviews. Indeed, increased insulin resistance is considered a normal consequence of all healthy pregnancies [13]. As there is currently no consensus on the ideal bacterial composition and dose of probiotics for the management of glucose tolerance, the microbial components of the probiotics used in the GDM trials may not have been sufficient to effect FBG levels.

Two RCTs included in this review investigated the effect of probiotic supplementation on maternal lipid levels in GDM, with both reporting conflicting results [33,34]. While one study demonstrated that probiotic treatment may have mitigated the expected increase in total and LDL-cholesterol during pregnancy [33], the other trial reported significant reductions in VLDL-cholesterol and triglyceride, while a decrease in LDL-cholesterol approached significance [34]. Beneficial gut bacteria have been hypothesized to positively influence lipid metabolism by producing secondary bile acids which are unavailable for enterohepatic recirculation. The liver must then synthesize replacement bile acids from circulating cholesterol [47]. In the present review, a pooled analysis of LDL-cholesterol data from both studies in women with GDM was not significant. Trials of longer duration (>8 weeks) may have generated outcomes with larger effect sizes.

Three of the four studies included in this review [34–36] reported significant reductions in insulin resistance (as measured by HOMA-IR) following probiotic supplementation in women diagnosed with GDM. This did not appear to result in subsequent decreases in FBG, gestational weight gain or a reduced requirement for blood glucose-lowering medication in the intervention group, but further studies of longer duration should explore this. When all four studies were combined, there was a significant reduction in insulin resistance (MD = −0.69; 95% CI −1.24, −0.14, p = 0.01). The studies which found significant reductions in insulin resistance used *Bifidobacterium* spp. in their probiotic [34–36], whereas the study with non-significant findings did not [33]. *Bifidobacterium* spp. have been reported to play a protective role in the prevention of metabolic perturbations by reducing LPS-induced oxidative stress and low grade chronic inflammation [48].

The current management for GDM involves lifestyle changes through dietary modification and physical activity, and pharmacological intervention with metformin and/or insulin if required in order to achieve target blood glucose levels [49–51]. Metformin reduces hyperglycemia by increasing insulin sensitivity and reducing excessive hepatic gluconeogenesis [49]. Both insulin and metformin are considered safe for use in pregnancy, but can be associated with unwanted side effects such as gastrointestinal disturbances and hypoglycemia [52,53]. Metformin contributes to a healthy gut microbiome by increasing the growth of *Akkermansia muciniphila* and *Lactobacillus* spp. in murine studies, but further research in humans is required to confirm this [54]. Metformin-induced expansion of the *Akkermansia muciniphila* population has been shown to modulate glucose homeostasis in obese mice fed a high fat diet [55]. *Akkermansia muciniphilia* is a mucin-degrading bacterium important for the regulation of the thickness of the mucin layer lining the host gastrointestinal tract, thus protecting the integrity of the gut barrier [56]. Human studies are now required to determine whether metformin-induced improvements in gut microbial diversity contribute to improvements in glucose tolerance. The studies included in this review were not affected by participant use of metformin, as the women required to commence metformin or insulin during the course of the trials were excluded from the final analyses.

All of the RCTs in this review were determined to have a low risk of bias, with most authors publishing their study protocol in a clinical trials registry with pre-specified primary and secondary outcomes prior to study commencement. However, a limitation of these trials were their short duration and small sample sizes. Constraints associated with this systematic review include the substantial interstudy statistical heterogeneity observed, and the use of probiotics of differing microbial composition between trials. The metabolic benefits of probiotics may be strain specific, so the optimal species, dose and duration of treatment in GDM requires further elucidation.

5. Conclusions

The present review found that while probiotic supplementation resulted in a significant reduction in insulin resistance in pregnant women with GDM, there was no significant effect on fasting blood glucose or LDL-cholesterol levels. Further high quality studies using defined doses of specific bacterial species are required to confirm these findings and their clinical relevance before their routine use can be recommended in this patient group.

Author Contributions: All authors contributed to the design of the review, literature searching, risk of bias assessment, writing and editing of the paper.

References

1. Kunz, C.; Kuntz, S.; Rudloff, S. Intestinal flora. *Adv. Exp. Med. Biol.* **2009**, *639*, 67–79. [PubMed]
2. O'Hara, A.M.; Shanahan, F. The gut flora as a forgotten organ. *EMBO Rep.* **2006**, *7*, 688–693. [CrossRef] [PubMed]
3. Sekirov, I.; Finlay, B.B. The role of the intestinal microbiota in enteric infection. *J. Physiol.* **2009**, *587*, 4159–4167. [CrossRef] [PubMed]
4. Jia, W.; Li, H.; Zhao, L.; Nicholson, J.K. Gut microbiota: A potential new territory for drug targeting. *Nat. Rev. Drug Discov.* **2008**, *7*, 123–129. [CrossRef] [PubMed]
5. Walker, A.W.; Ince, J.; Duncan, S.H.; Webster, L.M.; Holtrop, G.; Ze, X.; Brown, D.; Stares, M.D.; Scott, P.; Bergerat, A.; et al. Dominant and diet-responsive groups of bacteria within the human colonic microbiota. *ISME J.* **2011**, *5*, 220–230. [CrossRef] [PubMed]
6. Dethlefsen, L.; Eckburg, P.B.; Bik, E.M.; Relman, D.A. Assembly of the human intestinal microbiota. *Trends Ecol. Evol.* **2006**, *21*, 517–523. [CrossRef] [PubMed]
7. Backhed, F.; Ding, H.; Wang, T.; Hooper, L.V.; Koh, G.Y.; Nagy, A.; Semenkovich, C.F.; Gordon, J.I. The gut microbiota as an environmental factor that regulates fat storage. *Proc. Natl. Acad. Sci. USA* **2004**, *101*, 15718–15723. [CrossRef] [PubMed]
8. Koren, O.; Goodrich, J.K.; Cullender, T.C.; Spor, A.; Laitinen, K.; Backhed, H.K.; Gonzalez, A.; Werner, J.J.; Angenent, L.T.; Knight, R.; et al. Host remodeling of the gut microbiome and metabolic changes during pregnancy. *Cell* **2012**, *150*, 470–480. [CrossRef] [PubMed]
9. Diamant, M.; Blaak, E.E.; de Vos, W.M. Do nutrient-gut-microbiota interactions play a role in human obesity, insulin resistance and type 2 diabetes? *Obes. Rev.* **2011**, *12*, 272–281. [CrossRef] [PubMed]

10. DiGiulio, D.B.; Callahan, B.J.; McMurdie, P.J.; Costello, E.K.; Lyell, D.J.; Robaczewska, A.; Sun, C.L.; Goltsman, D.S.; Wong, R.J.; Shaw, G.; et al. Temporal and spatial variation of the human microbiota during pregnancy. *Proc. Natl. Acad. Sci. USA* **2015**, *112*, 11060–11065. [CrossRef] [PubMed]
11. Tilg, H.; Moschen, A.R. Food, immunity, and the microbiome. *Gastroenterology* **2015**, *148*, 1107–1119. [CrossRef] [PubMed]
12. Gohir, W.; Whelan, F.J.; Surette, M.G.; Moore, C.; Schertzer, J.D.; Sloboda, D.M. Pregnancy-related changes in the maternal gut microbiota are dependent upon the mother's periconceptional diet. *Gut. Microbes* **2015**, *6*, 310–320. [CrossRef] [PubMed]
13. Wang, Q.; Wurtz, P.; Auro, K.; Makinen, V.P.; Kangas, A.J.; Soininen, P.; Tiainen, M.; Tynkkynen, T.; Jokelainen, J.; Santalahti, K.; et al. Metabolic profiling of pregnancy: Cross-sectional and longitudinal evidence. *BMC Med.* **2016**, *14*, 205. [CrossRef] [PubMed]
14. Hadar, E.; Hod, M. Gestational diabetes and pregnancy outcome: Do we need an update on diagnostic criteria? *Nutr. Metab. Cardiovasc. Dis.* **2009**, *19*, 75–76. [CrossRef] [PubMed]
15. Huynh, J.; Dawson, D.; Roberts, D.; Bentley-Lewis, R. A systematic review of placental pathology in maternal diabetes mellitus. *Placenta* **2015**, *36*, 101–114. [CrossRef] [PubMed]
16. Bellamy, L.; Casas, J.P.; Hingorani, A.D.; Williams, D. Type 2 diabetes mellitus after gestational diabetes: A systematic review and meta-analysis. *Lancet* **2009**, *373*, 1773–1779. [CrossRef]
17. Huynh, J.; Xiong, G.; Bentley-Lewis, R. A systematic review of metabolite profiling in gestational diabetes mellitus. *Diabetologia* **2014**, *57*, 2453–2464. [CrossRef] [PubMed]
18. Schneider, S.; Hoeft, B.; Freerksen, N.; Fischer, B.; Roehrig, S.; Yamamoto, S.; Maul, K. Neonatal complications and risk factors among women with gestational diabetes mellitus. *Acta Obstet. Gyn. Scand.* **2011**, *90*, 231–237. [CrossRef] [PubMed]
19. Shah, B.R.; Retnakaran, R.; Booth, G.L. Increased risk of cardiovascular disease in young women following gestational diabetes mellitus. *Diabetes Care* **2008**, *31*, 1668–1669. [CrossRef] [PubMed]
20. Vohr, B.R.; Boney, C.M. Gestational diabetes: The forerunner for the development of maternal and childhood obesity and metabolic syndrome? *J. Matern. Fetal Neonat. Med.* **2008**, *21*, 149–157. [CrossRef] [PubMed]
21. Davey, R.X. Gestational diabetes mellitus: A review from 2004. *Curr. Diabetes Rev.* **2005**, *1*, 203–213. [CrossRef] [PubMed]
22. Bertoldo, M.J.; Faure, M.; Dupont, J.; Froment, P. Impact of metformin on reproductive tissues: An overview from gametogenesis to gestation. *Ann. Transl. Med.* **2014**, *2*, 55. [PubMed]
23. Mobini, R.; Tremaroli, V.; Stahlman, M.; Karlsson, F.; Levin, M.; Ljungberg, M.; Sohlin, M.; Berteus Forslund, H.; Perkins, R.; Backhed, F.; et al. Metabolic effects of Lactobacillus reuteri DSM 17938 in people with type 2 diabetes: A randomized controlled trial. *Diabetes Obes. Metabl.* **2017**, *19*, 579–589. [CrossRef] [PubMed]
24. Soleimani, A.; Zarrati Mojarrad, M.; Bahmani, F.; Taghizadeh, M.; Ramezani, M.; Tajabadi-Ebrahimi, M.; Jafari, P.; Esmaillzadeh, A.; Asemi, Z. Probiotic supplementation in diabetic hemodialysis patients has beneficial metabolic effects. *Kidney Int.* **2017**, *91*, 435–442. [CrossRef] [PubMed]
25. Sanders, M.E. Probiotics: Definition, sources, selection, and uses. *Clin. Infect. Dis.* **2008**, *46*, S58–S61. [CrossRef] [PubMed]
26. Lye, H.S.; Kuan, C.Y.; Ewe, J.A.; Fung, W.Y.; Liong, M.T. The improvement of hypertension by probiotics: Effects on cholesterol, diabetes, renin, and phytoestrogens. *Int. J. Mol. Sci.* **2009**, *10*, 3755–3775. [CrossRef] [PubMed]
27. Zhang, H.; DiBaise, J.K.; Zuccolo, A.; Kudrna, D.; Braidotti, M.; Yu, Y.; Parameswaran, P.; Crowell, M.D.; Wing, R.; Rittmann, B.E.; et al. Human gut microbiota in obesity and after gastric bypass. *Proc. Natl. Acad. Sci. USA* **2009**, *106*, 2365–2370. [CrossRef] [PubMed]
28. Laitinen, K.; Poussa, T.; Isolauri, E. Probiotics and dietary counselling contribute to glucose regulation during and after pregnancy: A randomised controlled trial. *Brit. J. Nutr.* **2009**, *101*, 1679–1687. [CrossRef] [PubMed]
29. Luoto, R.; Laitinen, K.; Nermes, M.; Isolauri, E. Impact of maternal probiotic-supplemented dietary counselling on pregnancy outcome and prenatal and postnatal growth: A double-blind, placebo-controlled study. *Brit. J. Nutr.* **2010**, *103*, 1792–1799. [CrossRef] [PubMed]
30. Moher, D.; Liberati, A.; Tetzlaff, J.; Altman, D.G. Preferred reporting items for systematic reviews and meta-analyses: The PRISMA statement. *J. Clin. Epidemiol.* **2009**, *62*, 1006–1012. [CrossRef] [PubMed]

31. Rijkers, G.T.; Bengmark, S.; Enck, P.; Haller, D.; Herz, U.; Kalliomaki, M.; Kudo, S.; Lenoir-Wijnkoop, I.; Mercenier, A.; Myllyluoma, E.; et al. Guidance for substantiating the evidence for beneficial effects of probiotics: Current status and recommendations for future research. *J. Nutr.* **2010**, *140*, 671S–676S. [CrossRef] [PubMed]
32. Higgins, J.P.; Altman, D.G.; Gotzsche, P.C.; Juni, P.; Moher, D.; Oxman, A.D.; Savovic, J.; Schultz, K.F.; Weeks, L.; Sterne, J.A. The Cochrane Collaboration's tool for assessing risk of bias in randomised trials. *BMJ* **2011**, *343*, d5928. [CrossRef] [PubMed]
33. Lindsay, K.L.; Brennan, L.; Kennelly, M.A.; Maguire, O.C.; Smith, T.; Curran, S.; Coffey, M.; Foley, M.E.; Hatunic, M.; Shanahan, F.; et al. Impact of probiotics in women with gestational diabetes mellitus on metabolic health: A randomized controlled trial. *Am. J. Obstet. Gyn.* **2015**, *212*, 496.e1–496.e11. [CrossRef] [PubMed]
34. Karamali, M.; Dadkhah, F.; Sadrkhanlou, M.; Jamilian, M.; Ahmadi, S.; Tajabadi-Ebrahimi, M.; Jafari, P.; Asemi, Z. Effects of probiotic supplementation on glycaemic control and lipid profiles in gestational diabetes: A randomized, double-blind, placebo-controlled trial. *Diabetes Metab.* **2016**, *42*, 234–241. [CrossRef] [PubMed]
35. Jafarnejad, S.; Saremi, S.; Jafarnejad, F.; Arab, A. Effects of a Multispecies Probiotic Mixture on Glycemic Control and Inflammatory Status in Women with Gestational Diabetes: A Randomized Controlled Clinical Trial. *J. Nutr. Metab.* **2016**, *2016*, 5190846. [CrossRef] [PubMed]
36. Dolatkhah, N.; Hajifaraji, M.; Abbasalizadeh, F.; Aghamohammadzadeh, N.; Mehrabi, Y.; Abbasi, M.M. Is there a value for probiotic supplements in gestational diabetes mellitus? A randomized clinical trial. *J. Health Popul. Nutr.* **2015**, *33*, 25. [CrossRef] [PubMed]
37. Zhu, Y.; Olsen, S.F.; Mendola, P.; Yeung, E.H.; Vaag, A.; Bowers, K.; Liu, A.; Bao, W.; Li, S.; Madsen, C.; et al. Growth and obesity through the first 7 years of life in association with levels of maternal glycemia during pregnancy: A prospective cohort study. *Am. J. Clin. Nutr.* **2016**, *103*, 794–800. [CrossRef] [PubMed]
38. Gregor, M.F.; Hotamisligil, G.S. Inflammatory mechanisms in obesity. *Ann. Rev. Immunol.* **2011**, *29*, 415–445. [CrossRef] [PubMed]
39. Sekirov, I.; Russell, S.L.; Antunes, L.C.; Finlay, B.B. Gut microbiota in health and disease. *Physiol. Rev.* **2010**, *90*, 859–904. [CrossRef] [PubMed]
40. Kellow, N.J.; Coughlan, M.T.; Reid, C.M. Metabolic benefits of dietary prebiotics in human subjects: A systematic review of randomised controlled trials. *Brit. J. Nutr.* **2014**, *111*, 1147–1161. [CrossRef] [PubMed]
41. Jayashree, B.; Bibin, Y.S.; Prabhu, D.; Shanthirani, C.S.; Gokulakrishnan, K.; Lakshmi, B.S.; Mohan, V.; Balasubramanyam, M. Increased circulatory levels of lipopolysaccharide (LPS) and zonulin signify novel biomarkers of proinflammation in patients with type 2 diabetes. *Mol. Cell Biochem.* **2014**, *388*, 203–210. [CrossRef] [PubMed]
42. Cani, P.D.; Amar, J.; Iglesias, M.A.; Poggi, M.; Knauf, C.; Bastelica, D.; Neyrinck, A.M.; Fava, F.; Chabo, C.; Waget, A.; et al. Metabolic endotoxemia initiates obesity and insulin resistance. *Diabetes* **2007**, *56*, 1761–1772. [CrossRef] [PubMed]
43. Barrett, H.L.; Dekker Nitert, M.; Conwell, L.S.; Callaway, L.K. Probiotics for preventing gestational diabetes. *Cochrane Database Syst. Rev.* **2014**. [CrossRef]
44. Samah, S.; Ramasamy, K.; Lim, S.M.; Neoh, C.F. Probiotics for the management of type 2 diabetes mellitus: A systematic review and meta-analysis. *Diabetes Res. Clin. Pract.* **2016**, *118*, 172–182. [CrossRef] [PubMed]
45. Li, C.; Li, X.; Han, H.; Cui, H.; Peng, M.; Wang, G.; Wang, Z. Effect of probiotics on metabolic profiles in type 2 diabetes mellitus: A meta-analysis of randomized, controlled trials. *Medicine* **2016**, *95*, e4088. [CrossRef] [PubMed]
46. Ruan, Y.; Sun, J.; He, J.; Chen, F.; Chen, R.; Chen, H. Effect of Probiotics on Glycemic Control: A Systematic Review and Meta-Analysis of Randomized, Controlled Trials. *PLoS ONE* **2015**, *10*, e0132121. [CrossRef] [PubMed]
47. Tuohy, K.M.; Fava, F.; Viola, R. 'The way to a man's heart is through his gut microbiota'—Dietary pro- and prebiotics for the management of cardiovascular risk. *Proc. Nutr. Soc.* **2014**, *73*, 172–185. [CrossRef] [PubMed]
48. Cani, P.D.; Delzenne, N.M. Interplay between obesity and associated metabolic disorders: New insights into the gut microbiota. *Curr. Opin. Pharmacol.* **2009**, *9*, 737–743. [CrossRef] [PubMed]

49. Feng, Y.; Yang, H. Metformin—A potentially effective drug for gestational diabetes mellitus: A systematic review and meta-analysis. *J. Matern. Fetal Neonat. Med.* **2016**. [CrossRef] [PubMed]
50. Moses, R.G.; Barker, M.; Winter, M.; Petocz, P.; Brand-Miller, J.C. Can a low-glycemic index diet reduce the need for insulin in gestational diabetes mellitus? A randomized trial. *Diabetes Care* **2009**, *32*, 996–1000. [CrossRef] [PubMed]
51. McGrath, R.T.; Glastras, S.J.; Hocking, S.; Fulcher, G.R. Use of metformin earlier in pregnancy predicts supplemental insulin therapy in women with gestational diabetes. *Diabetes Res. Clin. Pract.* **2016**, *116*, 96–99. [CrossRef] [PubMed]
52. Rowan, J.A.; Hague, W.M.; Gao, W.; Battin, M.R.; Moore, M.P. Metformin versus insulin for the treatment of gestational diabetes. *N. Eng. J. Med.* **2008**, *358*, 2003–2015. [CrossRef] [PubMed]
53. Gui, J.; Liu, Q.; Feng, L. Metformin vs insulin in the management of gestational diabetes: A meta-analysis. *PLoS ONE* **2013**, *8*, e64585. [CrossRef] [PubMed]
54. Lee, H.; Ko, G. Effect of metformin on metabolic improvement and gut microbiota. *Appl. Environ. Microbiol.* **2014**, *80*, 5935–5943. [CrossRef] [PubMed]
55. Shin, N.R.; Lee, J.C.; Lee, H.Y.; Kim, M.S.; Whon, T.W.; Lee, M.S.; Bae, J.W. An increase in the Akkermansia spp. population induced by metformin treatment improves glucose homeostasis in diet-induced obese mice. *Gut* **2014**, *63*, 727–735. [CrossRef] [PubMed]
56. Zhou, Z.Y.; Ren, L.W.; Zhan, P.; Yang, H.Y.; Chai, D.D.; Yu, Z.W. Metformin exerts glucose-lowering action in high-fat fed mice via attenuating endotoxemia and enhancing insulin signaling. *Acta Pharmacol.* **2016**, *37*, 1063–1075. [CrossRef] [PubMed]

8

Exploring the Impact of Food on the Gut Ecosystem Based on the Combination of Machine Learning and Network Visualization

Hideaki Shima [1], Shizuka Masuda [1], Yasuhiro Date [2,3], Amiu Shino [2], Yuuri Tsuboi [2], Mizuho Kajikawa [1], Yoshihiro Inoue [4], Taisei Kanamoto [1] and Jun Kikuchi [2,3,5,*]

1 The Laboratory of Microbiology, Showa Pharmaceutical University, Machida, Tokyo 194-8543, Japan; shima@ac.shoyaku.ac.jp (H.S.); a12108@ug.shoyaku.ac.jp (S.M.); kajikawa@ac.shoyaku.ac.jp (M.K.); kanamoto@ac.shoyaku.ac.jp (T.K.)

2 RIKEN Center for Sustainable Resource Science, 1-7-22 Suehiro-cho, Tsurumi-ku, Yokohama, Kanagawa 230-0045, Japan; yasuhiro.date@riken.jp (Y.D.); amiu.shino@riken.jp (A.S.); yuuri.tsuboi@riken.jp (Y.T.)

3 Graduate School of Medical Life Science, Yokohama City University, 1-7-29 Suehiro-cho, Tsurumi-ku, Yokohama, Kanagawa 230-0045, Japan

4 Laboratory of Pharmaceutical Sciences and Education, Showa Pharmaceutical University, Machida, Tokyo 194-8543, Japan; inoue@ac.shoyaku.ac.jp

5 Graduate School of Bioagricultural Sciences, Nagoya University, 1 Furo-cho, Chikusa-ku, Nagoya, Aichi 464-0810, Japan

* Correspondence: jun.kikuchi@riken.jp

Abstract: Prebiotics and probiotics strongly impact the gut ecosystem by changing the composition and/or metabolism of the microbiota to improve the health of the host. However, the composition of the microbiota constantly changes due to the intake of daily diet. This shift in the microbiota composition has a considerable impact; however, non-pre/probiotic foods that have a low impact are ignored because of the lack of a highly sensitive evaluation method. We performed comprehensive acquisition of data using existing measurements (nuclear magnetic resonance, next-generation DNA sequencing, and inductively coupled plasma-optical emission spectroscopy) and analyses based on a combination of machine learning and network visualization, which extracted important factors by the Random Forest approach, and applied these factors to a network module. We used two pteridophytes, *Pteridium aquilinum* and *Matteuccia struthiopteris*, for the representative daily diet. This novel analytical method could detect the impact of a small but significant shift associated with *Matteuccia struthiopteris* but not *Pteridium aquilinum* intake, using the functional network module. In this study, we proposed a novel method that is useful to explore a new valuable food to improve the health of the host as pre/probiotics.

Keywords: gut ecosystem; food intake; metabolic response; machine learning; network analysis

1. Introduction

The gastrointestinal tract has a wide variety of functions, mainly in food digestion and nutrient absorption as well as in the development of systemic immunity, regulation of behavior, and targeting of drug delivery [1–3]. Gastrointestinal functions are directly and/or indirectly augmented by the gut microbiota [4–7]. However, dysbiosis can occur, which involves the disruption of proper microbial function; a typical case of this results from consuming an unbalanced diet, resulting in undesirable conditions in the host, such as inflammatory bowel disease and obesity [8–10]. Therefore, it is important to obtain a detailed understanding of the interaction between the gastrointestinal tract and intestinal microbiota.

The intestinal microbiota consists of many bacterial species, whose composition and metabolic function responds to the daily diet; probiotics and prebiotics positively impact the health of an individual [11,12]. Additionally, specific bacteria play a role in digesting specific molecules and providing metabolites to the host in cooperation with other bacteria, which are regulated by diet [13–15]. Any component of the daily diet and additional food have the potential of developing a pre/probiotic effect, thus emphasizing the need of a precise evaluation method to determine the impact of food on the intestinal microbiota; this information can be utilized to regulate the intestinal microbiota by controlling the daily diet (pre/probiotics), meal frequency, and time of food intake [16–18].

Many researchers have attempted to clarify effect of microbiota to host responses using mice, because the results obtained from such studies could be applied to humans [19,20]. Although many researchers have attempted to determine the factors that impact the intestinal microbiota, including antibiotics, pre/probiotics, and food intake, the data obtained from the microbiota analysis are affected by daily diet, stress, environment, and individual characteristics, including gene-based factors [11,15,21–23]. To overcome these problems, intestinal microbiota and host responses were measured by multiple methods, including next-generation DNA sequencing (NGS), nuclear magnetic resonance (NMR), mass spectrometry (MS), and biochemical analyses [10,24–28]. However, the data subjected to a multivariate analysis, including principal component analysis (PCA), correlation analysis, factor analysis, clustering analysis, and network analysis [26,27,29,30], remain potential options for further improvement of data mining.

In this research, we selected *Pteridium aquilinum* and *Matteuccia struthiopteris* as the representative components of the daily diet. *P. aquilinum* is consumed in Japan, Korea, and China, while *M. struthiopteris* is widely consumed in the Northern hemisphere; both plants are pteridophytes, which may have varied nutrient compositions from those of land plants and seaweed. This suggests that pteridophytes have a comparatively simple nutrient profile compared with higher plants, thus enabling easy evaluation [31]. In addition, *P. aquilinum* and *M. struthiopteris* may be beneficial prebiotics in daily diet because of their easy availability (Figure S1) [31]. We chose Random Forest, which is a machine learning tool, superior to classification by decision tree, to identify important factors associated with the impact of food, such as age and geography, on intestinal microbiota composition and applied these important factors to the network community of heterogeneous measurement data (Figure 1) [32–34]. This combination of machine learning and network visualization methods works well in identifying significant factors that are difficult to detect by other analytical approaches. A flow chart of the analysis protocol is presented in supplementary Figure S2, which indicates the novel part of this study.

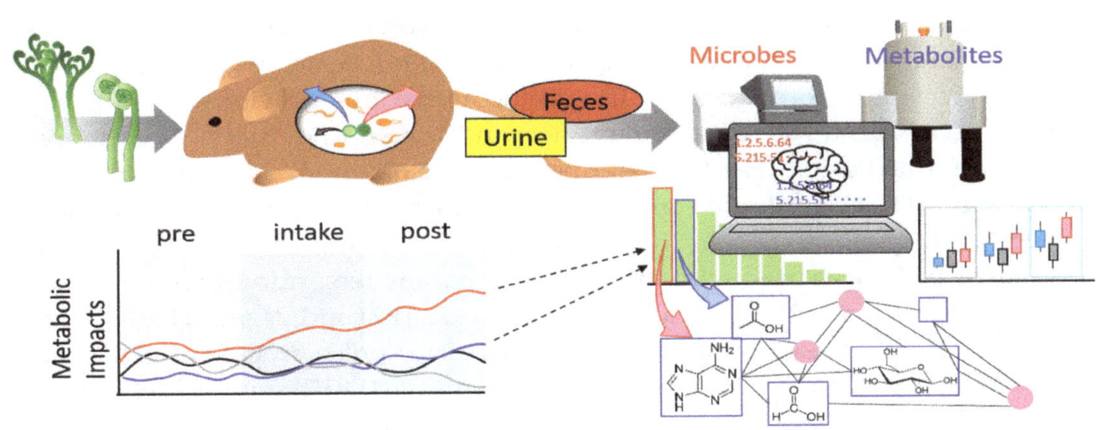

Figure 1. Schematic illustration of the novel method for exploring the impact of food, as proposed in this study. Mice were fed additional food and samples were collected (urine, feces). The samples were measured by multiple methods (e.g., NGS for the microbiome, NMR for the metabolome). These multiple data were analyzed by machine learning and important factors of response to food intake were determined. Furthermore, we calculated the network of normalized multiple data. Finally, combined functional network and important factors revealed masked impacts of food intake.

2. Materials and Methods

2.1. Animals

Male C57BL/6NCrl mice (3 weeks old) were obtained from Oriental Yeast (Tokyo, Japan) and habituated to the conditions in the animal facility before the start of the experiment (at 8 weeks old). All animal experiments were carried out in accordance with the Guidelines for the Laboratory Animal Facility of Showa Pharmaceutical University (ethic code number: P-2015-10).

2.2. Food Preparation

P. aquilinum and *M. struthiopteris*, used in this study, were developed in Yamagata Prefecture. *P. aquilinum* was boiled in 3% $NaHCO_3$ water and then soaked for at least 3 h in the same solution. Soaked *P. aquilinum* was rinsed thrice in sterile water and soaked in new sterile water for over 3 h. *M. struthiopteris* was boiled in 2% NaCl solution for 1 min and then soaked in cool water. These materials were then freeze-dried and crushed.

2.3. Animal Experiment and Sample Collection

We fixed the food-intake period (2 weeks) and the pre/post-food-intake periods. Cellulose (Wako), dried *P. aquilinum*, and *M. struthiopteris* were re-suspended (50 mg/mL) in 0.9% NaCl solution. Next, 400 μL of these solutions were orally administered to mice three times every other day in a week. Biological samples (feces, urine) were collected on the same day of food intake. A total of 216 fecal and 183 urinary samples were collected from mice ($n = 4$ for each group) throughout the experimental period for metabolic and microbial analyses. These samples were stored at −80 °C until sample preparation for analysis.

2.4. NMR Measurements

For the characterization of the components of *P. aquilinum* and *M. struthiopteris*, freeze-dried powder was suspended in 1 mL of KPi/D_2O solvent with 1 mmol/L sodium 2, 2-dimethyl-2-silapentane-5-sulfonate (DSS) and heated at 65 °C for 15 min with shaking (1400 rpm). After centrifugation, the supernatants of water- and methanol-soluble components were collected for NMR measurements. For the extraction of macromolecular components, 100 mg of the powder was rinsed with hexafluoroacetone (HFA) and ultrapure water, with a subsequent milling step, in accordance with a slightly modified version of the protocol in a previous study [35]. The milled samples were dissolved in 600 μL of DMSO-d_6/pyridine-d_5 (4:1) and the supernatant was used for NMR measurements. The collected urine and feces were prepared for NMR measurements, in accordance with the protocol used in a previous study [36]. All samples were measured by AVANCE II 700 MHz Bruker BioSpin (Bruker, Rheinstetten, Germany), metabolite annotations were performed using ^{1}H-^{13}C heteronuclear single quantum coherence (HSQC), HSQC-total correlation spectroscopy (TOCSY), double-quantum single-quantum (DQ-SQ), and two-dimensional (2D) ^{1}H-^{1}H *J*-resolved NMR spectroscopy. In the HSQC NMR measurements, the Bruker standard pulse program "hsqcetgpsisp2.2" was used with the following parameters: number of data points, 1024 (F2) and 256 (F1); number of scans, 128; spectral widths, 9803.922 (F2) and 24,649.248 (F1) Hz; and D1, 1 s. In the HSQC-TOCSY NMR measurements, the Bruker standard pulse program "hsqcdietgpsisp.2" was used with the following parameters: number of data points, 2048 (F2) and 256 (F1); number of scans, 128; and spectral widths, 9803.922 (F2) and 28,170.570 (F1) Hz. In the DQ-SQ NMR measurements, the Bruker standard pulse program "dqseagp90" was used with the following parameters: number of data points, 16,384 (F2) and 512 (F1); number of scans, 64; spectral widths, 9803.0922 (F2) and 14,003.065 (F1) Hz; and D1, 1 s. In the 2D *J*-resolved NMR measurements, the Bruker standard pulse program "jresgpprqf" was used with the following parameters: number of data points, 16,384 (F2) and 32 (F1); number of scans, 8; spectral widths, 12,500 (F2) and 50 (F1) Hz; and D1, 2 s. In addition, metabolic profiling for feces and urine was also performed using 2D *J*-resolved NMR with skyline projection [37]. The detected peaks in NMR spectra were annotated using SpinAssign (http://dmar.riken.jp/spinassign/)

and SpinCouple (http://dmar.riken.jp/spincpl/) programs, as well as the Human Metabolome Database (http://www.hmdb.ca/) [38–40].

2.5. Inductively Coupled Plasma-Optical Emission Spectroscopy (ICP-OES) Measurement

A sufficient amount of each of 138 urinary samples was diluted approximately 100 times and measured by ICP-OES (SPECTRO BLUE FMX26 EOP; SPECTRO, Tokyo, Japan). As the operating parameters, main argon pressure, plasma power, plasma gas flow, auxiliary gas flow, nebulizer gas flow, and pump speed were set to 6.5 bar, 1400 W, 12 L/min, 1 L/min, 1 L/min, and 30 rpm, respectively.

2.6. Fecal Microbiome Analysis

Fecal microbes were disrupted using 5 mm stainless beads and a medicine spoonful of 0.3 mm zirconia beads in 200 μL of SDS-TE buffer (10 mmol/L Tris-HCl, 1 mmol/L EDTA, 2% SDS) using a vortex mixer for a total of 60 s. Disrupted feces were subjected to three freeze–thaw cycles and then centrifuged (10,000× *g*, 4 °C, 5 min), after which 100 μL of the supernatant was transferred to a new tube. DNA was extracted by phenol:chloroform:isoamyl alcohol (25:24:1) from the supernatant. Extracted DNA was dissolved in TE buffer and stored at −80 °C until microbiome analysis. The region encoding 16S rRNA was amplified using PCR with a TaKaRa Ex Taq HS kit (TaKaRa Bio, Shiga, Japan) and a primer set (Table S1) [41]. DNA was amplified by the following program: preheating at 94 °C for 4 min; 25 cycles of denaturation at 94 °C for 30 s, annealing at 55 °C for 30 s, and extension at 72 °C for 2 min; and a final terminal extension at 72 °C for 10 min. The 16S rRNA gene amplicon was purified using AMPure XP (Beckman Coulter, Brea, CA, USA) with the manufacturer's protocol. The purified double-stranded DNA concentration was determined by Picogreen (Thermo Fisher Scientific, Waltham, MA, USA) and sequencing of prepared library was performed using a MiSeq sequencer (Illumina Inc., San Diego, CA, USA) following the manufacturer's instructions. Obtained DNA sequence data were analyzed by QIIME (http://qiime.org/) and detected bacteria are listed in Table S2 [42]. These bacterial data were handled as percentages in the following analysis. The sequences that passed the QIIME of 16S rRNA OTU had a mean of 5619.26, and SD of 1653.89.

2.7. Data Analysis

Peaks of one-dimensional skyline projection (^{1}H-NMR) data were picked up by rNMR on the "R" platform [43,44]. The peak-picking data and other microbial and elemental data were normalized by unit variance. PCA, Random Forest, and network analyses were performed using the packages "muma," "randomForest," and "igraph" on the R platform, respectively [45–47]. These packages were used with their default settings. Calculated network data were depicted by Cytoscape (http://www.cytoscape.org/) [48]. The top 30 important factors were extracted from the mean decrease in accuracy of the Random Forest analysis. These factors were applied to calculate the community. The important factors of the included community were statistically analyzed. Statistical significance was determined using the Holm method, in which the false discovery rate was intermediate between Benjamini–Hochberg method and Bonferroni method [49,50].

2.8. Data Deposition

DNA sequences of the study have been deposited in DDBJ (http://www.ddbj.nig.ac.jp/). The accession number was DRA006349.

3. Results and Discussion

3.1. Sample Measurement and Multivariate Analysis

NMR measurements of the components of *P. aquilinum* and *M. struthiopteris* revealed that the plants contained some sugar groups and organic acids, chlorogenic acid, shikimate, and quinate (Figure S3a,b), the metabolites of which are derived from the shikimate pathway [51]. In particular, chlorogenic acid was reported to reduce blood pressure, indicating that the plants have the possibility of improving health [52]. Additionally, the plants have almost the same high-molecular-weight components, except for olefin and starch (Figure S4a,b). Next, the contents of urine and feces from throughout the experimental period were annotated and used to create a PCA score plot, which is widely used to obtain an overview of multivariate data for easy visualization (Table S3, Figures S5 and S6, Figure 2a–c). Although the PCA score of feces from cellulose-treated mice moved slightly in the PC2 negative direction from the pre to post period (Figure 2a), the PCA scores of *P. aquilinum* and *M. struthiopteris* transitioned from the PC1 negative to the positive side (Figure 2b,c). This suggested that *P. aquilinum* and *M. struthiopteris* intake had a greater impact than cellulose intake, which may have arisen from the plants' sugar groups and organic acids. However, we were unable to determine the exact causal factor from the PCA score loading, as there was substantial noise. In addition, we measured intestinal microbiota by MiSeq and analyzed the data using PCA. The results of the microbiome data from all groups were not clearly separated among the groups (Figure 2d–f). Furthermore, we estimated the Firmicutes/Bacteroidetes ratio, which are major phyla in the gut and indicators of host life-style [12], to be almost the same (mean = 1.13, SD = 0.42, for the whole experimental period). These results suggest that additional food intake of six times every other day for two weeks could not make a major difference to gut microbiota composition. The urinary profiles based on NMR and elements by ICP-OES indicated a complex dispersion on the PCA score plot (Figure S7a–f). These results appear to demonstrate that PCA was unsuitable for exploring the impact of food in this case.

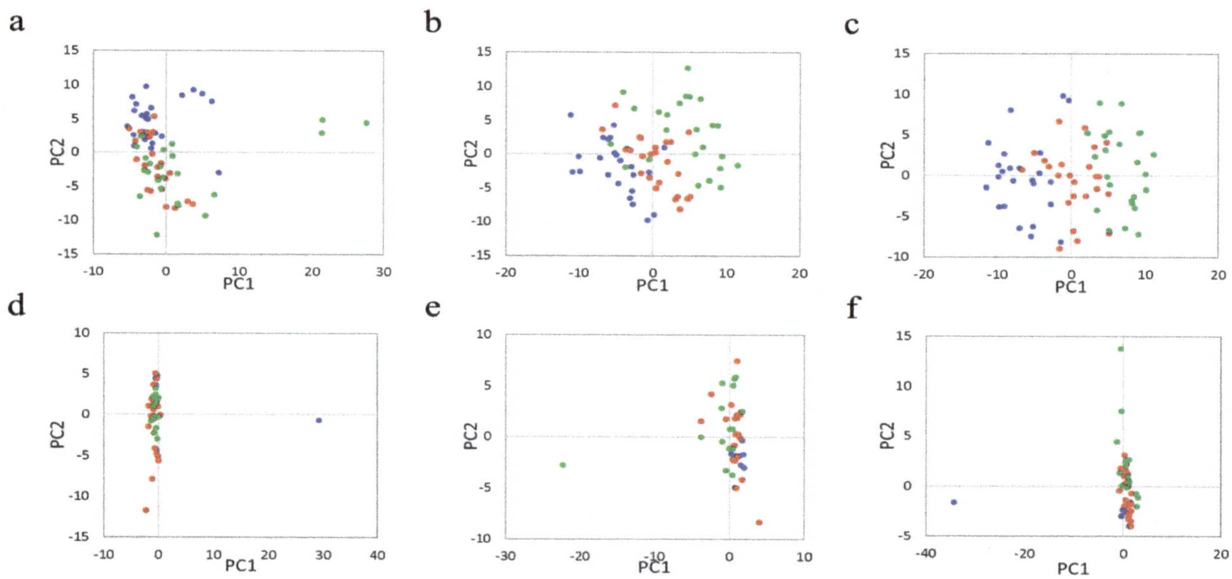

Figure 2. Principal component analysis of fecal metabolites and the microbiome. Red, blue, and green spheres represent single data points from pretreatment, during treatment, and posttreatment, respectively. Upper panels indicate the results of fecal NMR measurement analyzed by PCA. The data for the experimentally treated mouse groups (**a**–**c**) were from the administration of cellulose, *Pteridium aquilinum*, and *Matteuccia struthiopteris*, respectively; (**d**–**f**) show PCA score plots of the MiSeq data for each group; (**d**–**f**) show the results for the microbiota of mice treated with cellulose, *P. aquilinum*, and *M. struthiopteris*, respectively. The data analysis was performed using the package "muma" in R [45].

3.2. Selection of Important Variables by Determining the Food Impact

Although the impact of additional food intake was detected using fecal metabolite PCA, others indicated complex dispersion. It was suggested that the same composition microbiota shifted to another state of metabolism or that treated mice responses of food intake were masked by other factors, such as mouse-specific characteristics and stress [22]. We managed to mine the data on the impact of food by machine learning using Random Forest, which was applied to all datasets and was used to create a multi-dimensional plot, indicating that each group had a specific factor that separated it from the others (Figure 3a, Figures S8a and S9a); we then selected the factors important for this separation, with careful cross-validation, to avoid over-training, using the Random Forest package (Figure 3b, Figures S8b and S9b). Random Forest revealed differences that were undetectable on PCA. The representative factors were clustered in the functional network module of the following network analysis (Figure 3c, Figures S8c and S9c). In addition, urinary ICP-OES data could not be separated using Random Forest analysis. These results indicate that urinary elements were not affected by food intake in this case.

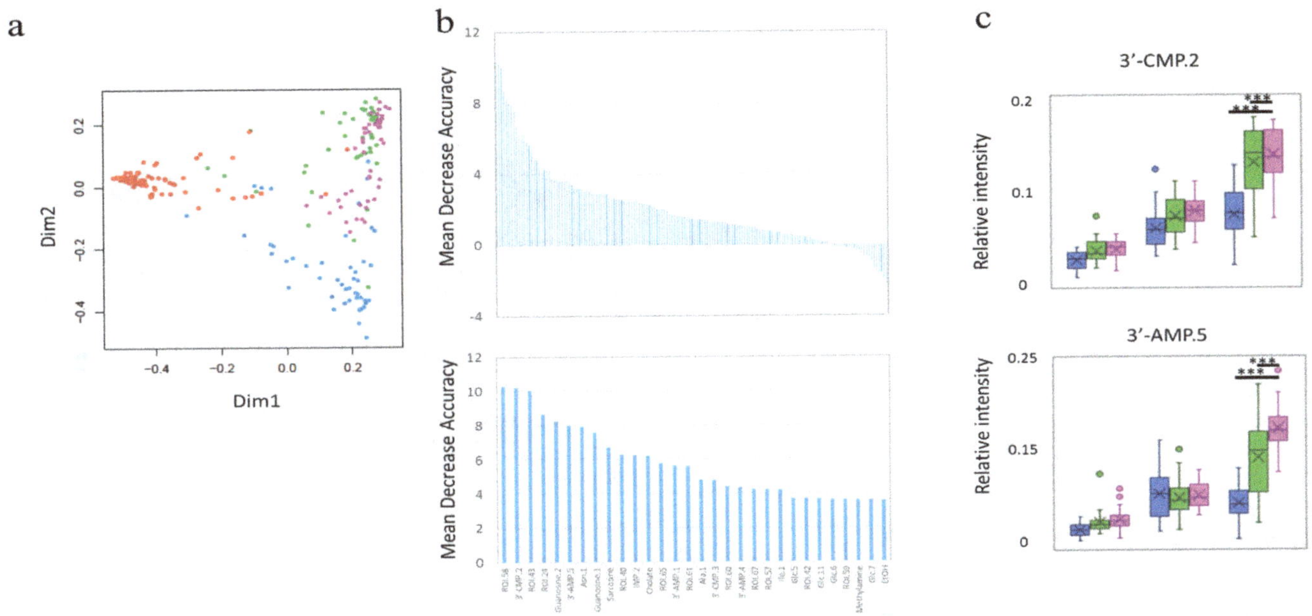

Figure 3. The results of Random Forest for fecal metabolites. Multi-dimensional score (MDS) plots (**a**) and important factors separating the groups (**b**) upper panel indicates all important factors and lower panel indicates the top 30 most important factors with annotation. In (**a**), red, blue, green, and purple circles represent single data points from the pre-treatment period for all groups, and the cellulose-, *Pteridium aquilinum*-, and *Matteuccia struthiopteris*-treated groups, respectively. (**c**) Shows a boxplot of representative important factors that can be applied on the network module. The upper panel and lower panel depict the results for 3′-CMP.2 and 3′-AMP.5, respectively. Blue, green, and purple boxes represent cellulose-, *P. aquilinum*-, and *M. struthiopteris*-treated groups, respectively. *** $p < 0.001$ calculated by the Holm method.

3.3. *Application of Important Factors to Network Modules for Separation*

We were able to detect important variables from the multivariate data by Random Forest and then attempted to find important variables in the network modules concerning the impact of additional food intake. We calculated the Spearman rank correlation coefficient with the combined dataset of the group treated with both *Pteridium aquilinum* and *Matteuccia struthiopteris* (metabolites of urine and feces and microbiome), performed analyses based on the correlation coefficients, using the R [45] package "igraph", and then described the network community, using Cytoscape (Figure 4, Figures S10 and S11). The purine/pyrimidine network of *M. struthiopteris* indicated that the impact of *M. struthiopteris* intake affected the microbiota, metabolites, and host metabolism. Dietary purine/pyrimidine was important to avoid an allergic state and to develop gastrointestinal systems [53,54]. The bacterium that was an important factor in the *M. struthiopteris*-treated group, from the genus-associated purine/pyrimidine metabolism community, was *Prevotella*, which is a gram-negative bacterium, reported to be associated with fiber [15]. In addition, the genus *Akkermansia*, which is known to affect metabolism and reduce obesity and inflammation [55,56], responded to *M. struthiopteris* intake. Another community, including glucose signal-associated bacterium, was described (Figures S10b and S11c); however, important bacterium and important glucose signals were indirectly connected. Furthermore, the community did not associate with urinary metabolites. The results suggested that the impact of *M. struthiopteris* intake affects the purine/pyrimidine network more than glucose network. The important community and its associated bacterium *Akkermansia* were reported to be useful for health, so the impact of *M. struthiopteris* intake may involve a prebiotic-like effect of shifting nucleotide availability. Our method, involving a combination of machine learning and network visualization, detected a less significant food impact, which may help in the identification of prebiotics and probiotics that could be useful in the daily diet.

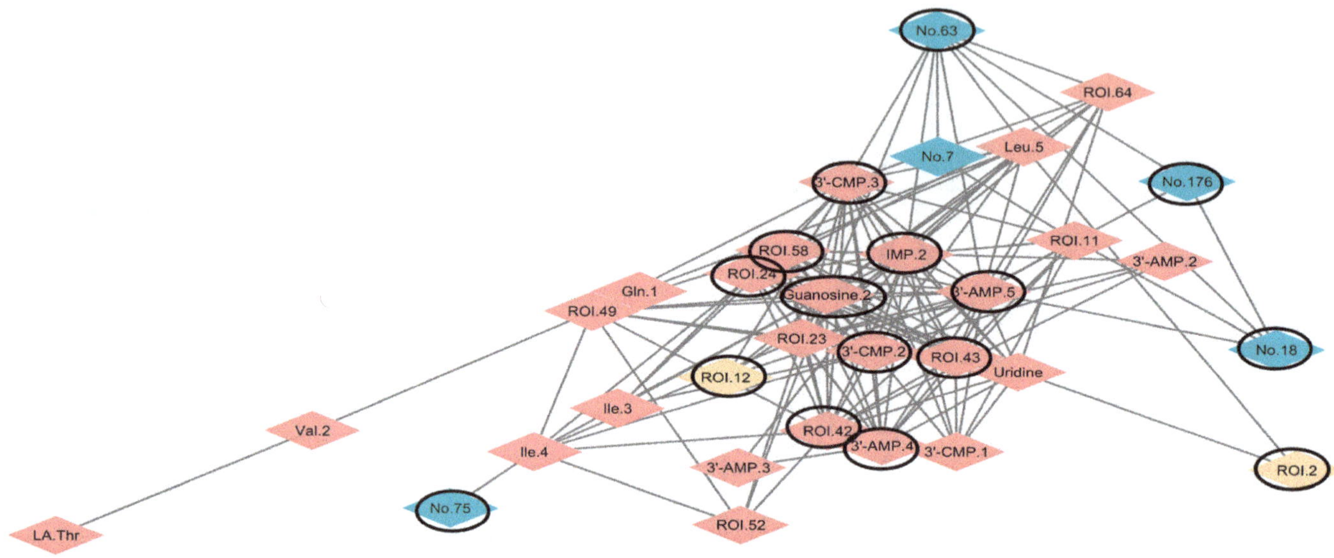

Figure 4. Purine/pyrimidine network with important bacteria and urinary metabolites of *Matteuccia struthiopteris*-treated mice based on the combined data set. The depicted network is based on calculations using the igraph package with Cytoscape. Blue, red, and light-yellow diamonds represent bacteria, fecal metabolites, and urinary metabolites, respectively (Tables S2 and S3). Black-line-circled diamonds represent factors selected by Random Forest as factors important for separating the groups.

4. Conclusions

In this paper, we selected two pteridophytes, which may have led to varied nutrient compositions between land plants and seaweed, as targets to study the impact of food on the gut ecosystem in mice. These pteridophytes may be beneficial prebiotics in the daily diet because of their easy availability. We proposed a novel methodology for exploring the impact of food on the gut ecosystem based on a combination of machine learning and network visualization. We obtained total of 490 variables by multiple measurements from non-invasive, time-course sampled urine and feces, and finally detected two important network modules, based on 30 selected variables of importance, based on Random Forest calculations. This novel analytical method could detect the impact of a small, but significant, shift associated with *Matteuccia struthiopteris* intake, using the functional purine/pyrimidine network module.

Supplementary Materials
Figure S1: Tree diagram of plant components based on data set obtained by NMR measurement, Figure S2: Flow chart of the analysis procedure in this study, Figure S3: ^{1}H-^{13}C HSQC NMR spectra of *Pteridium aquilinum* and *Matteuccia struthiopteris* extracted by KPi/D_2O solvent, Figure S4: ^{1}H-^{13}C HSQC NMR spectra of *Pteridium aquilinum* and *Matteuccia struthiopteris* components extracted by DMSO-d_6/pyridine-d_5 (4:1) solvent, Figure S5: Annotation of metabolites in urine NMR spectra, Figure S6: Annotation of metabolites in fecal NMR spectra, Figure S7: Principal component analysis of urinary metabolites and ions, Figure S8: The results of Random Forest for the fecal microbiome, Figure S9: The results of Random Forest for urinary metabolites, Figure S10: Network community correlation coefficients for *Matteuccia struthiopteris*-treated mice based on the combined data set, Figure S11: Network community correlation coefficients for *Pteridium aquilinum*-treated mice based on the combined data set, Table S1: Information on primers used for performing microbiome analysis, Table S2: List of sequential numbers for bacterial detection by MiSeq analysis, Table S3: List of annotated metabolites and unknown signals from NMR measurements.

Acknowledgments: This research was supported by a Sasakawa Scientific Research Grant from The Japan Science Society.

Author Contributions: H.S., Y.I. and J.K. conceived the experiments; H.S., S.M., Y.D. and J.K. designed the experiments; H.S., Y.D., M.K. and T.K. modified the experiments; H.S., S.M., A.S., Y.T. and Y.I. performed the experiments; H.S., S.M., Y.D., A.S., Y.T. and J.K. analyzed the data and created the Figures. H.S., Y.D. and J.K. wrote the paper.

References

1. Furusawa, Y.; Obata, Y.; Fukuda, S.; Endo, T.A.; Nakato, G.; Takahashi, D.; Nakanishi, Y.; Uetake, C.; Kato, K.; Kato, T.; et al. Commensal microbe-derived butyrate induces the differentiation of colonic regulatory T cells. *Nature* **2013**, *504*, 446–450. [CrossRef] [PubMed]
2. Sudo, N.; Chida, Y.; Aiba, Y.; Sonoda, J.; Oyama, N.; Yu, X.N.; Kubo, C.; Koga, Y. Postnatal microbial colonization programs the hypothalamic-pituitary-adrenal system for stress response in mice. *J. Physiol.* **2004**, *558*, 263–275. [CrossRef] [PubMed]
3. Shima, H.; Watanabe, T.; Fukuda, S.; Fukuoka, S.I.; Ohara, O.; Ohno, H. A novel mucosal vaccine targeting Peyer's patch M cells induces protective antigen-specific IgA responses. *Int. Immunol.* **2014**, *26*, 619–625. [CrossRef] [PubMed]
4. Ivanov, I.I.; Atarashi, K.; Manel, N.; Brodie, E.L.; Shima, T.; Karaoz, U.; Wei, D.; Goldfarb, K.C.; Santee, C.A.; Lynch, S.V.; et al. Induction of intestinal Th17 cells by segmented filamentous bacteria. *Cell* **2009**, *139*, 485–498. [CrossRef] [PubMed]
5. Fukuda, S.; Toh, H.; Hase, K.; Oshima, K.; Nakanishi, Y.; Yoshimura, K.; Tobe, T.; Clarke, J.M.; Topping, D.L.; Suzuki, T.; et al. Bifidobacteria can protect from enteropathogenic infection through production of acetate. *Nature* **2011**, *469*, 543–547. [CrossRef] [PubMed]
6. Atarashi, K.; Tanoue, T.; Ando, M.; Kamada, N.; Nagano, Y.; Narushima, S.; Suda, W.; Imaoka, A.; Setoyama, H.; Nagamori, T.; et al. Th17 Cell Induction by Adhesion of Microbes to Intestinal Epithelial Cells. *Cell* **2015**, *163*, 367–380. [CrossRef] [PubMed]
7. Wei, X.; Yang, Z.; Rey, F.E.; Ridaura, V.K.; Davidson, N.O.; Gordon, J.I.; Semenkovich, C.F. Fatty acid synthase modulates intestinal barrier function through palmitoylation of mucin 2. *Cell Host Microbe* **2012**, *11*, 140–152. [CrossRef] [PubMed]
8. Elson, C.O.; Cong, Y.; McCracken, V.J.; Dimmitt, R.A.; Lorenz, R.G.; Weaver, C.T. Experimental models of inflammatory bowel disease reveal innate, adaptive, and regulatory mechanisms of host dialogue with the microbiota. *Immunol. Rev.* **2005**, *206*, 260–276. [CrossRef] [PubMed]
9. Ridaura, V.K.; Faith, J.J.; Rey, F.E.; Cheng, J.; Duncan, A.E.; Kau, A.L.; Griffin, N.W.; Lombard, V.; Henrissat, B.; Bain, J.R.; et al. Gut microbiota from twins discordant for obesity modulate metabolism in mice. *Science* **2013**, *341*, 1241214. [CrossRef] [PubMed]
10. Lin, H.; An, Y.P.; Hao, F.H.; Wang, Y.L.; Tang, H.R. Correlations of fecal metabonomic and microbiomic changes induced by high-fat diet in the pre-obesity state. *Sci. Rep.* **2016**, *6*, 21618. [PubMed]
11. Jandhyala, S.M.; Talukdar, R.; Subramanyam, C.; Vuyyuru, H.; Sasikala, M.; Nageshwar Reddy, D. Role of the normal gut microbiota. *World J. Gastroenterol.* **2015**, *21*, 8787–8803. [CrossRef] [PubMed]
12. Arumugam, M.; Raes, J.; Pelletier, E.; Le Paslier, D.; Yamada, T.; Mende, D.R.; Fernandes, G.R.; Tap, J.; Bruls, T.; Batto, J.M.; et al. Enterotypes of the human gut microbiome. *Nature* **2011**, *473*, 174–180. [CrossRef] [PubMed]
13. Hehemann, J.H.; Correc, G.; Barbeyron, T.; Helbert, W.; Czjzek, M.; Michel, G. Transfer of carbohydrate-active enzymes from marine bacteria to Japanese gut microbiota. *Nature* **2010**, *464*, 908–912. [CrossRef] [PubMed]
14. Sugahara, H.; Odamaki, T.; Fukuda, S.; Kato, T.; Xiao, J.Z.; Abe, F.; Kikuchi, J.; Ohno, H. Probiotic Bifidobacterium longum alters gut luminal metabolism through modification of the gut microbial community. *Sci. Rep.* **2015**, *5*, 13548. [CrossRef] [PubMed]
15. Wu, G.D.; Chen, J.; Hoffmann, C.; Bittinger, K.; Chen, Y.Y.; Keilbaugh, S.A.; Bewtra, M.; Knights, D.; Walters, W.A.; Knight, R.; et al. Linking long-term dietary patterns with gut microbial enterotypes. *Science* **2011**, *334*, 105–108. [CrossRef] [PubMed]

16. Hatori, M.; Panda, S. Response of peripheral rhythms to the timing of food intake. *Methods Enzymol.* **2015**, *552*, 145–161. [PubMed]
17. Mattson, M.P.; Allison, D.B.; Fontana, L.; Harvie, M.; Longo, V.D.; Malaisse, W.J.; Mosley, M.; Notterpek, L.; Ravussin, E.; Scheer, F.A.; et al. Meal frequency and timing in health and disease. *Proc. Natl. Acad. Sci. USA* **2014**, *111*, 16647–16653. [CrossRef] [PubMed]
18. Zarrinpar, A.; Chaix, A.; Yooseph, S.; Panda, S. Diet and feeding pattern affect the diurnal dynamics of the gut microbiome. *Cell Metab.* **2014**, *20*, 1006–1017. [CrossRef] [PubMed]
19. Chaix, A.; Zarrinpar, A.; Miu, P.; Panda, S. Time-restricted feeding is a preventative and therapeutic intervention against diverse nutritional challenges. *Cell Metab.* **2014**, *20*, 991–1005. [CrossRef] [PubMed]
20. Gill, S.; Panda, S. A smartphone app reveals erratic diurnal eating patterns in humans that can be modulated for health benefits. *Cell Metab.* **2015**, *22*, 789–798. [CrossRef] [PubMed]
21. Jernberg, C.; Löfmark, S.; Edlund, C.; Jansson, J.K. Long-term impacts of antibiotic exposure on the human intestinal microbiota. *Microbiology* **2010**, *156*, 3216–3223. [CrossRef] [PubMed]
22. Rea, K.; Dinan, T.G.; Cryan, J.F. The microbiome: A key regulator of stress and neuroinflammation. *Neurobiol. Stress* **2016**, *4*, 23–33. [CrossRef] [PubMed]
23. Fanaro, S.; Chierici, R.; Guerrini, P.; Vigi, V. Intestinal microflora in early infancy: Composition and development. *Acta Paediatr. Suppl.* **2003**, *92*, 48–55. [CrossRef]
24. Aw, W.; Fukuda, S. Toward the comprehensive understanding of the gut ecosystem via metabolomics-based integrated omics approach. In *Seminars in Immunopathology*; Springer: Berlin, Germany, 2015.
25. Kaplan, C.W.; Astaire, J.C.; Sanders, M.E.; Reddy, B.S.; Kitts, C.L. 16S ribosomal DNA terminal restriction fragment pattern analysis of bacterial communities in feces of rats fed Lactobacillus acidophilus NCFM. *Appl. Environ. Microbiol.* **2001**, *67*, 1935–1939. [CrossRef] [PubMed]
26. Wu, J.F.; Yang, L.; Li, S.F.; Huang, P.; Liu, Y.; Wang, Y.L.; Tang, H.R. Metabolomics insights into the modulatory effects of long-term low calorie intake in mice. *J. Proteome Res.* **2016**, *15*, 2299–2308. [CrossRef] [PubMed]
27. Tian, Y.; Xu, T.P.; Huang, J.; Zhang, L.M.; Xu, S.; Xiong, B.; Wang, Y.L.; Tang, H.R. Tissue metabonomic phenotyping for diagnosis and prognosis of human colorectal cancer. *Sci. Rep.* **2016**, *6*, 20790. [CrossRef] [PubMed]
28. Markley, J.L.; Bruschweiler, R.; Edison, A.S.; Eghbalnia, H.R.; Powers, R.; Raftery, D.; Wishart, D.S. The future of NMR-based metabolomics. *Curr. Opin. Biotechnol.* **2017**, *43*, 34–40. [CrossRef] [PubMed]
29. Worley, B.; Powers, R. MVAPACK: A complete data handling package for NMR metabolomics. *ACS Chem. Biol.* **2014**, *9*, 1138–1144. [CrossRef] [PubMed]
30. Kim, Y.J.; Huh, I.; Kim, J.Y.; Park, S.; Ryu, S.H.; Kim, K.B.; Kim, S.; Park, T.; Kwon, O. Integration of traditional and metabolomics biomarkers identifies prognostic metabolites for predicting responsiveness to nutritional intervention against oxidative stress and inflammation. *Nutrients* **2017**, *9*, 233. [CrossRef] [PubMed]
31. Itouga, M.; Hayatsu, M.; Sato, M.; Tsuboi, Y.; Komatsu-Kato, Y.; Toyooka, K.; Suzuki, S.; Nakatsuka, S.; Kawakami, S.; Kikuchi, J.; et al. Characterization of the moss *Funaria hygrometrica protonema* cells as a lead (Pb) adsorbent. *PLoS ONE* **2017**, in press.
32. Breiman, L. Random forests. *Mach. Learn.* **2001**, *45*, 5–32. [CrossRef]
33. Shiokawa, Y.; Misawa, T.; Date, Y.; Kikuchi, J. Application of market basket analysis for the visualization of transaction data based on human lifestyle and spectroscopic measurements. *Anal. Chem.* **2016**, *88*, 2714–2719. [CrossRef] [PubMed]
34. Yatsunenko, T.; Rey, F.E.; Manary, M.J.; Trehan, I.; Dominguez-Bello, M.G.; Contreras, M.; Magris, M.; Hidalgo, G.; Baldassano, R.N.; Anokhin, A.P.; et al. Human gut microbiome viewed across age and geography. *Nature* **2012**, *486*, 222–227. [CrossRef] [PubMed]
35. Date, Y.; Sakata, K.; Kikuchi, J. Chemical profiling of complex biochemical mixtures from various seaweeds. *Polym. J.* **2012**, *44*, 888–894. [CrossRef]
36. Date, Y.; Nakanishi, Y.; Fukuda, S.; Nuijima, Y.; Kato, T.; Umehara, M.; Ohno, H.; Kikuchi, J. In vitro evaluation method for screening of candidate prebiotic foods. *Food Chem.* **2014**, *152*, 251–260. [CrossRef] [PubMed]
37. Mekuchi, M.; Sakata, K.; Yamaguchi, T.; Koiso, M.; Kikuchi, J. Trans-omics approaches used to characterise fish nutritional biorhythms in leopard coral grouper (*Plectropomus leopardus*). *Sci. Rep.* **2017**, *7*, 9372. [CrossRef] [PubMed]

38. Chikayama, E.; Sekiyama, Y.; Okamoto, M.; Nakanishi, Y.; Tsuboi, Y.; Akiyama, K.; Saito, K.; Shinozaki, K.; Kikuchi, J. Statistical indices for simultaneous large-scale metabolite detections for a single NMR spectrum. *Anal. Chem.* **2010**, *82*, 1653–1658. [CrossRef] [PubMed]
39. Kikuchi, J.; Tsuboi, Y.; Komatsu, K.; Gomi, M.; Chikayama, E.; Date, Y. SpinCouple: Development of a Web Tool for Analyzing Metabolite Mixtures via Two-Dimensional J-Resolved NMR Database. *Anal. Chem.* **2016**, *88*, 659–665. [CrossRef] [PubMed]
40. Wishart, D.S.; Jewison, T.; Guo, A.C.; Wilson, M.; Knox, C.; Liu, Y.; Djoumbou, Y.; Mandal, R.; Aziat, F.; Dong, E. HMDB 3.0—The human metabolome database in 2013. *Nucleic Acids Res.* **2012**, *41*, D801–D807. [CrossRef] [PubMed]
41. Caporaso, J.G.; Lauber, C.L.; Walters, W.A.; Berg-Lyons, D.; Huntley, J.; Fierer, N.; Owens, S.M.; Betley, J.; Fraser, L.; Bauer, M. Ultra-high-throughput microbial community analysis on the Illumina HiSeq and MiSeq platforms. *ISME J.* **2012**, *6*, 1621–1624. [CrossRef] [PubMed]
42. Caporaso, J.G.; Kuczynski, J.; Stombaugh, J.; Bittinger, K.; Bushman, F.D.; Costello, E.K.; Fierer, N.; Peña, A.G.; Goodrich, J.K.; Gordon, J.I. QIIME allows analysis of high-throughput community sequencing data. *Nat. Methods* **2010**, *7*, 335–336. [CrossRef] [PubMed]
43. Lewis, I.A.; Schommer, S.C.; Markley, J.L. rNMR: Open source software for identifying and quantifying metabolites in NMR spectra. *Magn. Reson. Chem.* **2009**, *47*, S123–S126. [CrossRef] [PubMed]
44. R Core Team. *R Language Definition*; R Foundation for Statistical Computing: Vienna, Austria, 2000.
45. Gaude, E.; Chignola, F.; Spiliotopoulos, D.; Spitaleri, A.; Ghitti, M.; Garcìa-Manteiga, J.M.; Mari, S.; Musco, G. muma, An R package for metabolomics univariate and multivariate statistical analysis. *Curr. Metabol.* **2013**, *1*, 180–189. [CrossRef]
46. Csardi, G.; Nepusz, T. The igraph software package for complex network research. *Int. J. Complex Syst.* **2006**, *1695*, 1–9.
47. Liaw, A.; Wiener, M. Classification and regression by random Forest. *R News* **2002**, *2*, 18–22.
48. Shannon, P.; Markiel, A.; Ozier, O.; Baliga, N.S.; Wang, J.T.; Ramage, D.; Amin, N.; Schwikowski, B.; Ideker, T. Cytoscape: A software environment for integrated models of biomolecular interaction networks. *Genome Res.* **2003**, *13*, 2498–2504. [CrossRef] [PubMed]
49. Holm, S. A simple sequentially rejective multiple test procedure. *Scand. J. Stat.* **1979**, *6*, 65–70.
50. Benjamini, Y.; Hochberg, Y. Controlling the false discovery rate: A practical and powerful approach to multiple testing. *J. R. Stat. Soc. Ser. B (Methodol.)* **1995**, *57*, 289–300.
51. Draths, K.; Knop, D.R.; Frost, J. Shikimic acid and quinic acid: Replacing isolation from plant sources with recombinant microbial biocatalysis. *J. ACS* **1999**, *121*, 1603–1604. [CrossRef]
52. Onakpoya, I.; Spencer, E.; Thompson, M.; Heneghan, C. The effect of chlorogenic acid on blood pressure: A systematic review and meta-analysis of randomized clinical trials. *J. Hum. Hypertens.* **2015**, *29*, 77–81. [CrossRef] [PubMed]
53. Sudo, N.; Aiba, Y.; Oyama, N.; Yu, X.N.; Matsunaga, M.; Koga, Y.; Kubo, C. Dietary nucleic acid and intestinal microbiota synergistically promote a shift in the Th1/Th2 balance toward Th1-skewed immunity. *Int. Arch. Allergy Immunol.* **2004**, *135*, 132–135. [CrossRef] [PubMed]
54. Carver, J. Dietary nucleotides: Effects on the immune and gastrointestinal systems. *Acta Paediatr. Suppl.* **1999**, *88*, 83–88. [CrossRef] [PubMed]
55. Everard, A.; Belzer, C.; Geurts, L.; Ouwerkerk, J.P.; Druart, C.; Bindels, L.B.; Guiot, Y.; Derrien, M.; Muccioli, G.G.; Delzenne, N.M.; et al. Cross-talk between Akkermansia muciniphila and intestinal epithelium controls diet-induced obesity. *Proc. Natl. Acad. Sci. USA* **2013**, *110*, 9066–9071. [CrossRef] [PubMed]
56. Caesar, R.; Tremaroli, V.; Kovatcheva-Datchary, P.; Cani, P.D.; Bäckhed, F. Crosstalk between gut microbiota and dietary lipids aggravates WAT inflammation through TLR signaling. *Cell Metabol.* **2015**, *22*, 658–668. [CrossRef] [PubMed]

9

Impact of High-Dose Multi-Strain Probiotic Supplementation on Neurocognitive Performance and Central Nervous System Immune Activation of HIV-1 Infected Individuals

Giancarlo Ceccarelli [1,*], Jason M. Brenchley [2], Eugenio Nelson Cavallari [1], Giuseppe Corano Scheri [1], Mariangela Fratino [3], Claudia Pinacchio [1], Ivan Schietroma [1], Saeid Najafi Fard [1], Carolina Scagnolari [4], Ivano Mezzaroma [5], Vincenzo Vullo [1] and Gabriella d'Ettorre [1]

1 Department of Public Health and Infectious Diseases, University of Rome "Sapienza", Rome (Italy) and Azienda Policlinico Umberto I, 00161 Rome, Italy; eugenionelson.cavallari@uniroma1.it (E.N.C.); giuseppe.coranoscheri@uniroma1.it (G.C.S.); claudiapinacchio@gmail.com (C.P.); schietroma.ivan@gmail.com (I.S.); saeid.najafifard@gmail.com (S.N.F.); vincenzo.vullo@uniroma1.it (V.V.); gabriella.dettorre@uniroma1.it (G.d.E.)

2 Laboratory of Parasitic Diseases, National Institute of Allergy and Infectious Diseases, NIH, Bethesda, MD 20892, USA; jbrenchl@niaid.nih.gov

3 Department of Neurology, University of Rome "Sapienza", 00185 Rome, Italy; marifra@hotmail.it

4 Department of Molecular Medicine, Laboratory of Virology, University of Rome "Sapienza", 00185 Rome, Italy; carolina.scagnolari@uniroma1.it

5 Department of Clinical Medicine, University of Rome "Sapienza", 00185 Rome, Italy; ivano.mezzaroma@uniroma1.it

* Correspondence: giancarlo.ceccarelli@uniroma1.it

Abstract: Background: Gut microbiota has metabolic activity which influences mucosal homeostasis, local and systemic immune responses, and other anatomical systems (i.e., brain). The effects of dysbiosis are still poorly studied in Human Immunodeficiency Virus-1 (HIV-1) positive subjects and insufficient data are available on the impairment of the gut-brain axis, despite neurocognitive disorders being commonly diagnosed in these patients. This study evaluated the impact of a probiotic supplementation strategy on intrathecal immune activation and cognitive performance in combined antiretroviral therapy (cART) treated HIV-1 infected subjects. **Methods:** Thirty-five HIV-1 infected individuals were included in this study. At baseline (T0) a battery of tests was administered, to evaluate neurocognitive function and a lumbar puncture was performed to determine neopterin concentration in cerebrospinal fluid (CSF), as a marker of Central Nervous System (CNS) immune activation. Subsequently, a subgroup of participants underwent a 6-month course of multi-strain probiotics supplementation; this intervention group was evaluated, after probiotic treatment, with a second lumbar puncture and with repeated neurocognitive tests. **Results:** At T0, all participants showed impaired results in at least one neurocognitive test and elevated neopterin concentrations in CSF. After supplementation with probiotics (T6), the interventional group presented a significant decrease in neopterin concentration and a significant improvement in several neurocognitive tests. In contrast, no significant modifications were observed in the neurocognitive performance of controls between T0 and T6. The CNS Penetration Effectiveness Score of antiretroviral therapy did not show an influence from any of the investigated variables. **Conclusions:** Multi-strain probiotic supplementation seems to exert a positive effect on neuroinflammation and neurocognitive impairment in HIV-1 infected subjects, but large trials are needed to support the concept that modulation of the gut microbiota can provide specific neurological benefits in these patients.

Keywords: HIV; asymptomatic neurocognitive impairment; immune activation; central nervous system; neopterin; probiotic; supplementation; multi-strain; dysbiosis; gut-brain axis

1. Introduction

Following the widespread use of combined antiretroviral therapy (cART) the prevalence of severe neurocognitive impairments, among HIV-1 infected individuals, considerably decreased, while the prevalence of milder extents of HIV-1 associated neurocognitive disorders, such as Asymptomatic Neurocognitive Impairment, persisted at a stable rate among this population [1]. Wider evidence shows that changes in the qualitative and quantitative composition of the gut's microbiome can affect the modulation of the gut-brain axis, thus resulting in the onset of behavioral and neurocognitive alterations [2]. For these reasons, the use of probiotics represents a novel potential approach to manage conditions, such as stress-related behaviors, and to ameliorate cognitive function in several pathological settings [3,4].

HIV-1 infected patients usually suffer from two conditions that negatively affect neurocognitive function: the alteration of the normal gut flora composition (dysbiosis), with the overgrowth of detrimental bacterial strains [5] and elevated cerebrospinal fluid (CSF) concentrations of neopterin, a biomarker of Central Nervous System (CNS) immune activation [6]. Neopterin—a biochemical product of the guanosine triphosphate pathway—is a recognized marker of monocyte activation, and an association between its expression and the development of HIV-associated neurocognitive disorders (HAND), Acquired Immuno-Deficiency Sindrome (AIDS) dementia complex, and HIV encephalitis have been proposed [7–10]. The expression of neopterin has been found to be higher in HIV-1-positive patients, compared to healthy people, and in naïve HIV-1-positive patients, compared to those on effective cART [10,11]. In this study, we evaluated the impact of a 6 month course of high dose multi-strain probiotic supplementation on CSF immune activation and neurocognitive impairment of HIV-1 positive patients.

2. Materials and Methods

2.1. Study Design, Recruitment, Study Eligibility Criteria and Ethics Statement

The present study included 35 HIV infected individuals, enrolled at the HIV Outpatient Clinic of the Department of Public Health and Infectious Diseases of University of Rome "Sapienza". The study protocol was approved by the internal committee of the Department of Public Health and Infectious Diseases of "Sapienza" University of Rome and by the Ethics Committee of Policlinico Umberto I Hospital, Rome (ethical approval code Rif# 2970). All participants agreed to the enrolment by signing a written informed consent form.

The design of the study is shown in Figure 1. Inclusion criteria for the enrolment in the study were: age >18 years old, a stable and effective (plasma HIV RNA <37 copies/mL) cART regimen for at least 6 months prior to enrolment. Exclusion criteria were: education below primary school, Mini Mental State Examination <26, any impairment in daily living activities, as defined in the Instrumental Activities of Daily Living scale, previous history or actual diagnosis of any neurologic or psychiatric condition, positive Polymerase Chain Reaction (PCR) on CSF for any of the following pathogens: Cytomegalovirus (CMV), Epstein-Barr virus (EBV), Herpes simplex virus-1 (HSV-1), Herpes simplex virus-2 (HSV-2), Varicella-zoster virus (VZV), Human herpesvirus-8 (HHV-8), BK virus (BKV), JC virus (JCV). At baseline (T0) all participants underwent (I) a lumbar puncture, to assess HIV-RNA, PCR for CMV, EBV, HSV-1, HSV-2, VZV, HHV-8, BKV, JCV, and neopterin concentration in CSF, (II) an array of neuropsychological tests.

Subsequently, we divided the enrolled patients into two groups, on the basis of their neuroinflammation levels (interventional group with higher level of CSF neopterin and control group with lower levels of CSF neopterin). Nine participants with higher levels of CSF neopterin (interventional group) underwent a six month course of supplementation with oral probiotics (2 sachets, each containing 450×10^9 billion bacteria, twice a day); the selected probiotic was a commercially available product with the following composition: *Lactobacillus plantarum* DSM 24730, *Streptococcus thermophilus* DSM 24731, *Bifidobacterium breve* DSM 24732, *Lactobacillus paracasei* DSM 24733, *Lactobacillus delbrueckii* subsp. *bulgaricus* DSM 24734, *Lactobacillus acidophilus* DSM 24735, *Bifidobacterium longum* DSM 24736, and *Bifidobacterium infantis* DSM 24737 (Vivomixx®, Dupont, Madison, WI, USA).

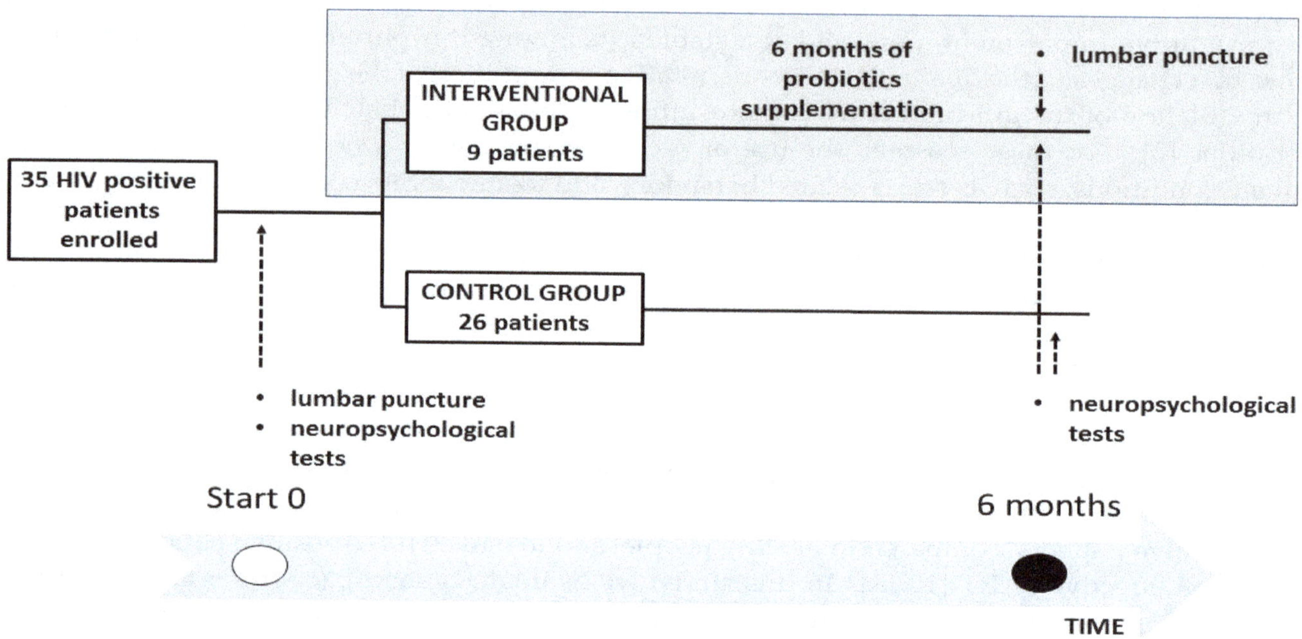

Figure 1. The design of the study. (Abbreviations. HIV: Human Immunodeficiency Virus).

At the end of the supplementation period (T6) participants from the intervention group underwent a second lumbar puncture and a second neurocognitive assessment battery, while controls (the remaining 26 subjects) were assessed with a second assay of neurocognitive tests (a parallel version of the Rey Auditory Verbal Learning Test (RAVLT) was administered at T6; parallel versions with Italian validation for the other tests are not available).

2.2. *Neuropsychological Test Battery*

Neuropsychological tests, administered by a trained neuropsychologist, explored verbal areas, language, attention, working memory, abstraction, executive, learning memory, processing speed of information, sensory-perceptual and motor skills. The tests included the Rey–Osterrieth Complex Figure Test (ROCF), to evaluate participants' recognition and recall skills for non-verbal contents, the Rey Auditory Verbal Learning Test (RAVLT) to evaluate short term auditory-verbal memory, rate of learning and retention of information, the Test of Weights and Measures Estimation (STEP), to evaluate abstraction skills, the Visual Search Test (Attention Matrices Test) to evaluate attention skills, the Verbal Fluency test (FAB), to evaluate executive functions and the ability to switch between different tasks, the Test of Phonological and Semantic Verbal Fluency (respectively PVF and SVF) to evaluate phonological and semantic supplies and the ability to access them, Raven's Standard Progressive Matrices (SPM), to evaluate abstract reasoning and problem solving capabilities, the Digit Span test, to evaluate short term memory and executive functions, the Corsi Block Tapping Test (CBTT) to evaluate short term spatial memory and executive functions, the Aachener Aphasia Test (AAT), to evaluate the presence of aphasia among study participants, the Trail Making Test A and B (TMT A and TMT B), to evaluate visual-spatial attention and motor skills. On average, the neuropsychological evaluation required 45 min for the operator.

2.3. Evaluation of Neopterin Levels by ELISA Assay

CSF was collected by lumbar puncture, and cell-free centrifuged supernatant samples were stored at −80 °C. CSF neopterin levels were determined by a commercially available solid phase enzyme-linked immunosorbent assay (ELISA), based on the basic principle of a competitive ELISA (IBL International GmbH, Hamburg, Germany). The upper normal reference value was previously determined to be 5 nmol/L (upper limit of the 99% confidence interval) [12].

2.4. Bacterial DNA Isolation from Fecal Samples

Faecal samples from patients enrolled in the intervention group, were collected at T0 and T6, in order to evaluate adherence to the treatment and the efficacy of the multi-strain probiotic supplementation in changing the microbiota composition. For this reason, the QIAamp DNA Stool Mini Kit (Qiagen, Hilden, Germany) was used according to the manufacturer's instructions: 200 mg of frozen samples were suspended in 1.4 mL of ASL lysis buffer from the stool kit, added with glass beads (150–212 μm, Sigma–Aldrich, St. Louis, MO, USA), and homogenized. The suspension was incubated at 95 °C for 5 min, DNA was purified and eluted in 200 μL of AE buffer and the samples obtained were stored at −20 °C. Finally, bacterial DNA from faecal samples was extracted and quantified by a real-time PCR, performed to evaluate Bifidobacteria levels. Briefly, PCR amplification and detection were performed on optical-grade 96-well plates, using the Applied Biosystems 7500 Real-Time PCR instrument (Applied Biosystems, Inc., Norwalk, CT, USA). The reaction mixture (25 μL) was composed of SensiMix SYBR Low-ROX (BIOLINE, Taunton, MA, USA), 500 nM primers for *Bifidobacterium* genus, and 2.5 μL of template DNA. A melting curve analysis was made after amplification, to distinguish target amplicons from aspecific non-target PCR products. Standard curves were made by using 10-fold dilutions of DNA, extracted from *Bifidobacterium breve*. All samples were analyzed in duplicate in two independent real-time PCR assays.

2.5. Statistical Analysis

A Wilcoxon test for paired samples and Pearson's correlation coefficient were applied for data analysis, using SPSS version 24 for Windows (IBM, New York, NY, USA). Graphics were done using GraphPad Prism software, version 5.0 (GraphPad Software Inc., La Jolla, CA, USA). Differences were considered statistically significant when $p < 0.05$.

3. Results

3.1. Demographic and Clinical Characteristics of HIV-1-Positive Patients

All 35 HIV-1 infected individuals enrolled were Caucasian. The majority of our population was represented by males (94%), the median age of participants was 48 years old (IQR: 38–54) and the median duration of time from diagnosis was 14 years (IQR: 7–23). All included subjects had finished at least the primary course of school education.

Individuals enrolled in the study had been taking cART therapy for a median of 14 years (IQR: 8–19) and they had been on a stable and effective ARV regimen for at least 1 year at the time of inclusion (all participants showed plasma HIV RNA <37 copies/mL at enrollment). Antiretroviral therapy did not change and anti-inflammatory drugs were not used during the follow-up. The median value, in regard to cluster of differentiation 4 (CD4) nadir, was 250 cell/μL (IQR: 45–400) while the median value of the actual CD4 count was 566 cell/μL (IQR: 397–714).

The CNS Penetration-Effectiveness score (CPE) of ARV regimens included in the study was calculated according to the classification proposed by Letendere et al. and the median CPE score of our population was 7 (IQR: 7–8).

3.2. *Correlations between Neuroinflammation and Neuropsychological Impairment*

At baseline (T0), all participants underwent a lumbar puncture to evaluate their HIV-1 viral load and the extent of neuro-inflammation (determined through the concentration of neopterin) into CSF. All subjects enrolled in the study showed an HIV-RNA in CSF <37 copies/mL and the median concentration of neopterin in CSF was 23.4 nmol/L (10.5–65.2). Participants also showed negative polimerase-chain reaction (PCR) tests on CSF for CMV, EBV, HSV-1, HSV-2, VZV, HHV-8, BKV and JCV.

At baseline, all participants showed a normal performance on the Mini-Mental State Examination (MMSE) and no impairment on the instrumental activities of daily living (IADL) scale. Neuropsychological tests, administered at T0, with the aim of assessing the neurocognitive performance, showed that all subjects presented an altered result in at least one test exploring the executive functions, moreover most participants presented with a pathological impairment in at least two different domains.

In our population, we did not observe a correlations between the CPE score and neopterin concentration in CSF ($r = 0.220$; $p = 0.271$); the CPE score did not show any correlations with the results of any of the proposed neurocognitive tests either. On the contrary, at T0, neopterin was inversely correlated with the results for the following tests: forward Corsi Block Tapping Test ($r = -0.474$; $p = 0.004$), backward Corsi Block Tapping Test ($r = -0.468$; $p = 0.005$), forward Digit test ($r = -0.480$; $p = 0.004$) and Verbal Fluency test ($r = -0.361$; $p = 0.033$). Neopterin showed slight inverse correlations with Raven's Standard Progressive Matrices test ($r = -0.308$; $p = 0.071$), the time estimation during the Test of Weights and Measures Estimation ($r = -0.295$; $p = 0.085$) and the Test of Weights and Measures total score ($r = -0.294$; $p = 0.087$).

3.3. *Results of Probiotic Supplementation: Reduction of Neuroinflammation and Recovery of Neuropsychological Impairment*

A subgroup of nine subjects (intervention group), including the individuals presenting with the highest extent of neuro-inflammation from the 35 patients enrolled, underwent a 6 months course with a high dose of oral probiotics supplementation (the main characteristics of this subpopulation are shown in Table 1). The main characteristics of this subpopulation of nine people, compared with the control group of the remaining 26 subjects, are shown in Table 1.

Table 1. Sub-study population (supplemented with multi-strain probiotics) and control group main characteristics (expressed as median values; interquartile range is reported between brackets).

Characteristics	Probiotics Supplementation Group	Control Group	*p*-Value
N of subjects	9	26	
Males	9	24	
Females	0	2	
Age	45 (35–52.5)	43 (38.2–53)	0.097
Years from diagnosis	14 (5–19.5)	12.5 (7–23)	0.593
Years on ARV treatment	14 (6.5–16)	12.5 (7–20)	0.373
T CD4 nadir	180 cell/μL (40–438)	288 cell/μL (57–407)	0.678
T CD4 at enrollment	651 cell/μL (563–883)	526 cell/μL (340–663)	0.515
CPE score	7 (7–7.25)	7 (7–8)	0.527
HIV-RNA in CSF	<37 copies/mL	<37 copies/mL	-
Neopterin in CSF	34.14 nmol/L (22.5–65.2)	12.3 nmol/L (10.1–14.8)	0.008

Abbreviations. ARV: antiretroviral; CD4: cluster of differentiation 4; CPE: Central Nervous System Penetration Effectiveness; CSF: cerebrospinal fluid.

The median neopterin concentration in CSF at T0 in this subpopulation was 34.14 nmol/L (IQR: 22.53–65.2), showing no significant difference in comparison to the median value of the entire population ($p = 0.655$), but significantly higher than the median value of the control group ($p = 0.008$) Before probiotic supplementation (T0), we did not find significant differences in neurocognitive performances between the two subgroups, despite the differences in neopterin levels. (Table 2). No statistically significant difference in CSF neopterin levels were found between the two groups ($p > 0.05$) at T0; higher levels were found in patients with the impairment of at least two neurocognitive domains, than in those with a single neurocognitive domain impairment.

Table 2. Baseline neurocognitive tests results (expressed as median values; interquartile range is reported between brackets).

Neurocognitive Tests	Probiotics Supplementation Group (T0)	Control Group (T0)	*p*-Value
Rey–Osterrieth Complex Figure immediate recall (*more is better*)	16.6 (15.9–17.8)	13.1 (8.5–22.0)	0.860
Rey–Osterrieth Complex Figure delayed recall (*more is better*)	15.5 (14.3–17.8)	11.6 (6.3–19.9)	0.280
Rey Auditory Verbal Learning Test immediate recall (*more is better*)	46.0 (29.4–47.4)	30.6 (27.9–40.0)	0.214
Rey Auditory Verbal Learning Test delayed recall (*more is better*)	9.2 (5.6–10.9)	5.2 (3.5–8.0)	0.360
Rey Auditory Verbal Learning Test recognition (*more is better*)	98.0 (90.0–100.0)	96.0 (92.0–98.0)	0.400
Verbal Fluency (*more is better*)	15.0 (13.7–16.0)	15.9 (13.9–18.0)	0.314
Phonological Verbal Fluency (*more is better*)	30.0 (23.6–39.2)	26.7 (21.6–35.1)	0.906
Semantic Verbal Fluency (*more is better*)	47.0 (33.5–57.5)	39.0 (33.0–42.0)	0.173
Visual Search Test (*more is better*)	46.2 (45.1–60.0)	46.7 (40.2–50.6)	0.374
Test of Weights and Measures Estimation—Time (*more is better*)	19.0 (13.0–23.5)	22.0 (19.0–24.0)	0.074
Test of Weights and Measures Estimation—Weight (*more is better*)	19.0 (14.0–20.5)	19.0 (16.5–21.0)	0.933
Test of Weights and Measures Estimation—Total (*more is better*)	38.0 (30.5–46.5)	40.0 (36.5–43.5)	0.594
Raven's Standard Progressive Matrices (*more is better*)	27.5 (22.6–31.6)	28.3 (25.7–31.8)	0.327
Verbal Span forward (*more is better*)	5.0 (3.5–5.7)	5.2 (4.9–6.0)	0.065
Verbal Span backward (*more is better*)	5.0 (4.0–5.0)	4.0 (3.0–4.5)	0.161
Corsi Block Tapping Test forward (*more is better*)	4.7 (4.0–5.2)	5.5 (4.7–6.0)	0.078
Corsi Block Tapping Test backward (*more is better*)	4.0 (3.0–4.0)	5.0 (4.0–6.0)	0.196
Aachener Aphasia Test (*more is better*)	9.0 (9.0–9.0)	9.0 (9.0–9.0)	1.000
Trail Making Test A (s) (*less is better*)	50.0 (44.0–62.0)	50.0 (41.0–67.0)	0.575
Trail Making Test B (s) (*less is better*)	115.0 (93.0–142.0)	97.0 (77.5–144.5)	0.086

At the end of supplementation (T6), in the intervention group, we observed that the results of viral replication in CSF remained stably suppressed (HIV-RNA in CSF resulted <37 copies/mL in all subjects at T6) and the neopterin concentration in CSF significantly decreased at T6 when compared to T0 values (T6 24.11 nmol/L vs. T0 34.14 nmol/L; $p = 0.011$). The results of the neuropsychological tests at T0 and T6 among participants who underwent probiotics supplementation are shown in Table 3; an improvement in overall neurocognitive performance was observed in the majority of our population, with a significant improvement revealed in multiple tests—immediate copy of the Rey–Osterrieth Complex Figure ($p = 0.0089$), delayed copy of the Rey–Osterrieth Complex Figure ($p = 0.0039$), immediate recall during the Rey Auditory Verbal Learning Test ($p = 0.027$), delayed recall during the Rey Auditory Verbal Learning Test ($p = 0.042$), time estimation during the Test of Time and Weights Estimation ($p = 0.043$), weight estimation during the Test of Time and Weights Estimation ($p = 0.035$), Phonological Verbal Fluency Test ($p = 0.027$), Trail Making Test A ($p = 0.0502$) and forward Corsi Block Tapping Test ($p = 0.057$). A direct correlation with neopterin concentration in CSF was observed at T6 with the results for the Trail Making Test B ($r = 0.741$; $p = 0.022$); in contrast an inverse correlation was observed between neopterin and the forward Corsi Block Tapping Test ($r = -0.793$; $p = 0.011$). A slight inverse correlation was also observed between Raven's Standard Progressive Matrices test and neopterin in CSF ($r = -0.644$; $p = 0.061$). CPE scores did not show any correlation with neopterin or any of the provided neurocognitive tests, at T6. No difference was observed in the CD4 count between T0 and T6 among these individuals (674 cell/μL vs. 682 cell/μL; $p = 0.959$).

Neurocognitive performance was also evaluated among the 26 individuals who did not undergo supplementation with probiotics; this was assessed by a second administration of the assay of neuropsychological tests at T6 (results are shown in Table 3). No difference between T0 and T6 was observed for neurocognitive performance among this group of participants.

Table 3. Neurocognitive tests results after supplementation with probiotics (expressed as median values; interquartile range is reported between brackets).

Performed Neurocognitive Tests	Probiotics Supplementation Group (T0 vs. T6)	Control Group (T0 vs. T6)	Probiotics Supplementation Group vs. Control Group (T6 vs.T6)
Rey–Osterrieth Complex Figure immediate recall (*more is better*)	16.6 vs. 22.0 ($p = 0.007$)	13.1 vs. 14.7 ($p = 0.603$)	22.0 (19.0–23.7) vs. 14.7 (8.8–20.3) ($p = 0.011$)
Rey-Osterrieth Complex Figure delayed recall (*more is better*)	15.5 vs. 22.4 ($p = 0.008$)	11.6 vs. 12.6 ($p = 0.369$)	22.4 (22.0–25.5) vs. 12.6 (5.7–19.1) ($p = 0.011$)
Rey Auditory Verbal Learning Test immediate recall (*more is better*)	46.0 vs. 53.0 ($p = 0.028$)	30.6 vs. 32.5 ($p = 0.619$)	53.0 (49.3–55.6) vs. 32.5 (28.7–37.5) ($p = 0.008$)
Rey Auditory Verbal Learning Test delayed recall (*more is better*)	9.2 vs. 12.0 ($p = 0.034$)	5.2 vs. 5.3 ($p = 0.241$)	12 .0 (10.7–13.8) vs. 5.3 (4.3–8.0) ($p = 0.008$)
Rey Auditory Verbal Learning Test recognition (*more is better*)	98.0 vs. 99.0 ($p = 0.176$)	96.0 vs. 96.0 ($p = 0.575$)	99.0 (97.0–100.0) vs. 96.0 (92.0–98.0) ($p = 0.013$)
Verbal Fluency (*more is better*)	15.0 vs. 15.9 ($p = 0.233$)	15.9 vs. 15.3 ($p = 0.152$)	15.9 (14.1–18.0) vs. 15.3 (13.7–16.8) ($p = 0.594$)
Phonological Verbal Fluency (*more is better*)	30.0 vs. 44.0 ($p = 0.028$)	26.7 vs. 25.9 ($p = 0.271$)	44.0 (42.5–45.0) vs. 25.9 (21.6–36.1) ($p = 0.021$)
Semantic Verbal Fluency (*more is better*)	47.0 vs. 49.0 ($p = 0.373$)	39 vs. 38.0 ($p = 0.396$)	49.0 (46.0–49.0) vs. 38.0 (33.5–43.5) ($p = 0.123$)

Table 3. *Cont.*

Performed Neurocognitive Tests	Probiotics Supplementation Group (T0 vs. T6)	Control Group (T0 vs. T6)	Probiotics Supplementation Group vs. Control Group (T6 vs.T6)
Visual Search Test (*more is better*)	46.2 vs. 49.0 (p = 0.859)	46.7 vs. 46.7 (p = 1.000)	49.0 (45.6–50.0) vs. 46.7 (40.2–50.6) (p = 0.722)
Test of Weights and Measures Estimation—Time (*more is better*)	19.0 vs. 23.0 (p = 0.038)	22.0 vs. 22.0 (p = 0.776)	23.0 (21.0–23.5) vs. 22.0 (18.0–25.0) (p = 0.512)
Test of Weights and Measures Estimation—Weight (*more is better*)	19.0 vs. 21.0 (p = 0.027)	19 vs. 20.0 (p = 0.843)	21.0 (20.5–23.5) vs. 20.0 (15.5–21.5) (p = 0.08)
Test of Weights and Measures Estimation—Total (*more is better*)	38.0 vs. 45.0 (p = 0.138)	40.0 vs. 40.0 (p = 0.776)	45.0 (41.5–46.0) vs. 40.0 (35.5–44.0) (p = 0.02)
Raven's Standard Progressive Matrices (*more is better*)	25.7 vs. 30.0 (p = 0.208)	28.3 vs. 28.3 (p = 0.939)	30.0 (28.5–33.5) vs. 28.3 (25.2–31.6) (p = 0.374)
Verbal Span forward (*more is better*)	5.0 vs. 5.0 (p = 0.121)	5.2 vs. 5.2 (p = 0.632)	5.0 (5.0–6.0) vs. 5.2 (4.6–6.0) (p = 0.551)
Verbal Span backward (*more is better*)	5.0 vs. 5.0 (p = 1.000)	4.0 vs. 4.0 (p = 0.344)	5.0 (4.0–5.0) vs. 4.0 (3.75–5.0) (p = 0.206)
Corsi Block Tapping Test forward (*more is better*)	4.7 vs. 5.2 (p = 0.049)	5.5 vs. 5.2 (p = 0.980)	5.2 (5.0–5.5) vs. 5.2 (5.0–6.0) (p = 0.888)
Corsi Block Tapping Test backward (*more is better*)	4.0 vs. 4.0 (p = 0.180)	5.0 vs. 5.0 (p = 0.317)	4.0 (4.0–4.5) vs. 5.0 (4.0–5.0) (p = 0.102)
Aachener Aphasia Test (*more is better*)	9.0 vs. 9.0 (p = 1.000)	9.0 vs. 9.0 (p = 1.000)	9.0 (9.0–9.0) vs. 9.0 (9.0–9.0) (p = 1.000)
Trail Making Test A (s) (*less is better*)	50.0 vs. 43.0 (p = 0.041)	50.0 vs. 51.0 (p = 0.747)	43.0 (39.0–53.0) vs. 51.0 (40.5–65.5) (p = 0.674)
Trail Making Test B (s) (*less is better*)	115.0 vs. 120.0 (p = 0.726)	97.0 vs. 98.0 (p = 0.279)	120.0 (76.0–138.0) vs. 98.0 (78.5–146.0) (p = 0.138)

3.4. Adherence to Probiotic Supplementation and Safety of the Treatment

Adherence to the probiotic supplementation was documented by the increase in Bifidobacteria spp. in fecal samples collected at T6, compared to their basal level (T0). No side effects were observed over the course of 6 months of treatment in all patients.

4. Discussion

In recent years, the interdependence between the microbiome, gut and brain has been highlighted. The disruption of the gut mucosa barrier and intestinal dysbiosis—both conditions commonly observed in HIV-1 infected patients—play a pivotal role in the pathogenesis of HIV infection [13] and several studies have shown the beneficial effects of probiotics on the intestinal barrier, systemic immune activation and tryptophan metabolism of on HIV-1 infected patients [14,15].

At T0, in the overall analysis of the 35 patients enrolled, we observed that higher neopterin levels in CSF were correlated with a poorer result in the neurocognitive tests. No correlation was observed between the CNS Penetration Effectiveness (CPE) score and the neopterin concentration in CSF, nor between the CPE score and neurocognitive performance, suggesting a possible low impact of cART on the treatment of neuroinflammation and neurocognitive impairment.

When we divided the enrolled patients into two groups (intervention group and control group) on the basis of their neuroinflammation levels, we observed that, at T0, both groups showed similar results in neurocognitive performances (Table 2), despite their different neopterin concentrations observed in CSF; taken together, these data suggest that the levels of neuroinflammation are not the only determinant of the neurocognitive impairment in HIV-1 infected patients. On the other hand, to investigate the role of dysbiosis on neuroinflammation and cognitive performance, we assigned nine participants (with highest levels of neuroinflammation shown by their levels of neopterin in CSF, which were higher than the control group) from our study population, to start supplementation with oral probiotics for 6 months (interventional group).

At the end of the supplementation period, we observed a reduction in CNS immune activation and an improvement in cognitive performance in the intervention group, thus suggesting a possible role of probiotics in the treatment of the intrathecal immune activation and cognitive impairment of HIV infected individuals. In fact, at T6, the intervention group showed improved results in comparison to controls in the following tests: immediate recall of ROCF, delayed recall of ROCF, immediate recall of RAVLT, delayed recall of RAVLT, recognition of RAVLT, FAB, STEP weight and STEP total; improvements were also observed within the intervention group between T0 and T6, while, on the other hand, controls showed no advances (Table 3).

Also, the neopterin concentration decreased after supplementation with probiotics, but the reduction in the neopterin concentration cannot be explained by better suppression of HIV replication in CSF, given the fact that HIV-RNA results were undetectable in all participants at T0 and T6. On the other hand, the alteration of the gut mucosa barrier that occurs during HIV-1 infection allows a large amount of bacterial-derived products (such as lipopolysaccharides) to enter into the general circulation, thus causing systemic immune activation. Experimental evidence has shown that lipopolysaccharides can alter the blood-brain barrier permeability [16], possibly leading to leakage of the serum pro-inflammatory milieu into the CSF, precipitating local inflammation. In this sense, several studies have shown that the gut microbiota and its products play central regulatory roles in this bidirectional relationship between the enteric and the central nervous system and on gut-brain axis [17–22]. The administration of probiotics to correct dysbiosis reduces microbial translocation, systemic inflammation and, possibly, the subsequent blood-brain barrier permeability, thus exerting an ameliorative effect on intrathecal immune activation and cognitive function.

For these reasons, probiotic supplementation could represent an innovative therapeutic resource, enhancing the direct-indirect effects of the gut environment on the CNS, through the rebalance of the microbiota composition.

5. Conclusions

The results of this study were limited by the small sample size of patients analyzed and by the possible influence of the operator and repeated tests on neuropsychological performances. To minimize these practice effects, we used parallel/alternate forms of tests, but we are aware that it does not fully eliminate concerns about this topic. Further limits were the lack of CSF samples at T6 in the control group and of plasmatic/serological markers of immune activation. The significance of our results was restricted by the inclusion of only patients with ANI (Asymptomatic Neurocognitive Impairment). Moreover, a possible limitation is the role of ANI that is, at present, being debated.

Despite these limitations, justified by the complexity of the procedures and ethical issues, our findings suggest that supplementation with probiotics could represent a novel strategy to manage neurocognitive impairment in cART treated HIV-1 infected patients, but larger studies are needed prior to introducing this intervention into everyday clinical practice.

Acknowledgments: We thank all the participants for the study.

Author Contributions: Giancarlo Ceccarelli, study concept and design, interpretation of data and critical revision of manuscript for intellectual content; Eugenio Nelson Cavallari, study concept and design, acquisition, analysis and interpretation of data; Ivan Schietroma, study concept and design, acquisition, analysis and interpretation of data; Giuseppe Corano Scheri, study concept and design, acquisition, analysis and interpretation of data; Saeid Najafi Fard, study concept, acquisition of data; Claudia Pinacchio, study design, acquisition of data;

Mariangela Fratino, study concept, acquisition, analysis and interpretation of data; Carolina Scagnolari, study design, critical revision of manuscript for intellectual content; Ivano Mezzaroma, study design, interpretation of data, critical revision of manuscript for intellectual content; Vincenzo Vullo, and Jason M. Brenchley study supervision, critical revision of manuscript for intellectual content; Gabriella d'Ettorre, study concept and design, interpretation of data, study supervision, critical revision of manuscript for intellectual content.

References

1. Heaton, R.K.; Franklin, D.R.; Ellis, R.J.; McCutchan, J.A.; Letendre, S.L.; LeBlanc, S.; Corkran, S.H.; Duarte, N.A.; Clifford, D.B.; Woods, S.P.; et al. HIV-associated neurocognitive disorders before and during the era of combination antiretroviral therapy: Differences in rates, nature, and predictors. *J. Neurovirol.* **2011**, *17*, 3–16. [CrossRef] [PubMed]
2. Dinan, T.G.; Stilling, R.M.; Stanton, C.; Cryan, J.F. Collective unconscious: How gut microbes shape human behavior. *J. Psychiatr. Res.* **2015**, *63*, 1–9. [CrossRef] [PubMed]
3. Akbari, E.; Asemi, Z.; Daneshvar Kakhaki, R.; Bahmani, F.; Kouchaki, E.; Tamtaji, O.R.; Hamidi, G.A.; Salami, M. Effect of Probiotic Supplementation on Cognitive Function and Metabolic Status in Alzheimer's Disease: A Randomized, Double-Blind and Controlled Trial. *Front. Aging Neurosci.* **2016**, *8*, 256. [CrossRef] [PubMed]
4. Huang, R.; Wang, K.; Hu, J. Effect of Probiotics on Depression: A Systematic Review and Meta-Analysis of Randomized Controlled Trials. *Nutrients* **2016**, *8*, 483. [CrossRef] [PubMed]
5. Zilberman-Schapira, G.; Zmora, N.; Itav, S.; Bashiardes, S.; Elinav, H.; Elinav, E. The gut microbiome in human immunodeficiency virus infection. *BMC Med.* **2016**, *14*, 83. [CrossRef] [PubMed]
6. Hagberg, L.; Cinque, P.; Gisslen, M.; Brew, B.J.; Spudich, S.; Bestetti, A.; Price, R.W.; Fuchs, D. Cerebrospinal fluid neopterin: An informative biomarker of central nervous system immune activation in HIV-1 infection. *AIDS Res. Ther.* **2010**, *7*, 15. [CrossRef] [PubMed]
7. Griffin, D.E.; McArthur, J.C.; Cornblath, D.R. Neopterin and interferon-gamma in serum and cerebrospinal fluid of patients with HIV-associated neurologic disease. *Neurology* **1991**, *41*, 69–74. [CrossRef] [PubMed]
8. Sönnerborg, A.B.; von Stedingk, L.V.; Hansson, L.O.; Strannegård, O.O. Elevated neopterin and β2-microglobulin levels in blood and cerebrospinal fluid occur early in HIV-1 infection. *AIDS* **1989**, *3*, 277–283. [CrossRef] [PubMed]
9. Fuchs, D.; Chiodi, F.; Albert, J.; Asjö, B.; Hagberg, L.; Hausen, A.; Norkrans, G.; Reibnegger, G.; Werner, E.R.; Wachter, H. Neopterin concentrations in cerebrospinal fluid and serum of individuals infected with HIV-1. *AIDS* **1989**, *3*, 285–288. [CrossRef] [PubMed]
10. Eden, A.; Price, R.W.; Spudich, S.; Fuchs, D.; Hagberg, L.; Gisslén, M. Immune activation of the central nervous system is still present after >4 years of effective HAART. *J. Infect. Dis.* **2007**, *196*, 1779–1783. [CrossRef] [PubMed]
11. Yilmaz, A.; Yiannoutsos, C.T.; Fuchs, D.; Price, R.W.; Crozier, K.; Hagberg, L.; Spudich, S.; Gisslén, M. Cerebrospinal fluid neopterin decay characteristics after initiation of antiretroviral therapy. *J. Neuroinflamm.* **2013**, *10*, 10–62. [CrossRef] [PubMed]
12. Viaccoz, A.; Ducray, F.; Tholance, Y.; Barcelos, G.K.; Thomas-Maisonneuve, L.; Ghesquières, H.; Meyronet, D.; Quadrio, I.; Cartalat-Carel, S.; Louis-Tisserand, G.; et al. CSF neopterin level as a diagnostic marker in primary central nervous system lymphoma. *Neuro Oncol.* **2015**, *17*, 1497–1503. [CrossRef] [PubMed]
13. Tincati, C.; Douek, D.; Marchetti, G. Gut barrier structure, mucosal immunity and intestinal microbiota in the pathogenesis and treatment of HIV infection. *AIDS Res. Ther.* **2016**, *13*, 19. [CrossRef] [PubMed]
14. D'ettorre, G.; Rossi, G.; Scagnolari, C.; Andreotti, M.; Giustini, N.; Serafino, S.; Schietroma, I.; Scheri, G.C.; Fard, S.N.; Trinchieri, V. Probiotic supplementation promotes a reduction in T-cell activation, an increase in Th17 frequencies, and a recovery of intestinal epithelium integrity and mitochondrial morphology in ART-treated HIV-1-positive patients. *Immun. Inflamm. Dis.* **2017**, *20*. [CrossRef] [PubMed]
15. Scagnolari, C.; Corano Scheri, G.; Selvaggi, C.; Schietroma, I.; Fard, S.N.; Mastrangelo, A.; Giustini, N.; Serafino, S.; Pinacchio, C.; Pavone, P. Probiotics Differently Affect Gut-Associated Lymphoid Tissue Indolamine-2,3-Dioxygenase mRNA and Cerebrospinal Fluid Neopterin Levels in Antiretroviral-Treated HIV-1 Infected Patients: A Pilot Study. *Int. J. Mol. Sci.* **2016**, *17*, 1639. [CrossRef] [PubMed]

16. Banks, W.A.; Gray, A.M.; Erickson, M.A.; Salameh, T.S.; Damodarasamy, M.; Sheibani, N.; Meabon, J.S.; Wing, E.E.; Morofuji, Y.; Cook, D.G. Lipopolysaccharide-induced blood-brain barrier disruption: Roles of cyclooxygenase, oxidative stress, neuroinflammation, and elements of the neurovascular unit. *J. Neuroinflamm.* **2015**, *12*, 223. [CrossRef] [PubMed]
17. Ceccarelli, G.; Fratino, M.; Selvaggi, C.; Giustini, N.; Serafino, S.; Schietroma, I.; Corano Scheri, G.; Pavone, P.; Passavanti, G.; Alunni Fegatelli, D.; et al. A pilot study on the effects of probiotic supplementation on neuropsychological performance and microRNA-29a-c levels in antiretroviral-treated HIV-1-infected patients. *Brain Behav.* **2017**, *7*, e00756. [CrossRef] [PubMed]
18. Ceccarelli, G.; Vullo, V.; d'Ettorre, G. Single-strain vs. multi-strain probiotic supplementation strategy against rheumatoid arthritis. *Arthritis Rheumatol.* **2017**. [CrossRef] [PubMed]
19. D'ettorre, G.; Ceccarelli, G.; Giustini, N.; Serafino, S.; Calantone, N.; de Girolamo, G.; Bianchi, L.; Bellelli, V.; Ascoli-Bartoli, T.; Marcellini, S. Probiotics Reduce Inflammation in Antiretroviral Treated, HIV-Infected Individuals: Results of the "Probio-HIV" Clinical Trial. *PLoS ONE* **2015**, *10*, e0137200. [CrossRef] [PubMed]
20. Scheri, G.C.; Fard, S.N.; Schietroma, I.; Mastrangelo, A.; Pinacchio, C.; Giustini, N.; Serafino, S.; de Girolamo, G.; Cavallari, E.N.; Statzu, M. Modulation of Tryptophan/Serotonin Pathway by Probiotic Supplementation in Human Immunodeficiency Virus-Positive Patients: Preliminary Results of a New Study Approach. *Int. J. Tryptophan Res.* **2017**. [CrossRef]
21. O'Hara, A.M.; Shanahan, F. The gut flora as a forgotten organ. *EMBO Rep.* **2006**, *7*, 688–693. [CrossRef] [PubMed]
22. Thomas, L.V.; Suzuki, K.; Zhao, J. Probiotics: A proactive approach to health. A symposium report. *Br. J. Nutr.* **2015**, *114* (Suppl. 1), S1–S15. [CrossRef] [PubMed]

10

Probiotic, Prebiotic and Brain Development

Tomás Cerdó [1,2], Alicia Ruíz [2,3], Antonio Suárez [3] and Cristina Campoy [1,2,4,5,*]

1 Department of Paediatrics, School of Medicine, University of Granada, 18016 Granada, Spain; tcr@ugr.es
2 EURISTIKOS Excellence Centre for Paediatric Research, Biomedical Research Centre, University of Granada, 18016 Granada, Spain; aliruizrodriguez@ugr.es
3 Department of Biochemistry and Molecular Biology 2, Biomedical Research Centre, University of Granada, 18016 Granada, Spain; asuarez@ugr.es
4 Spanish Network of Biomedical Research in Epidemiology and Public Health (CIBERESP), Carlos III Institute, 18016 Granada, Spain
5 Department of Paediatrics, Faculty of Medicine, University of Granada, Av. de la Investigación, 11, 18016 Granada, Spain
* Correspondence: ccampoy@ugr.es

Abstract: Recently, a number of studies have demonstrated the existence of a link between the emotional and cognitive centres of the brain and peripheral functions through the bi-directional interaction between the central nervous system and the enteric nervous system. Therefore, the use of bacteria as therapeutics has attracted much interest. Recent research has found that there are a variety of mechanisms by which bacteria can signal to the brain and influence several processes in relation to neurotransmission, neurogenesis, and behaviour. Data derived from both in vitro experiments and in vivo clinical trials have supported some of these new health implications. While recent molecular advancement has provided strong indications to support and justify the role of the gut microbiota on the gut–brain axis, it is still not clear whether manipulations through probiotics and prebiotics administration could be beneficial in the treatment of neurological problems. The understanding of the gut microbiota and its activities is essential for the generation of future personalized healthcare strategies. Here, we explore and summarize the potential beneficial effects of probiotics and prebiotics in the neurodevelopmental process and in the prevention and treatment of certain neurological human diseases, highlighting current and future perspectives in this topic.

Keywords: microbiota; prebiotics; probiotics; health; disease

---

1. Introduction

The micro-organisms that inhabit the human gastrointestinal tract (GI) have been implicated in the development and functioning of a number of basic physiological processes, such as digestion, immunity, and the maintenance of homeostasis. The GI microbiota may also play a role in multiple diseases, ranging from inflammation to obesity [1,2]. Recently, many studies have shown that gut microbiota play a very important role in the development and function of the central nervous system (CNS) through specific channels, such as metabolic, neuroendocrine, and immune pathways [3]. In particular, these researchers have found bi-directional communication between the brain and the gut microbiota, denominated the microbiota–gut–brain axis [4–6].

Although the molecular mechanisms by which the gut microbiota communicate with the brain are not yet clear, the link between both components is currently attributed to immune signals and the vagus nerve. Cellular components produced by gut microbiota, such as lipopolysaccharide (LPS), peptidoglycan, and flagellin, are recognized by pattern-recognition receptors (PRRs), such as Toll-like receptors (TLRs), NOD-like receptors (NLRs), or RIG-1-like receptors (RLRs), on epithelial and immune cells, producing cytokines, hormones, and other molecular signals, which will act as neurotransmitters within the CNS [7]. Several studies have found that, in the densely innervated gut, the vagus nerve is involved in the bi-directional communication of the microbiota–gut–brain axis [8,9], while others have shown vagus-independent effects [10,11]. Either way, a supplementing nutrition therapy with specific probiotic commensals and prebiotics can alter the excitability of enteric nervous system (ENS) sensory neurons [12–14]. Prebiotics-induced growth of probiotic members within the *Bifidobacterium* and *Lactobacillus* genera show multiple beneficial effects on host immunity and physiology [15]. Moreover, strong effects of *Bifidobacterium* and *Lactobacillus* spp. on the brain–gut axis have been reported [16].

This review summarizes current knowledge on the influence of the establishment of the gut microbiota in critical neurodevelopmental windows, and discusses recent findings on the interactions between the gut microbiota and the host's brain–gut axis communications. In addition, current research on the effects of the administration of probiotics and prebiotics in specific neurological disorders is reviewed. Finally, recommendations for future research on this topic are also discussed.

2. Establishment of Intestinal Microbiota during Early Neurodevelopmental Windows

Gut microbiota establish a beneficial cohabitation with the host that will prime for health later in life [17]. The assembly of the gut microbiota occurs during the first three years of life, starting from birth, where there is a rapid rate of colonization and expansion of gut bacteria dominated by *Actinobacteria* and *Proteobacteria* that shifts towards one dominated by *Firmicutes* and *Bacteroidetes*, increasing compositional diversity and stability while maturing into an adult-like state [18]. This process coincides in time with the intense synaptogenesis and pruning in the cerebral cortex during early life [18–20], ending in adolescence [21]. Therefore, perturbations of gut microbiota colonization and maturation by environmental factors may influence brain development. The dynamics of the microbial ecosystem's maturation during this critical period of CNS development is influenced by several environmental factors, such as mother-to-child bacterial transfer, mode of delivery, and type of feeding. The mother-to-child transfer of commensal bacteria in the uterus has been shown to influence an infant's immune system development [22,23]. Until recently, the idea that foetuses were sterile in the uterus and that the microbial colonization of the new-born started during and after birth had been widely accepted [24]. However, nowadays, this belief has been challenged by evidence of microbes in placenta and other tissues surrounding the foetus, such as umbilical cord blood after vaginal and caesarean birth [25–27]. Several studies have analysed the meconium of new-born babies and showed the presence of bacterial populations, including *Enterococcus*, *Lactococcus*, *Escherichia*, *Leuconostoc*, and *Streptococcus*, though at low levels, concluding that gut colonization occurs mainly after birth [28]. Based on these findings, prenatal probiotic intervention has been shown to modulate the expression of TLR-related genes in the placenta and foetal GI tract and to reduce atopic dermatitis [29,30]. Thus, prenatal and postnatal maternal oral probiotic therapy may represent an effective method of intervention to prevent pathologies such as allergy [31], atopic diseases [32], and neurodevelopmental disorders, reviewed below. Still, the origin of the microbiota colonizing the placenta is unknown and results have to be carefully interpreted, because, in samples with low microbial biomass, such as those from placenta, the risk of contamination is high when using high-throughput sequencing methods based on DNA amplification [29]. Further studies are needed to discern whether foetuses have contact with bacteria before birth or are colonized during and after parturition.

Regardless of mother-to-child transmission within the intrauterine environment, two different modes of maternal–infant transmission during delivery have been proposed: (a) horizontal, in which microbes are taken up from the environment for infants born by caesarean section; and (b) vertical, in which vaginal microbes are transferred during parturition to the infants [33]. Infants delivered by Caesarean section are more likely to suffer several diseases, such as asthma, obesity, or allergies, in adulthood [34]. Interestingly, a study carried out by Jasarevic et al. using a mouse model of early prenatal stress found that changes in the vaginal microbiome were associated with shifts in the abundance of *Lactobacillus* in the expression of maternal stress proteins related to vaginal immunity, in offspring metabolic profiles related to energy balance, and in the amino acid profiles of the developing brain [35].

The third strong environmental factor that influences an infant's gut microbial development as well as neurodevelopment is the type of feeding. In recent years, several studies have reported that breastfeeding and particularly full breastfeeding has beneficial effects on child neuropsychological development [36]. Human milk is the optimal feeding source, since it provides all the nutrition factors that an infant needs for healthy development. Human milk is not sterile, and, during breastfeeding, bacteria from mother's skin and mammary gland via maternal dendritic cells and macrophages [37] are transferred to the baby [38]. Breast-fed infants tend to contain a more uniform population of gut microbes dominated by *Bifidobacterium* and *Lactobacillus* [39], whereas formula-fed infants exhibit higher proportions of *Bacteroides, Clostridium, Streptococcus, Enterobacteria,* and *Veillonella* spp. [21]. Bacteria belonging to the *Bifidobacterium* genus present in human milk are early colonizers that characterize the gut microbial composition of healthy breast-fed new-born's [40] with beneficial functions for the host, such as the acceleration of the maturation of the immune response, the limitation of excessive inflammation, the improvement of the intestinal permeability, and an increase of acetate production [41]. In mice, *B. infantis* produces antidepressant-like effects and normalizes peripheral pro-inflammatory cytokine and tryptophan concentrations, both of which have been implicated in depression [42–44]. Moreover, breastfeeding has an additional role in the establishment of an infant's gut microbiota, since it contains bioactive molecules that are increasingly recognized as drivers of microbiota development and overall gut health [45]. Among the nutrients present in human milk, oligosaccharides constitute the third-most abundant class of molecules in terms of concentration after lactose and lipids. Nowadays, more than 200 different structures have been identified as human milk oligosaccharides (HMOs) [35]. HMOs can act as prebiotics, stimulating the growth of specific bacterial groups such as *Staphylococci* [46] and *Bifidobacteria* [47].

These results suggest that postnatal neurodevelopment and gut microbiota establishment co-occur, suggesting the intriguing possibility of a bi-directional regulation of each other's maturation [48]. Further studies are needed in order to clarify whether those differences in bacterial acquisition during early life lead to neurodevelopmental differences in infants.

3. Gut Microbiota–Brain Axis

The brain and the gut reciprocally influence each other by constant communication (Figure 1). The brain–gut–microbiota axis includes the CNS, the endocrine-immune system, the hypothalamus–pituitary–adrenal (HPA) axis, the autonomic nervous system, the ENS, and the gut microbiota [49]. This bi-directional communication enables signalling from the brain to influence motor, sensory, and secretory modalities of the GI tract, and conversely, signalling from the gut to affect brain function, most notably the hypothalamus and amygdala that are implicated in stress [50–52].

Though communication between brain and gut was realized in the middle of the nineteenth century [53], gut microorganisms had not been considered important for the development and function of the CNS or for brain diseases until recently, expanding the term to microbiome–gut–brain axis [54]. In humans, evidence of microbiome–gut–brain axis interactions have been obtained from the association of shifts in gut microbiota composition with central nervous disorders (i.e., autism spectrum disorder (ASD) and anxiety and depressive behaviours) and functional gastrointestinal disorders [54]. Most of the data demonstrating the role of the microbiota in the gut–brain axis have been obtained from germ-free animals [55]. Mice fed with prebiotics showed diminished stressor-induced anxiety-like behavior [56]. In a mouse model of ASD, Buffington et al. showed that a maternal high-fat diet reduced the number of oxytocin immunoreactive neurons in the hypothalamus and induced dysbiosis that was restored by a commensal *Lactobacillus reuteri* strain [57]. In a mouse model of Parkinson's disease, Sampson et al. highlighted a negative interaction in the microbiome–gut–brain axis because the absence of gut bacteria decreased aggregated misfolded α-synuclein levels and reduced the severity of the animals' abnormal movements. The authors showed that short chain fatty acids (SCFA), such as acetate, propionate, and butyrate, the end products of anaerobic fermentation of dietary fibre and starch, promoted a microglia-mediated immune response and increased α-synuclein aggregation, causing movement abnormalities [58]. Butyrate can cross the blood-brain barrier (BBB) and produce a dose-dependent increase in neuronal and glial nuclear histone H3 acetylation in mice due to its potential to inhibit histone deacetylation [59]. Another metabolite whose levels in the host are influenced by gut microbiota is tryptophan, the amino acid precursor of the neurotransmitter serotonin, and kynurenine, the main breakdown product of tryptophan catabolism [60]. Kynurenine intake during gestation and postnatal development, a time frame in which the maternal and offspring microbiota undergo major compositional and functional remodelling, produced neurochemical and cognitive deficits later in adulthood [61]. The prenatal inhibition of kynurenine synthesis modified hippocampal neuron morphology and changed neocortical and cerebellar protein expression that persisted into adulthood. In germ-free and in antibiotic-induced microbiota-depleted mice, despite increased circulating tryptophan levels, serotonin and kynurenin availabilities were decreased, suggesting that gut microbiota modulated kynurenin metabolism [62]. Distinct gut microbial species affect host physiology, producing diverse neuromolecules involved in mood regulation. *Lactobacillus* and *Bifidobacterium* spp. generate gamma-aminobutyric acid (GABA). *Candida, Streptococcus, Escherichia,* and *Enterococcus* spp. synthesise serotonin while *Bacillus* spp. produces dopamine [63].

Gut microbiota also influence the regulation of BBB integrity. The BBB is an active interface between systemic circulation and the CNS that maintains brain homeostasis by preventing the entry of potentially toxic or harmful substances and regulates the transport of nutrients and the removal of metabolites [64]. Braniste et al. (2014) [65] showed that the transplantation of gut microbiota into germ-free mice normalized BBB permeability and upregulated the expression of tight junction proteins. Therefore, gut microbiota have a key role in regulating BBB permeability, suggesting that the maternal gut microbiome influences an offspring's BBB integrity. Together with the results discussed in the previous section, these findings open an intriguing question on the mechanism by which a mother's gut microbiota cooperate in regulating BBB integrity and ultimately brain function development.

Gut microbiota have direct effects on the immune system, which constitutes another route of communication between gut microbes and the brain. The signalling molecules of the immune system, cytokines and chemokines, access the brain from the periphery via the vagus nerve or directly via the circumventricular organs [66]. The administration of rifaximin (a non-systemic, broad-spectrum antibiotic) to stressed rats increased the abundance of *Lactobacillus* in the ileum and the expression of the tight junction protein occludin while decreasing the expression of pro-inflammatory interleukin 17, interleukin 6, and tumour necrosis factor α mRNA [67].

Since many of the above effects have been observed during early life, it is plausible that an environmentally induced dysbiosis of infants' microbiota (e.g., mode of birth, maternal transmission of a suboptimal microbiota, antibiotics) may generate altered patterns of microbial metabolites with detrimental effects in human CNS development. Further research is needed to unravel these mechanisms and develop probiotics or prebiotics therapies that shape gut microbial composition and metabolism to ultimately modulate CNS development.

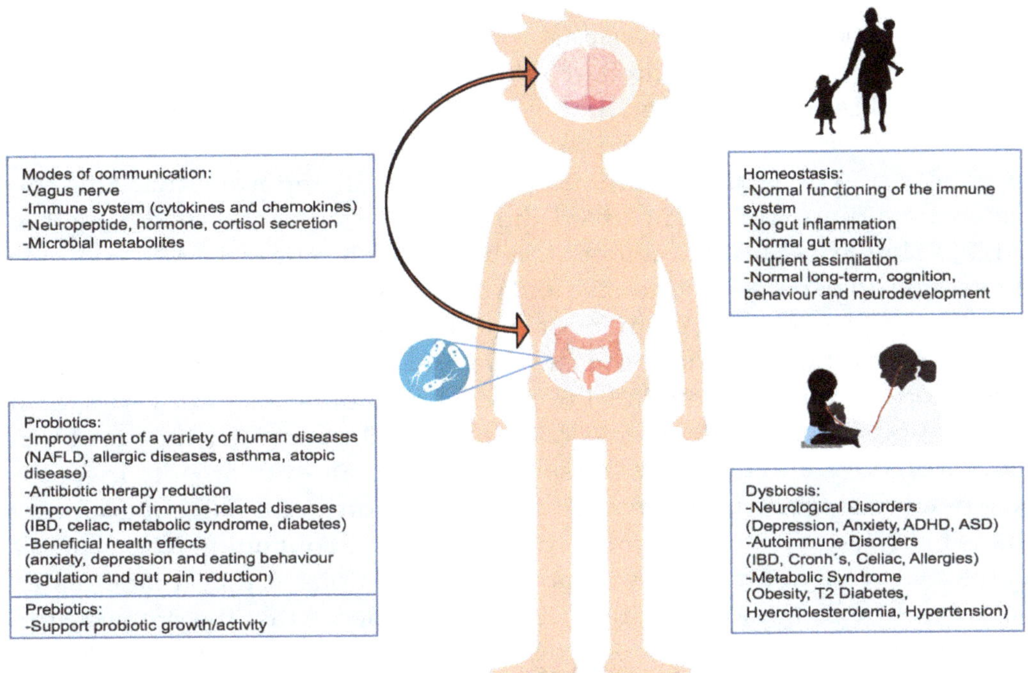

Figure 1. The gut microbiota–brain axis. The central part of the figure shows the bidirectional influence between the brain and gut microbiota. The left side of this figure shows modes of communication in the bidirectional crosstalk between gut microbiota and the brain and the possible influences of prebiotics and probiotics on human diseases. The right side of the figure shows the consequences of gut dysbiosis/homeostasis. Intestinal dysbiosis can adversely influence gut physiology, leading to inappropriate brain–gut axis signalling and associated consequences for CNS functions and disease states. Abbreviations: Non-Alcoholic Fatty Liver Disease (NAFLD), Inflammatory Bowel Disease (IBD), Attention deficit hyperactivity disorder (ADHD), Autism spectrum disorder (ASD).

4. Probiotics

In 2001, the Food and Agriculture Organization of the United Nations and the World Health Organization (FAO/WHO) proposed the following definition of probiotics: "live micro-organisms which, when administered in adequate amounts, confer a health benefit on the host" [68], which was reaffirmed in 2014 [69]. Probiotics, comprised by strains of *Lactobacilli*, *Bifidobacteria* and *Saccharomycetes* have been suggested to play a role in fighting human diseases, such as non-alcoholic fatty liver disease (NAFLD), allergy diseases, and asthma. They also promote protection against atopic disease in the infant during pregnancy and breastfeeding [32,70,71]. In addition, probiotics also reduce the duration of antibiotic therapy, and reduce symptom severity in immune-related diseases, such as inflammatory bowel diseases (IBDs), celiac disease, metabolic syndrome and diabetes [72,73].

The search for probiotics that can affect cognitive functions, known as psychobiotics, has increased in recent years (Table 1). Psychobiotics are defined as live organisms that, when ingested in adequate amounts, produce beneficial health effects to patients suffering from psychiatric illness [74]. Depression is currently a major psychiatric disorder in developed countries, and is characterized by a low mood or loss of interest and anxiety affecting appetite and sleep. Messaoudi et al. [75,76] reported a double-blind, placebo-controlled, randomized study where a multispecies probiotic containing *Lactobacillus helveticus* R0052 and *Bifidobacterium longum* R0175 (PF) was administered to healthy women for 30 days. This treatment resulted in a decrease in the global scores of the hospital anxiety and depression scale (HADs) and the global severity index of the Hopkins symptoms checklist (HSCL-90) due to the decrease of the sub-scores of somatization, depression, and anger–hostility spheres. In a cohort of 124 healthy humans, Benton et al. reported that the consumption of *Lactobacillus casei*-containing yogurt improved the self-reported mood of those whose mood was initially poor [77]. Similarly, Steenbergen et al. reported a significantly reduced overall cognitive reactivity to depression, in particular aggressive and ruminative thoughts, in forty healthy young adults that consumed either a probiotic supplement or placebo for 4 weeks [78]. Recently, Akkasheh et al. showed that the consumption of a probiotic supplement significantly decreased Beck Depression Inventory (BDI) scores, indicating overall improved symptoms, including mood, in 40 patients diagnosed with depression [79]. Conversely, Marcos et al. reported that probiotics decreased, respectively, levels of stress and anxiety assessed using the state-trait anxiety inventory (STAI) that remained unchanged in subjects under academic examination stress [80]. In a recent study carried out by Romijn et al. [81], administering a multispecies probiotic containing *L. helveticus* and *B. longum* in 79 participants that were not taking psychotropic medications at that moment and with at least moderate scores on self-report mood measures, found no evidence that the probiotic formulation was effective in treating low mood or in moderating the levels of inflammatory and other biomarkers. Improved cognitive function (neuropsychological and cognitive fatigue) was reported by Chung et al., which tested a *L. helveticus*-fermented milk in healthy 60–75 year olds, though no effects on stress or geriatric depression symptoms were observed [82].

Probiotics affect mood by their ability to modulate pain in the gut. A recent study reported that the administration of *Lactobacillus reuteri* DSM 17938 in the treatment of children with functional abdominal pain (FAP) and irritable bowel syndrome (IBS) is associated with a possible reduction of the intensity of pain [83]. In 35 patients suffering from chronic fatigue syndrome, Rao et al. showed that while the consumption of the probiotic improved anxiety scores, it had no effect on depressive symptoms [84]. Giannetti et al. also reported that a probiotic mixture of *B. infantis* M-63, *B. breve* M-16V, and *B longum* BB536 was associated with improvement in children with IBS, but not in children with functional dyspepsia (FD) [85]. In healthy women without gastrointestinal or psychiatric symptoms, the consumption of a fermented milk product containing *B. animalis* subsp. *lactis*, *Streptococcus thermophilus*, *Lactobacillus bulgaricus*, and *L. lactis* subsp. *lactis* resulted in robust alterations in activity in the brain regions that control the central processing of emotions and sensations, as observed by functional magnetic resonance imaging [86].

Table 1. Studies evaluating probiotics supplementation on central nervous system (CNS) disorders.

Study (Reference)	Cohort Population	Probiotic Used	Key Findings
Messaoudi et al. (2011) [75,76]	55 healthy human volunteers plus 25 subjects with urinary free cortisol (UFC) levels less than 50 ng/mL (less stressed subjects), 10 subjects received the probiotic and 15 placebo.	*Lactobacillus helveticus* R0052 and *Bifidobacterium longum* R0175 (PF)	Beneficial effects on anxiety and depression related behaviors in healthy human volunteers and volunteers with lower levels of cortisol
Benton et al. (2007) [77]	124 healthy adults volunteers were randomly allocated to a group that consumed, on a daily basis, a probiotic-containing milk drink or a placebo	*Lactobacillus casei* Shirota	The consumption of a probiotic-containing yoghurt improved the mood of those whose mood was initially poor. However, there was not an increased frequency of defaecation.
Steenbergen et al. (2015) [78]	40 healthy young adults were randomly assigned to receive a 4-week intervention of either placebo or multispecies probiotics in a triple-blind intervention assessment design.	*Bifidobacterium bifidum* W23, *Bifidobacterium lactis* W52, *Lactobacillus acidophilus* W37, *Lactobacillus brevis* W63, *Lactobacillus casei* W56, *Lactobacillus salivarius* W24, and *Lactococcus lactis* (W19 and W58)	Participants who received multispecies probiotics showed a significantly reduced overall cognitive reactivity to sad mood, which was largely accounted for by reduced rumination and aggressive thoughts.
Akkasheh et al. (2016) [79]	40 patients with a diagnosis of major depressive disorder (MDD) whose age ranged between 20 and 55 years were randomized.	*Lactobacillus acidophilus*, *Lactobacillus casei*, and *Bifidobacterium bifidum*.	Patients who received probiotic supplements had significantly decreased Beck Depression Inventory total scores
Marcos et al. (2004) [80]	136 university students were randomized.	*Lactobacillus delbrueckii* subsp. *bulgaricus* and *Streptococcus salivarius* subsp. *thermophilus* plus *Lactobacillus casei* DN-114001	There was no significant treatment effect on anxiety.
Romijn et al. (2017) [81]	79 participants not currently taking psychotropic medications with at least moderate scores on self-report mood measures. Participants were randomly allocated to receive a probiotic preparation or placebo.	*Lactobacillus helveticus* and *Bifidobacterium longum*	No significant difference was found between the probiotic and placebo groups on any psychological outcome measured.
Jadrešin et al. (2017) [83]	55 children with age between 4 and 18 years old, diagnosed as functional abdominal pain (FAP) or irritable bowel syndrome (IBS) were randomly allocated.	*Lactobacillus reuteri* DSM 17938	Administration of *L. reuteri* DSM 17938 was associated with a possible reduction of the intensity of pain and significantly more days without pain in children with FAP and IBS
Giannetti et al. (2016) [85]	48 children with IBS aged between 8 and 17.9 years and 25 with functional dyspepsia (FD) with age between 8 and 16.6 years were randomized.	*Bifidobacterium infantis* M-63, *breve* M-16V, and *longum* BB536	In children with IBS a mixture of *Bifidobacteria* is associated with improvement in abdominal pain (AP) and quality of life (QoL).
Kałużna-Czaplińska et al. (2012) [87]	22 autistic children.	*Lactobacillus acidophilus*	The probiotic supplementation let to a significant decrease in D-arabinitol (DA) and the ratio of D-/L-arabinitol (DA/LA) and to a significant improvement in ability of concentration and carrying out orders
West et al. (2013) [88]	33 ASD children.	Delpro® (*Lactocillus acidophilus*, *Lactobacillus casei*, *Lactobacillus delbruecki*, *Bifidobacteria longum*, *Bifidobacteria bifidum*)	88% reported a decrease in total autism treatment evaluation checklist (ATEC) score, an improvement of ASD symptoms. Participants also had significant improvements in all ATEC domains (speech/language/communication, sociability, sensory/cognitive awareness, and health/physical/behavior)

Table 1. *Cont.*

Study (Reference)	Cohort Population	Probiotic Used	Key Findings
Tomova et al. (2015) [89]	10 children with autism, 9 siblings and 10 healthy children.	"Children Dophilus" containing three strains of *Lactobacillus* (60%), two strains of *Bifidobacterium* (25%), and one strain of *Streptococcus* (15%)	Probiotic diet supplementation normalized the *Bacteroidetes/Firmicutes* ratio, *Desulfovibrio* spp. and the amount of *Bifidobacterium* spp. in feces of autistic children. No significant difference was found to reduce symptom severity in patients with autism.
Santocchi et al. (2016) [90]	100 preschoolers with ASD on the basis of a symptom severity index specific to gastrointestinal (GI) disorders. Patients with and without GI disorders were blind randomized to regular diet with probiotics or with placebo	"Vivomixx®" (one strain of *Streptococcus thermophilus* DSM 24731, three strains of *Bifidobacterium* (*Bifidobacterium breve* DSM 24732, *B. longum* DSM 24736, *B. infantis* DSM 24737), and four strains of *Lactobacillus* (*Lactobacillus acidophilus* DSM 24735, *Lactobacillus plantarum* DSM 24730, *Lactobacillus paracasei* DSM 24733, *Lactobacillus delbrueckii* subsp. *bulgaricus* DSM 24734))	Ongoing study
Dickerson et al. (2014) [91] and Tomasik et al. (2015) [92]	32 patients healthy and 33 patients with schizophrenia meeting DSM-IV criteria and with at least moderately severe psychotic symptoms	*Lactobacillus rhamnosus* strain GG and *Bifidobacterium animalis* subsp. *lactis* strain Bb12	No significant difference was found to reduce symptom severity in patients with schizophrenia. Probiotic regulate immune and intestinal epithelial cells through the IL-17 family of cytokines

Probiotics have been tested to normalize gut microbial composition and metabolism, enhance gut barrier, and relieve patients suffering from ASD. In 2012, Kaluzna-Czaplinska and Blaszczyk reported that the administration of *Lactobacillus acidophilus* in 22 ASD subjects decreased D-arabinitol concentration and the ratio of D-arabinitol to L-arabinitol in urine, and improved their ability to follow directions, as demonstrated through a comparison with data collected before the treatment [87]. Another study reported that a combination of *Lactobacillus acidophilus, L. casei, Lactobacillus delbrueckii, B. longum* and *Bifidobacterium bifidum*, formulated with the imunomodulator Del-Immune V (*Lactobacillus rhamnosus* V lysate), decreased the severity of ASD symptoms and improved GI symptoms in 33 children [88]. Moreover, a recent study of "Children Dophilus" (a combination of three species of *Lactobacillus*, two species of *Bifidobacterium* and one strain of *Streptococcus*) in 10 ASD children showed higher GI dysfunction in ASD children and siblings and a very strong association of the amount of *Desulfovibrio* spp. with the severity of autism. After the intervention, the *Bacteroidetes/Firmicutes* ratio, *Desulfovibrio* spp., and the amount of *Bifidobacterium* spp. were normalized in faeces of autistic children [89]. However, the effects of treatments with probiotics on children with ASD need to be evaluated through rigorous, controlled trials. In a recent clinical study currently in progress, Santocchi et al. are providing a multispecies probiotic (one strain of *S. thermophilus* DSM 24731, three strains of *Bifidobacterium* (*B. breve* DSM 24732, *B. longum* DSM 24736, and *B. infantis* DSM 24737), and four strains of *Lactobacillus* (*L. acidophilus* DSM 24735, *Lactobacillus plantarum* DSM 24730, *Lactobacillus paracasei* DSM 24733, and *L. delbrueckii* subsp. *bulgaricus* DSM 24734) to a group of 100 pre-schoolers with ASD. This study will try to provide new insights to clinical and neurophysiological patterns in response to a probiotic mixture in ASD patients [90].

Probiotics are also tested in the treatment of schizophrenia and bipolar disorder. One of the first trials of probiotic compounds in schizophrenia used a combined probiotic of *L. rhammosus* strain *GG* and *B. animals* subsp. *Lactis strain* Bb12. The results showed no significant difference in psychiatric symptom severity between probiotic and placebo supplementation [91]. However, other studies have found that probiotic supplementation significantly alters the levels of several serum proteins, including the von Willebrand factor and the brain-derived neurotrophic factor, and lowered the level of antibodies to the fungus *Candida albicans* [92,93].

Despite that the majority of the studies found positive results on symptoms in these neurological disorders, future studies are needed to identify potential probiotics for the effective modulation of these disorders as well as to define probiotics risk in therapeutic interventions. Gut microbial studies that use 16S rRNA gene sequencing to characterize bacteria must consider that highly similar bacteria (higher than 97% sequence identity) can have large differences in genomic sequences and profound differences in growth and metabolism. Hence, it is important to characterize probiotics to the strain level and apply next-generation sequencing techniques to analyse the functions encoded by their genome [94]. Therefore, the effects of one probiotic strain should not be generalized to others without confirmation in separate studies.

5. Prebiotics

Although the concept of a prebiotic was first defined in 1995 by Gibson, the current definition of a prebiotic is the one proposed by the International Scientific Association for Probiotics and Prebiotics (ISAPP): a substrate that is selectively utilized by host micro-organisms and confers a health benefit [95]. The group of substances recognized for their ability to influence gastrointestinal health comprise certain non-digestible oligosaccharides (NDOs), soluble fermentable fibres, and HMOs. NDOs are low molecular weight carbohydrates in nature that are intermediates between simple sugars and polysaccharides. The use of NDOs as prebiotics has rapidly increased because the enrichment of a diet with NDOs provides the opportunity to improve the gut microbial ecosystem, including bacterial populations, biochemical profiles, and physiological effects [96]. Fibre influences satiety by the following two mechanisms. One is by increasing the chewing time of fibre-rich foods, which promotes saliva and gastric acid production and increases gastric distension, triggering afferent vagal signals of fullness contributing to this end. The other mechanism is by slowing gastric emptying and decreasing the rate of glucose absorption in the small intestine. Consequently, the insulin response may also be attenuated; this is sometimes correlated with satiation and satiety [97]. Various hormones (i.e., ghrelin, the polypeptide YY, and the glucagon-like peptide) have been related to satiety, and are sent to the brain, where they regulate food intake and overall energy balance [98].

Though prebiotic therapies potentially could be beneficial for children with a genetic pre-disposition to develop ASD or attention deficit hyperactivity disorder because of their selective enhancement of *Lactobacilli* and *Bifidobacteria* growth [99], a small number of studies has examined the effect of these prebiotics on disorders related to CNS (Table 2). Inductive evidence that prebiotics modulated emotional satisfaction was provided by Hume et al., who investigated the effect of oligofructose-enriched inulin/d administration versus a placebo (maltodextrin) in a randomized, double-blind, placebo-controlled trial with 42 children (who were aged 7–12 and were overweight and obese) [100]. Prebiotic supplementation improved subjective appetite ratings, reducing energy intake in older but not in younger children.

In a cohort of healthy male and female subjects (n = 45), Schmidt et al. tested the intake of fructo-oligosaccharides (FOS) and Bimuno®-galactooligosaccharides (B-GOS), and reported that only B-GOS reduced the waking-cortisol response [101]. Exaggerated waking cortisol is a biomarker of emotional disturbances, such as depression [102]. Besides this, the subjects also provided measures of vigilance, or attention to negative stimuli, which is also a behavioral marker of anxiety and depression [103]. B-GOS attenuated vigilance, suggesting a reduction in anxiety and depression [104]. Van den berg et al. found no evidence that the use of short-chain galacto-oligosaccharides/long-chain fructo-oligosaccharides/pectin-derived acidic oligosaccharides in preterm infants at 24 months improves neurodevelopmental outcomes [105]. LeCouffe et al. studied the effect of an enteral supplementation of a prebiotic mixture (neutral and acidic oligosaccharides) in the neonatal period and found no effect on neurodevelopment [106], though lower *Bifidobacteria* counts are associated with serious neonatal infections and lower neurodevelopmental outcomes.

More studies are required to determine whether prebiotics exert a beneficial effect on neurodevelopmental disorders in infants, and to understand the mechanism of action, by stimulating certain bacterial taxa or bacterial activities within gut microbiota. Efficacy, safety, and dosing schedules should be established for each prebiotic product in long-term follow-up studies.

Table 2. Studies evaluating prebiotics and synbiotics supplementation on CNS disorders.

Study (Reference)	Cohort Population	Prebiotic Used	Key Findings
Prebiotics			
Hume et al. (2017) [100]	42 boys and girls, ages 7–12 years, with a body mass index (BMI) of ≥85th percentile	Oligofructose-enriched inulin/d	Prebiotic supplementation in children with overweight and obesity significantly increased feelings of fullness and reduced prospective food consumption in older but not in younger children
Schmidt et al. (2105) [101]	45 adults healthy volunteers	FOS and Bimuno®-galactooligosaccharides, B-GOS	B-GOS reduced waking-cortisol response and decreased attentional vigilance to negative versus positive information
van den Berg et al. (2016) [105]	77 preterm infants (gestational age <32 weeks and/or birth weight <1500 g), admitted to the level-III neonatal intensive care unit (NICU)	scGOS/lcFOS/pAOS	Neurodevelopmental outcomes were not different in the scGOS/lcFOS/pAOS and placebo group. Infections, lower bifidobacteria counts, and higher serum cytokine levels during the neonatal period were associated with lower neurodevelopmental outcomes at 24 months of age
LeCouffe et al. (2014) [106]	93 Infants, with a gestational age (GA) of less than 32 weeks and/or birth weight of less than 1500 g, participed in the study (prebiotic mixture group (n = 48) and placebo group (n = 45)	80% scGOS/lcFOS and 20% pAO	Short-term enteral supplementation of a prebiotic mixture in the neonatal period had no effect on neurodevelopmental outcome in preterm infants in the first year of life
Synbiotics			
Malaguarnera et al. (2007) [107]	60 cirrhotic patients (30 with synbiotics and 30 with placebo)	*Bifidobacterium longum* plus fructo-oligosaccharides	Patients with minimal hepatic encephalopathy (MHE) treated with *Bifidobacterium* + FOS, showed an improvement and a recovery of neuropsychological activities related to short-term memory, attention and computing ability, language, orientation ability, and cognitive activities
Firmansyah et al. (2011) [108]	393 healthy 12 month-old toddlers	The probiotic *Bifidobacterium longum* BL999 (ATCC: BAA 999) and *Lactobacillus rhamonosus*, LPR (CGMCC 1.3724), the prebiotics inulin (30%) and fructo-oligosaccharide (70%), and the LCPUFA, arachidonic acid (AA) and docosahexaenoic acid (DHA)	Changes in cognitive and adaptive behaviour scores between 12 and 16 months were higher but not significantly different in the synbiotics group compared with the control group

6. Synbiotics

The term synbiotic was primarily stated considering the benefits of a product that combines prebiotics and probiotics and in which the prebiotic compounds selectively favour the probiotic strains [109]. Several studies have shown positive synergistic effects for synbiotics on obesity, diabetes, non-alcoholic fatty liver disease, necrotizing enterocolitis in very low birth weight infants, and in the treatment of hepatic encephalopathy [110–114]. Despite these findings, few studies have tested the potential benefits of synbiotics on neurodevelopmental disorders (Table 2). Malaguarnera et al. reported that *B. longum* plus FOS improved cognitive function in the treatment of minimal hepatic encephalopathy (MHE) [107]. Firmansyah et al. provided milk containing synbiotics (BL999, LPR, and prebiotics) and LCPUFA to 393 healthy toddlers at 12 months-old for 12 months. The authors reported that the change in cognitive and adaptive behaviour scores between 12 and 16 months was higher but not significantly different in the synbiotics group compared with the control group [108]. Future work is needed to determine whether synbiotics may contribute to relieve neurological diseases and to explore the benefits of new potential synbiotics during critical time windows in an infant's CNS development and susceptibility to neurological disorders.

7. Future Perspectives

During the last decade, numerous in vivo and in vitro studies have explored the influence of probiotics and prebiotics in host physiology [115]. Their results showed that gut microbiota may modulate inflammation, adiposity, satiety, energy expenditure, and glucose metabolism. Most efforts have focused on studying the mechanisms by which certain probiotics regulate the colonization of and protect against pathogens through the activation of the mucosal immune system and competition for limited nutrients [116,117]. Alternate approaches such as recombinant probiotics expressing therapeutic biomolecules, faecal microbiota transplantation and phage therapy, need be explored for the manipulation of the gut ecosystem. A proof of concept was the experiment performed by Paton et al., where they created a recombinant probiotic by introducing glycosyltransferase genes from *Neisseria meningitidis* or *Campylobacter jejuni* in a harmless *Escherichia coli* strain (CWG308) to treat and prevent the diarrheal disease caused by enterotoxigenic *E. coli* strains [118]. The same group also developed a recombinant probiotic for the treatment and prevention of cholera [119]. A recent study showed that microbiota transfer therapy improves ASD symptoms in children, which persists for at least 8 weeks after the treatment ends [120]. And finally, phage therapy has become an interesting strategy to treat bacterial infections due to the rise of antibioticresistant microbial strains. The only approved phage therapy clinical trial in the human gut was carried out in 120 patients with diarrhoea caused by *E. coli*, who were infected by a coliphage mix. The treatment failed to solve diarrhoea, although no adverse effects of phage infection were observed [121]. Customized phage cocktails could be an alternative for future therapies. These phages would directly target pre-identified bacterial pathogens though the main drawback would be the high interindividual variation of the gut microbiome and legislative approval [122,123].

In conclusion, this review summarized the accumulating evidence on the modulation of gut microbial composition and metabolism as a potential strategy for neurological disorders and CNS development. Despite this wealth of information, the effect of probiotics and prebiotics is still largely unexplored, and numerous gaps and inconsistencies exist when the studies are compared. Differences in quantity of dose, type of strain, type of prebiotic, assessment of gut microbiota, duration of intervention, standardization of neurological measurements, variety and complexity of neurological symptoms, study design, and cohort size make it difficult to confirm evidence of efficacy. To this end, double-blind placebo in vivo studies that exploit the power of the latest robust high-throughput multi-omic technologies are required to identify the molecular mechanisms of the gut's microbial modulation of neurological disorders and CNS development and ultimately to design effective probiotic and prebiotic therapies.

Acknowledgments: This work was supported by the European Union's 7th Framework Programme under grant agreement No. 613979 (MyNewGut Project 2013/KB/613979) and by the Spanish Ministry of Economy and Competitiveness (MINECO) BFU2012-40254-C03-01. Tomás Cerdó participated in the Ph.D. Program in Biomedicine of the University of Granada and is a fellow of the FPI (BES-2013-065133) program at the Spanish Ministry of Economy and Competitiveness. This article will be part of the Ph.D. of Tomás Cerdó.

Author Contributions: T.C. and A.R. wrote the paper and contributed equally to this work. A.S. reviewed the paper and C.C. wrote, reviewed, and directed the article.

References

1. Rieder, R.; Wisniewski, P.J.; Alderman, B.L.; Campbell, S.C. Microbes and mental health: A review. *Brain Behav. Immun.* **2017**, *66*, 9–17. [CrossRef] [PubMed]
2. Cerdó, T.; Ruiz, A.; Jáuregui, R.; Azaryah, H.; Torres-Espínola, F.J.; García-Valdés, L.; Segura, M.T.; Suárez, A.; Campoy, C. Maternal obesity is associated with gut microbial metabolic potential in offspring during infancy. *J. Physiol. Biochem.* **2017**, 1–11. [CrossRef] [PubMed]
3. Vuong, H.; Yano, J.; Fung, T.; Hsiao, E. The microbiome and host behavior. *Annu. Rev. Neurosci.* **2017**, *40*, 21–49. [CrossRef] [PubMed]
4. Ross, S.M. Microbiota-gut-brain axis, part 1: An integrated system of immunological, neural, and hormonal signals. *Holist. Nurs. Pract.* **2017**, *31*, 133–136. [PubMed]
5. Hennessey, C.H.; Sladek, J.; Miller, E.; Kim, J.; Kaur, M.; Gareau, M.G. Intestinal dysbiosis during neonatal development alters the microbiota-gut-brain axis in adulthood. *FASEB J.* **2017**, *31*, 890–895.
6. Scott, K.A.; Ida, M.; Peterson, V.L.; Prenderville, J.A.; Moloney, G.M.; Izumo, T.; Murphy, K.; Murphy, A.; Ross, R.P.; Stanton, C.; et al. Revisiting metchnikoff: Age-related alterations in microbiota-gut-brain axis in the mouse. *Brain Behav. Immun.* **2017**, *65*, 20–32. [CrossRef] [PubMed]
7. Schroeder, B.O.; Bäckhed, F. Signals from the gut microbiota to distant organs in physiology and disease. *Nat. Med.* **2016**, *22*, 1079–1089. [CrossRef] [PubMed]
8. Bravo, J.A.; Forsythe, P.; Chew, M.V.; Escaravage, E.; Savignac, H.M.; Dinan, T.G.; Bienenstock, J.; Cryan, J.F. Ingestion of lactobacillus strain regulates emotional behavior and central gaba receptor expression in a mouse via the vagus nerve. *Proc. Natl. Acad. Sci. USA* **2011**, *108*, 16050–16055. [CrossRef] [PubMed]
9. Bercik, P.; Park, A.; Sinclair, D.; Khoshdel, A.; Lu, J.; Huang, X.; Deng, Y.; Blennerhassett, P.; Fahnestock, M.; Moine, D.; et al. The anxiolytic effect of bifidobacterium longum ncc3001 involves vagal pathways for gut–brain communication. *Neurogastroenterol. Motil.* **2011**, *23*, 1132–1139. [CrossRef] [PubMed]
10. Bercik, P.; Verdu, E.F.; Foster, J.A.; Macri, J.; Potter, M.; Huang, X.; Malinowski, P.; Jackson, W.; Blennerhassett, P.; Neufeld, K.A.; et al. Chronic gastrointestinal inflammation induces anxiety-like behavior and alters central nervous system biochemistry in mice. *Gastroenterology* **2010**, *139*, 2102–2112. [CrossRef] [PubMed]
11. Bercik, P.; Denou, E.; Collins, J.; Jackson, W.; Lu, J.; Jury, J.; Deng, Y.; Blennerhassett, P.; Macri, J.; McCoy, K.D.; et al. The intestinal microbiota affect central levels of brain-derived neurotropic factor and behavior in mice. *Gastroenterology* **2011**, *141*, 599–609. [CrossRef] [PubMed]
12. Kunze, W.A.; Mao, Y.K.; Wang, B.; Huizinga, J.D.; Ma, X.; Forsythe, P.; Bienenstock, J. Lactobacillus reuteri enhances excitability of colonic ah neurons by inhibiting calcium-dependent potassium channel opening. *J. Cell. Mol. Med.* **2009**, *13*, 2261–2270. [CrossRef] [PubMed]
13. McVey Neufeld, K.; Mao, Y.; Bienenstock, J.; Foster, J.; Kunze, W. The microbiome is essential for normal gut intrinsic primary afferent neuron excitability in the mouse. *Neurogastroenterol. Motil.* **2013**, *25*, 183. [CrossRef] [PubMed]
14. Cerdó, T.; García-Valdés, L.; Altmäe, S.; Ruíz, A.; Suárez, A.; Campoy, C. Role of microbiota function during early life on child's neurodevelopment. *Trends Food Sci. Technol.* **2016**, *57*, 273–288. [CrossRef]
15. Vandenplas, Y.; Zakharova, I.; Dmitrieva, Y. Oligosaccharides in infant formula: More evidence to validate the role of prebiotics. *Br. J. Nutr.* **2015**, *113*, 1339–1344. [CrossRef] [PubMed]
16. Zhou, L.; Foster, J.A. Psychobiotics and the gut–brain axis: In the pursuit of happiness. *Neuropsychiatr. Disease Treat.* **2015**, *11*, 715.

17. Borre, Y.E.; O'Keeffe, G.W.; Clarke, G.; Stanton, C.; Dinan, T.G.; Cryan, J.F. Microbiota and neurodevelopmental windows: Implications for brain disorders. *Trends Mol. Med.* **2014**, *20*, 509–518. [CrossRef] [PubMed]
18. Clemente, J.C.; Ursell, L.K.; Parfrey, L.W.; Knight, R. The impact of the gut microbiota on human health: An integrative view. *Cell* **2012**, *148*, 1258–1270. [CrossRef] [PubMed]
19. Tau, G.Z.; Peterson, B.S. Normal development of brain circuits. *Neuropsychopharmacology* **2010**, *35*, 147–168. [CrossRef] [PubMed]
20. Roca-Saavedra, P.; Mendez-Vilabrille, V.; Miranda, J.M.; Nebot, C.; Cardelle-Cobas, A.; Franco, C.M.; Cepeda, A. Food additives, contaminants and other minor components: Effects on human gut microbiota-a review. *J. Phys. Biochem.* **2017**, 1–15. [CrossRef] [PubMed]
21. Jost, T.; Lacroix, C.; Braegger, C.P.; Rochat, F.; Chassard, C. Vertical mother–neonate transfer of maternal gut bacteria via breastfeeding. *Environ. Microbiol.* **2014**, *16*, 2891–2904. [CrossRef] [PubMed]
22. Rudi, K.; Avershina, E. The composition of the gut microbiota throughout life, with an emphasis on early life. *Microb. Ecol. Health Dis.* **2015**, *26*, 26050.
23. Rautava, S. Early microbial contact, the breast milk microbiome and child health. *J. Dev. Orig. Health Dis.* **2016**, *7*, 5–14. [CrossRef] [PubMed]
24. Escherich, T. The intestinal bacteria of the neonate and breast-fed infant. *Rev. Infect. Dis.* **1988**, *10*, 1220–1225. [CrossRef] [PubMed]
25. Aagaard, K.; Ma, J.; Antony, K.M.; Ganu, R.; Petrosino, J.; Versalovic, J. The placenta harbors a unique microbiome. *Sci. Transl. Med.* **2014**, *6*. [CrossRef] [PubMed]
26. Zheng, J.; Xiao, X.; Zhang, Q.; Mao, L.; Yu, M.; Xu, J. The placental microbiome varies in association with low birth weight in full-term neonates. *Nutrients* **2015**, *7*, 6924–6937. [CrossRef] [PubMed]
27. Perez-Muñoz, M.E.; Arrieta, M.-C.; Ramer-Tait, A.E.; Walter, J. A critical assessment of the "sterile womb" and "in utero colonization" hypotheses: Implications for research on the pioneer infant microbiome. *Microbiome* **2017**, *5*, 48. [CrossRef] [PubMed]
28. Mueller, N.T.; Bakacs, E.; Combellick, J.; Grigoryan, Z.; Dominguez-Bello, M.G. The infant microbiome development: Mom matters. *Trends Mol. Med.* **2015**, *21*, 109–117. [CrossRef] [PubMed]
29. Rautava, S.; Collado, M.C.; Salminen, S.; Isolauri, E. Probiotics modulate host-microbe interaction in the placenta and fetal gut: A randomized, double-blind, placebo-controlled trial. *Neonatology* **2012**, *102*, 178–184. [CrossRef] [PubMed]
30. Toh, Z.Q.; Anzela, A.; Tang, M.L.; Licciardi, P.V. Probiotic therapy as a novel approach for allergic disease. *Front. Pharmacol.* **2012**, *3*, 171. [CrossRef] [PubMed]
31. Zhang, G.-Q.; Hu, H.-J.; Liu, C.-Y.; Zhang, Q.; Shakya, S.; Li, Z.-Y. Probiotics for prevention of atopy and food hypersensitivity in early childhood: A prisma-compliant systematic review and meta-analysis of randomized controlled trials. *Medicine* **2016**, *95*, e2562. [CrossRef] [PubMed]
32. Hansen, R.; Scott, K.P.; Khan, S.; Martin, J.C.; Berry, S.H.; Stevenson, M.; Okpapi, A.; Munro, M.J.; Hold, G.L. First-pass meconium samples from healthy term vaginally-delivered neonates: An analysis of the microbiota. *PLoS ONE* **2015**, *10*, e0133320. [CrossRef] [PubMed]
33. Bright, M.; Bulgheresi, S. A complex journey: Transmission of microbial symbionts. *Nat. Rev. Microbiol.* **2010**, *8*, 218–230. [CrossRef] [PubMed]
34. Jakobsson, H.E.; Abrahamsson, T.R.; Jenmalm, M.C.; Harris, K.; Quince, C.; Jernberg, C.; Björkstén, B.; Engstrand, L.; Andersson, A.F. Decreased gut microbiota diversity, delayed bacteroidetes colonisation and reduced th1 responses in infants delivered by caesarean section. *Gut* **2014**, *63*, 559–566. [CrossRef] [PubMed]
35. Jašarević, E.; Howerton, C.L.; Howard, C.D.; Bale, T.L. Alterations in the vaginal microbiome by maternal stress are associated with metabolic reprogramming of the offspring gut and brain. *Endocrinology* **2015**, *156*, 3265–3276. [CrossRef] [PubMed]
36. Jain, A.; Concato, J.; Leventhal, J.M. How good is the evidence linking breastfeeding and intelligence? *Pediatrics* **2002**, *109*, 1044–1053. [CrossRef] [PubMed]
37. Pacheco, A.R.; Barile, D.; Underwood, M.A.; Mills, D.A. The impact of the milk glycobiome on the neonate gut microbiota. *Annu. Rev. Anim. Biosci.* **2015**, *3*, 419–445. [CrossRef] [PubMed]
38. Hunt, K.M.; Foster, J.A.; Forney, L.J.; Schütte, U.M.; Beck, D.L.; Abdo, Z.; Fox, L.K.; Williams, J.E.; McGuire, M.K.; McGuire, M.A. Characterization of the diversity and temporal stability of bacterial communities in human milk. *PLoS ONE* **2011**, *6*, e21313. [CrossRef] [PubMed]

39. Zivkovic, A.M.; German, J.B.; Lebrilla, C.B.; Mills, D.A. Human milk glycobiome and its impact on the infant gastrointestinal microbiota. *Proc. Natl. Acad. Sci. USA* **2011**, *108*, 4653–4658. [CrossRef] [PubMed]
40. Urbaniak, C.; Cummins, J.; Brackstone, M.; Macklaim, J.M.; Gloor, G.B.; Baban, C.K.; Scott, L.; O'Hanlon, D.M.; Burton, J.P.; Francis, K.P.; et al. Microbiota of human breast tissue. *Appl. Environ. Microbiol.* **2014**, *80*, 3007–3014. [CrossRef] [PubMed]
41. Gueimonde, M.; Laitinen, K.; Salminen, S.; Isolauri, E. Breast milk: A source of bifidobacteria for infant gut development and maturation? *Neonatology* **2007**, *92*, 64–66. [CrossRef] [PubMed]
42. Underwood, M.A.; German, J.B.; Lebrilla, C.B.; Mills, D.A. Bifidobacterium longum subspecies infantis: Champion colonizer of the infant gut. *Pediatr. Res.* **2015**, *77*, 229. [CrossRef] [PubMed]
43. Desbonnet, L.; Garrett, L.; Clarke, G.; Kiely, B.; Cryan, J.; Dinan, T. Effects of the probiotic bifidobacterium infantis in the maternal separation model of depression. *Neuroscience* **2010**, *170*, 1179–1188. [CrossRef] [PubMed]
44. Desbonnet, L.; Garrett, L.; Clarke, G.; Bienenstock, J.; Dinan, T.G. The probiotic bifidobacteria infantis: An assessment of potential antidepressant properties in the rat. *J. Psychiatr. Res.* **2008**, *43*, 164–174. [CrossRef] [PubMed]
45. Maes, M.; Berk, M.; Goehler, L.; Song, C.; Anderson, G.; Gałecki, P.; Leonard, B. Depression and sickness behavior are janus-faced responses to shared inflammatory pathways. *BMC Med.* **2012**, *10*, 66. [CrossRef] [PubMed]
46. Bezirtzoglou, E.; Tsiotsias, A.; Welling, G.W. Microbiota profile in feces of breast-and formula-fed newborns by using fluorescence in situ hybridization (fish). *Anaerobe* **2011**, *17*, 478–482. [CrossRef] [PubMed]
47. Fallani, M.; Young, D.; Scott, J.; Norin, E.; Amarri, S.; Adam, R.; Aguilera, M.; Khanna, S.; Gil, A.; Edwards, C.A.; et al. Intestinal microbiota of 6-week-old infants across europe: Geographic influence beyond delivery mode, breast-feeding, and antibiotics. *J. Pediatr. Gastroenterol. Nutr.* **2010**, *51*, 77–84. [CrossRef] [PubMed]
48. Tognini, P. Gut microbiota: A potential regulator of neurodevelopment. *Front. Cell. Neurosci.* **2017**, *11*. [CrossRef] [PubMed]
49. Cong, X.; Henderson, W.A.; Graf, J.; McGrath, J.M. Early life experience and gut microbiome: The brain-gut-microbiota signaling system. *Adv. Neonatal Care Off. J. Natl. Assoc. Neonatal Nurses* **2015**, *15*, 314. [CrossRef] [PubMed]
50. Collins, S.M.; Bercik, P. Gut microbiota: Intestinal bacteria influence brain activity in healthy humans. *Nat. Rev. Gastroenterol. Hepatol.* **2013**, *10*, 326–327. [CrossRef] [PubMed]
51. Palma, G.; Collins, S.M.; Bercik, P.; Verdu, E.F. The microbiota–gut–brain axis in gastrointestinal disorders: Stressed bugs, stressed brain or both? *J. Physiol.* **2014**, *592*, 2989–2997. [CrossRef] [PubMed]
52. Collins, S.M.; Surette, M.; Bercik, P. The interplay between the intestinal microbiota and the brain. *Nat. Rev. Microbiol.* **2012**, *10*, 735–742. [CrossRef] [PubMed]
53. Cryan, J.F.; Dinan, T.G. Mind-altering microorganisms: The impact of the gut microbiota on brain and behaviour. *Nat. Rev. Neurosci.* **2012**, *13*, 701–712. [CrossRef] [PubMed]
54. Mayer, E.A.; Knight, R.; Mazmanian, S.K.; Cryan, J.F.; Tillisch, K. Gut microbes and the brain: Paradigm shift in neuroscience. *J. Neurosci.* **2014**, *34*, 15490–15496. [CrossRef] [PubMed]
55. Luczynski, P.; McVey Neufeld, K.-A.; Oriach, C.S.; Clarke, G.; Dinan, T.G.; Cryan, J.F. Growing up in a bubble: Using germ-free animals to assess the influence of the gut microbiota on brain and behavior. *Int. J. Neuropsychopharmacol.* **2016**, *19*. [CrossRef] [PubMed]
56. Tarr, A.J.; Galley, J.D.; Fisher, S.E.; Chichlowski, M.; Berg, B.M.; Bailey, M.T. The prebiotics 3′ sialyllactose and 6′ sialyllactose diminish stressor-induced anxiety-like behavior and colonic microbiota alterations: Evidence for effects on the gut–brain axis. *Brain Behav. Immun.* **2015**, *50*, 166–177. [CrossRef] [PubMed]
57. Buffington, S.A.; Di Prisco, G.V.; Auchtung, T.A.; Ajami, N.J.; Petrosino, J.F.; Costa-Mattioli, M. Microbial reconstitution reverses maternal diet-induced social and synaptic deficits in offspring. *Cell* **2016**, *165*, 1762–1775. [CrossRef] [PubMed]
58. Sampson, T.R.; Debelius, J.W.; Thron, T.; Janssen, S.; Shastri, G.G.; Ilhan, Z.E.; Challis, C.; Schretter, C.E.; Rocha, S.; Gradinaru, V.; et al. Gut microbiota regulate motor deficits and neuroinflammation in a model of parkinson's disease. *Cell* **2016**, *167*, 1469–1480. [CrossRef] [PubMed]

59. Minamiyama, M.; Katsuno, M.; Adachi, H.; Waza, M.; Sang, C.; Kobayashi, Y.; Tanaka, F.; Doyu, M.; Inukai, A.; Sobue, G. Sodium butyrate ameliorates phenotypic expression in a transgenic mouse model of spinal and bulbar muscular atrophy. *Hum. Mol. Genet.* **2004**, *13*, 1183–1192. [CrossRef] [PubMed]
60. Slominski, A.; Semak, I.; Pisarchik, A.; Sweatman, T.; Szczesniewski, A.; Wortsman, J. Conversion of l-tryptophan to serotonin and melatonin in human melanoma cells. *FEBS Lett.* **2002**, *511*, 102–106. [CrossRef]
61. Alexander, K.S.; Pocivavsek, A.; Wu, H.-Q.; Pershing, M.L.; Schwarcz, R.; Bruno, J.P. Early developmental elevations of brain kynurenic acid impair cognitive flexibility in adults: Reversal with galantamine. *Neuroscience* **2013**, *238*, 19–28. [CrossRef] [PubMed]
62. Khalil, O.S.; Pisar, M.; Forrest, C.M.; Vincenten, M.C.; Darlington, L.G.; Stone, T.W. Prenatal inhibition of the kynurenine pathway leads to structural changes in the hippocampus of adult rat offspring. *Eur. J. Neurosci.* **2014**, *39*, 1558–1571. [CrossRef] [PubMed]
63. Holzer, P.; Farzi, A. Neuropeptides and the microbiota-gut-brain axis. In *Microbial Endocrinology: The Microbiota-Gut-Brain Axis in Health and Disease*; Springer: New York, NY, USA, 2014; pp. 195–219.
64. Del Zoppo, G.J.; Mabuchi, T. Cerebral microvessel responses to focal ischemia. *J. Cereb. Blood Flow Metab.* **2003**, *23*, 879–894. [CrossRef] [PubMed]
65. Braniste, V.; Al-Asmakh, M.; Kowal, C.; Anuar, F.; Abbaspour, A.; Tóth, M.; Korecka, A.; Bakocevic, N.; Ng, L.G.; Kundu, P.; et al. The gut microbiota influences blood-brain barrier permeability in mice. *Sci. Transl. Med.* **2014**, *6*. [CrossRef] [PubMed]
66. Sherwin, E.; Rea, K.; Dinan, T.G.; Cryan, J.F. A gut (microbiome) feeling about the brain. *Curr. Opin. Gastroenterol.* **2016**, *32*, 96–102. [CrossRef] [PubMed]
67. Xu, D.; Gao, J.; Gillilland, M.; Wu, X.; Song, I.; Kao, J.Y.; Owyang, C. Rifaximin alters intestinal bacteria and prevents stress-induced gut inflammation and visceral hyperalgesia in rats. *Gastroenterology* **2014**, *146*, 484–496. [CrossRef] [PubMed]
68. Joint, F.A.O. Who expert consultation on evaluation of health and nutritional properties of probiotics in food including powder milk with live lactic acid bacteria. *Córdoba Argentina Oct.* **2001**, *1*, 1–4.
69. Hill, C.; Guarner, F.; Reid, G.; Gibson, G.R.; Merenstein, D.J.; Pot, B.; Morelli, L.; Canani, R.B.; Flint, H.J.; Salminen, S.; et al. Expert consensus document: The international scientific association for probiotics and prebiotics consensus statement on the scope and appropriate use of the term probiotic. *Nat. Rev. Gastroenterol. Hepatol.* **2014**, *11*, 506–514. [CrossRef] [PubMed]
70. Al-muzafar, H.M.; Amin, K.A. Probiotic mixture improves fatty liver disease by virtue of its action on lipid profiles, leptin, and inflammatory biomarkers. *BMC Complement. Altern. Med.* **2017**, *17*, 43. [CrossRef] [PubMed]
71. West, C.E.; Jenmalm, M.C.; Kozyrskyj, A.L.; Prescott, S.L. Probiotics for treatment and primary prevention of allergic diseases and asthma: Looking back and moving forward. *Expert Rev. Clin. Immunol.* **2016**, *12*, 625–639. [CrossRef] [PubMed]
72. Rayes, N.; Seehofer, D.; Hansen, S.; Boucsein, K.; Müller, A.R.; Serke, S.; Bengmark, S.; Neuhaus, P. Early enteral supply of lactobacillus and fiber versus selective bowel decontamination: A controlled trial in liver transplant recipients. *Transplantation* **2002**, *74*, 123–128. [CrossRef] [PubMed]
73. Ivanov, I.I.; Honda, K. Intestinal commensal microbes as immune modulators. *Cell Host Microbe* **2012**, *12*, 496–508. [CrossRef] [PubMed]
74. Dinan, T.G.; Stanton, C.; Cryan, J.F. Psychobiotics: A novel class of psychotropic. *Biol. Psychiatry* **2013**, *74*, 720–726. [CrossRef] [PubMed]
75. Messaoudi, M.; Violle, N.; Bisson, J.-F.; Desor, D.; Javelot, H.; Rougeot, C. Beneficial psychological effects of a probiotic formulation (lactobacillus helveticus r0052 and bifidobacterium longum r0175) in healthy human volunteers. *Gut Microbes* **2011**, *2*, 256–261. [CrossRef] [PubMed]
76. Messaoudi, M.; Lalonde, R.; Violle, N.; Javelot, H.; Desor, D.; Nejdi, A.; Bisson, J.-F.; Rougeot, C.; Pichelin, M.; Cazaubiel, M.; et al. Assessment of psychotropic-like properties of a probiotic formulation (lactobacillus helveticus r0052 and bifidobacterium longum r0175) in rats and human subjects. *Br. J. Nutr.* **2011**, *105*, 755–764. [CrossRef] [PubMed]
77. Benton, D.; Williams, C.; Brown, A. Impact of consuming a milk drink containing a probiotic on mood and cognition. *Eur. J. Clin. Nutr.* **2007**, *61*, 355–361. [CrossRef] [PubMed]

78. Steenbergen, L.; Sellaro, R.; van Hemert, S.; Bosch, J.A.; Colzato, L.S. A randomized controlled trial to test the effect of multispecies probiotics on cognitive reactivity to sad mood. *Brain Behav. Immun.* **2015**, *48*, 258–264. [CrossRef] [PubMed]
79. Akkasheh, G.; Kashani-Poor, Z.; Tajabadi-Ebrahimi, M.; Jafari, P.; Akbari, H.; Taghizadeh, M.; Memarzadeh, M.R.; Asemi, Z.; Esmaillzadeh, A. Clinical and metabolic response to probiotic administration in patients with major depressive disorder: A randomized, double-blind, placebo-controlled trial. *Nutrition* **2016**, *32*, 315–320. [CrossRef] [PubMed]
80. Marcos, A.; Wärnberg, J.; Nova, E.; Gómez, S.; Alvarez, A.; Alvarez, R.; Mateos, J.A.; Cobo, J.M. The effect of milk fermented by yogurt cultures plus lactobacillus casei dn-114001 on the immune response of subjects under academic examination stress. *Eur. J. Nutr.* **2004**, *43*, 381–389. [CrossRef] [PubMed]
81. Romijn, A.R.; Rucklidge, J.J.; Kuijer, R.G.; Frampton, C. A double-blind, randomized, placebo-controlled trial of lactobacillus helveticus and bifidobacterium longum for the symptoms of depression. *Aust. N. Z. J. Psychiatry* **2017**. [CrossRef] [PubMed]
82. Chung, Y.-C.; Jin, H.-M.; Cui, Y.; Kim, D.S.; Jung, J.M.; Park, J.-I.; Jung, E.-S.; Choi, E.-K.; Chae, S.-W. Fermented milk of lactobacillus helveticus idcc3801 improves cognitive functioning during cognitive fatigue tests in healthy older adults. *J. Funct. Foods* **2014**, *10*, 465–474. [CrossRef]
83. Jadrešin, O.; Hojsak, I.; Mišak, Z.; Kekez, A.J.; Trbojevic, T.; Ivkovic, L.; Kolacek, S. Lactobacillus reuteri dsm 17938 in the treatment of functional abdominal pain in children: Rct study. *J. Pediatr. Gastroenterol. Nutr.* **2017**, *64*, 925–929. [CrossRef] [PubMed]
84. Rao, A.V.; Bested, A.C.; Beaulne, T.M.; Katzman, M.A.; Iorio, C.; Berardi, J.M.; Logan, A.C. A randomized, double-blind, placebo-controlled pilot study of a probiotic in emotional symptoms of chronic fatigue syndrome. *Gut Pathog.* **2009**, *1*, 6. [CrossRef] [PubMed]
85. Giannetti, E.; Maglione, M.; Alessandrella, A.; Strisciuglio, C.; De Giovanni, D.; Campanozzi, A.; Miele, E.; Staiano, A. A mixture of 3 bifidobacteria decreases abdominal pain and improves the quality of life in children with irritable bowel syndrome: A multicenter, randomized, double-blind, placebo-controlled, crossover trial. *J. Clin. Gastroenterol.* **2017**, *51*, e5–e10. [CrossRef] [PubMed]
86. Tillisch, K.; Labus, J.; Kilpatrick, L.; Jiang, Z.; Stains, J.; Ebrat, B.; Guyonnet, D.; Legrain–Raspaud, S.; Trotin, B.; Naliboff, B.; et al. Consumption of fermented milk product with probiotic modulates brain activity. *Gastroenterology* **2013**, *144*, 1394–1401. [CrossRef] [PubMed]
87. Kałużna-Czaplińska, J.; Błaszczyk, S. The level of arabinitol in autistic children after probiotic therapy. *Nutrition* **2012**, *28*, 124–126. [CrossRef] [PubMed]
88. West, R.; Roberts, E.; Sichel, L.; Sichel, J. Improvements in gastrointestinal symptoms among children with autism spectrum disorder receiving the delpro®probiotic and immunomodulator formulation. *J. Prob. Health* **2013**, *1*, 2.
89. Tomova, A.; Husarova, V.; Lakatosova, S.; Bakos, J.; Vlkova, B.; Babinska, K.; Ostatnikova, D. Gastrointestinal microbiota in children with autism in slovakia. *Physiol. Behav.* **2015**, *138*, 179–187. [CrossRef] [PubMed]
90. Santocchi, E.; Guiducci, L.; Fulceri, F.; Billeci, L.; Buzzigoli, E.; Apicella, F.; Calderoni, S.; Grossi, E.; Morales, M.A.; Muratori, F. Gut to brain interaction in autism spectrum disorders: A randomized controlled trial on the role of probiotics on clinical, biochemical and neurophysiological parameters. *BMC Psychiatry* **2016**, *16*, 183. [CrossRef] [PubMed]
91. Dickerson, F.B.; Stallings, C.; Origoni, A.; Katsafanas, E.; Savage, C.L.; Schweinfurth, L.A.; Goga, J.; Khushalani, S.; Yolken, R.H. Effect of probiotic supplementation on schizophrenia symptoms and association with gastrointestinal functioning: A randomized, placebo-controlled trial. *Prim. Care Companion CNS Disord.* **2014**, *16*. [CrossRef] [PubMed]
92. Tomasik, J.; Yolken, R.H.; Bahn, S.; Dickerson, F.B. Immunomodulatory effects of probiotic supplementation in schizophrenia patients: A randomized, placebo-controlled trial. *Biomark. Insights* **2015**, *10*, 47. [CrossRef] [PubMed]
93. Severance, E.G.; Gressitt, K.L.; Stallings, C.R.; Katsafanas, E.; Schweinfurth, L.A.; Savage, C.L.; Adamos, M.B.; Sweeney, K.M.; Origoni, A.E.; Khushalani, S.; et al. Candida albicans exposures, sex specificity and cognitive deficits in schizophrenia and bipolar disorder. *NPJ Schizophr.* **2016**, *2*, 16018. [CrossRef] [PubMed]
94. Culligan, E.P.; Hill, C.; Sleator, R.D. Probiotics and gastrointestinal disease: Successes, problems and future prospects. *Gut Pathog.* **2009**, *1*, 19. [CrossRef] [PubMed]

95. Gibson, G.R.; Hutkins, R.W.; Sanders, M.E.; Prescott, S.L.; Reimer, R.A.; Salminen, S.J.; Scott, K.; Stanton, C.; Swanson, K.S.; Cani, P.D. The international scientific association for probiotics and prebiotics (isapp) consensus statement on the definition and scope of prebiotics. *Nat. Rev. Gastroenterol. Hepatol.* **2017**. [CrossRef] [PubMed]
96. Mussatto, S.I.; Mancilha, I.M. Non-digestible oligosaccharides: A review. *Carbohydr. Polym.* **2007**, *68*, 587–597. [CrossRef]
97. Slavin, J. Fiber and prebiotics: Mechanisms and health benefits. *Nutrients* **2013**, *5*, 1417–1435. [CrossRef] [PubMed]
98. Page, A.; Kentish, S. Plasticity of gastrointestinal vagal afferent satiety signals. *Neurogastroenterol. Motil.* **2016**. [CrossRef] [PubMed]
99. Theije, C.G.; Bavelaar, B.M.; Lopes da Silva, S.; Korte, S.M.; Olivier, B.; Garssen, J.; Kraneveld, A.D. Food allergy and food-based therapies in neurodevelopmental disorders. *Pediatr. Allergy Immunol.* **2014**, *25*, 218–226. [CrossRef] [PubMed]
100. Hume, M.P.; Nicolucci, A.C.; Reimer, R.A. Prebiotic supplementation improves appetite control in children with overweight and obesity: A randomized controlled trial. *Am. J. Clin. Nutr.* **2017**, *105*, 790–799. [CrossRef] [PubMed]
101. Schmidt, K.; Cowen, P.J.; Harmer, C.J.; Tzortzis, G.; Errington, S.; Burnet, P.W. Prebiotic intake reduces the waking cortisol response and alters emotional bias in healthy volunteers. *Psychopharmacology* **2015**, *232*, 1793–1801. [CrossRef] [PubMed]
102. Mannie, Z.N.; Harmer, C.J.; Cowen, P.J. Increased waking salivary cortisol levels in young people at familial risk of depression. *Am. J. Psychiatry* **2007**, *164*, 617–621. [CrossRef] [PubMed]
103. Beck, A.T. *Cognitive Therapy and the Emotional Disorders*; Penguin: London, UK, 1979.
104. Ironside, M.; O'Shea, J.; Cowen, P.J.; Harmer, C.J. Frontal cortex stimulation reduces vigilance to threat: Implications for the treatment of depression and anxiety. *Biol. Psychiatry* **2016**, *79*, 823–830. [CrossRef] [PubMed]
105. Van den Berg, J.P.; Westerbeek, E.A.; Bröring-Starre, T.; Garssen, J.; van Elburg, R.M. Neurodevelopment of preterm infants at 24 months after neonatal supplementation of a prebiotic mix: A randomized trial. *J. Pediatr. Gastroenterol. Nutr.* **2016**, *63*, 270–276. [CrossRef] [PubMed]
106. LeCouffe, N.E.; Westerbeek, E.A.; van Schie, P.E.; Schaaf, V.A.; Lafeber, H.N.; van Elburg, R.M. Neurodevelopmental outcome during the first year of life in preterm infants after supplementation of a prebiotic mixture in the neonatal period: A follow-up study. *Neuropediatrics* **2014**, *45*, 022–029. [CrossRef] [PubMed]
107. Malaguarnera, M.; Greco, F.; Barone, G.; Gargante, M.P.; Malaguarnera, M.; Toscano, M.A. Bifidobacterium longum with fructo-oligosaccharide (fos) treatment in minimal hepatic encephalopathy: A randomized, double-blind, placebo-controlled study. *Dig. Dis. Sci.* **2007**, *52*, 3259. [CrossRef] [PubMed]
108. Firmansyah, A.; Dwipoerwantoro, P.G.; Kadim, M.; Alatas, S.; Conus, N.; Lestarina, L.; Bouisset, F.; Steenhout, P. Improved growth of toddlers fed a milk containing synbiotics. *Asia Pac. J. Clin. Nutr.* **2011**, *20*, 69–76. [PubMed]
109. Schrezenmeir, J.; de Vrese, M. Probiotics, prebiotics, and synbiotics—Approaching a definition. *Am. J. Clin. Nutr.* **2001**, *73*, 361s–364s. [PubMed]
110. Islek, A.; Sayar, E.; Yilmaz, A.; Baysan, B.O.; Mutlu, D.; Artan, R. The role of bifidobacterium lactis b94 plus inulin in the treatment of acute infectious diarrhea in children. *Turk. J. Gastroenterol.* **2014**, *25*, 628–633. [CrossRef] [PubMed]
111. Asemi, Z.; Khorrami-Rad, A.; Alizadeh, S.-A.; Shakeri, H.; Esmaillzadeh, A. Effects of synbiotic food consumption on metabolic status of diabetic patients: A double-blind randomized cross-over controlled clinical trial. *Clin. Nutr.* **2014**, *33*, 198–203. [CrossRef] [PubMed]
112. Steed, H.; Macfarlane, G.T.; Blackett, K.L.; Bahrami, B.; Reynolds, N.; Walsh, S.V.; Cummings, J.H.; Macfarlane, S. Clinical trial: The microbiological and immunological effects of synbiotic consumption—A randomized double-blind placebo-controlled study in active crohn's disease. *Aliment. Pharmacol. Ther.* **2010**, *32*, 872–883. [CrossRef] [PubMed]
113. Dilli, D.; Aydin, B.; Fettah, N.D.; Özyazıcı, E.; Beken, S.; Zenciroğlu, A.; Okumuş, N.; Özyurt, B.M.; İpek, M.Ş.; Akdağ, A. The propre-save study: Effects of probiotics and prebiotics alone or combined on necrotizing enterocolitis in very low birth weight infants. *J. Pediatr.* **2015**, *166*, 545–551. [CrossRef] [PubMed]

114. Eslamparast, T.; Poustchi, H.; Zamani, F.; Sharafkhah, M.; Malekzadeh, R.; Hekmatdoost, A. Synbiotic supplementation in nonalcoholic fatty liver disease: A randomized, double-blind, placebo-controlled pilot study. *Am. J. Clin. Nutr.* **2014**, *99*, 535–542. [CrossRef] [PubMed]
115. Daliri, E.B.-M.; Lee, B.H. New perspectives on probiotics in health and disease. *Food Sci. Hum. Wellness* **2015**, *4*, 56–65. [CrossRef]
116. Kamada, N.; Chen, G.Y.; Inohara, N.; Núñez, G. Control of pathogens and pathobionts by the gut microbiota. *Nat. Immunol.* **2013**, *14*, 685–690. [CrossRef] [PubMed]
117. Christensen, K.V.; Morch, M.G.; Morthorst, T.H.; Lykkemark, S.; Olsen, A. Microbiota, probiotic bacteria and ageing. In *Ageing: Lessons from C. elegans*; Springer: New York, NY, USA, 2017; pp. 411–429.
118. Paton, A.W.; Jennings, M.P.; Morona, R.; Wang, H.; Focareta, A.; Roddam, L.F.; Paton, J.C. Recombinant probiotics for treatment and prevention of enterotoxigenic escherichia coli diarrhea. *Gastroenterology* **2005**, *128*, 1219–1228. [CrossRef] [PubMed]
119. Focareta, A.; Paton, J.C.; Morona, R.; Cook, J.; Paton, A.W. A recombinant probiotic for treatment and prevention of cholera. *Gastroenterology* **2006**, *130*, 1688–1695. [CrossRef] [PubMed]
120. Kang, D.-W.; Adams, J.B.; Gregory, A.C.; Borody, T.; Chittick, L.; Fasano, A.; Khoruts, A.; Geis, E.; Maldonado, J.; McDonough-Means, S. Microbiota transfer therapy alters gut ecosystem and improves gastrointestinal and autism symptoms: An open-label study. *Microbiome* **2017**, *5*, 10. [CrossRef] [PubMed]
121. Sarker, S.A.; Sultana, S.; Reuteler, G.; Moine, D.; Descombes, P.; Charton, F.; Bourdin, G.; McCallin, S.; Ngom-Bru, C.; Neville, T.; et al. Oral phage therapy of acute bacterial diarrhea with two coliphage preparations: A randomized trial in children from bangladesh. *EBioMedicine* **2016**, *4*, 124–137. [CrossRef] [PubMed]
122. Mirzaei, M.K.; Maurice, C.F. Menage a trois in the human gut: Interactions between host, bacteria and phages. *Nat. Rev. Microbiol.* **2017**, *15*, 397–408. [CrossRef] [PubMed]
123. Cooper, C.J.; Mirzaei, M.K.; Nilsson, A.S. Adapting drug approval pathways for bacteriophage-based therapeutics. *Front. Microbiol.* **2016**, *7*. [CrossRef] [PubMed]

11

Probiotic Supplementation in Preterm: Feeding Intolerance and Hospital Cost

Flavia Indrio [1,*], Giuseppe Riezzo [2], Silvio Tafuri [3], Maria Ficarella [1], Barbara Carlucci [4], Massimo Bisceglia [5], Lorenzo Polimeno [6] and Ruggiero Francavilla [1]

1. Department of Pediatric, Aldo Moro University of Bari, Ospedale Pediatrico Giovanni XXIII via Amendola 276, 70125 Bari, Italy; maria.ficarella@hotmail.com (M.F.); rfrancavilla@gmail.com (R.F.)
2. Laboratory of Nutritional Physiopathology, National Institute for Digestive Diseases, Istituto di Ricerca e Cura a Carattere Scientifico (I.R.C.C.S.), Saverio de Bellis, 70013 Castellana Grotte (BA), Italy; griezzo@gmail.com
3. Department of Biomedical Sciences and Human Oncology, Section of Hygiene, Aldo Moro University of Bari, 70125 Bari, Italy; silvio.tafuri@uniba.it
4. Division of Neonatology, Ospedale Perrino, 72100 Brindisi, Italy; bcalucci@lbero.it
5. Department of Pediatrics, Neonatology Division San Giovanni di Dio Hospital, 88900 Crotone, Italy; m.bisceglia@tin.it
6. Department of Organ Transplantation, Gastroenterology Section, University Aldo Moro Bari, 70125 Bari, Italy; lorenzo.polimeno@uniba.it

* Correspondence: f.indrio@neonatologia.uniba.it

Abstract: We hypothesized that giving the probiotic strain *Lactobacillus reuteri* (*L. reuteri*) DSM 17938 to preterm, formula-fed infants would prevent an early traumatic intestinal inflammatory insult modulating intestinal cytokine profile and reducing the onset of feeding intolerance. Newborn were randomly allocated during the first 48 h of life to receive either daily probiotic (10^8 colony forming units (CFUs) of *L. reuteri* DSM 17938) or placebo for one month. All the newborns underwent to gastric ultrasound for the measurement of gastric emptying time. Fecal samples were collected for the evaluation of fecal cytokines. Clinical data on feeding intolerance and weight gain were collected. The costs of hospital stays were calculated. The results showed that the newborns receiving *L. reuteri* DSM 17938 had a significant decrease in the number of days needed to reach full enteral feeding ($p < 0.01$), days of hospital stay ($p < 0.01$), and days of antibiotic treatment ($p < 0.01$). Statistically significant differences were observed in pattern of fecal cytokine profiles. The anti-inflammatory cytokine interleukin (IL)-10, was increased in newborns receiving *L. reuteri* DSM 17938. Pro-inflammatory cytokines: IL-17, IL-8, and tumor necrosis factor (TNF)-alpha levels were increased in newborns given placebo. Differences in the gastric emptying and fasting antral area (FAA) were also observed. Our study demonstrates an effective role for *L. reuteri* DSM 17938 supplementation in preventing feeding intolerance and improving gut motor and immune function development in bottle-fed stable preterm newborns. Another benefit from the use of probiotics is the reducing cost for the Health Care service.

Keywords: preterm newborn; feeding intolerance; probiotic

---

1. Introduction

During the third trimester of pregnancy and in the first days after birth, important processes of intestinal maturation take place. Although anatomical differentiation of the human gut is usually achieved within 20 weeks of gestation, the functional maturation of the gastrointestinal tract occurs later and requires organized peristalsis and coordinated sucking and swallowing reflexes that are not established until 29–30 weeks and 32–34 weeks of gestations, respectively [1]. Sensory-motor gastrointestinal functions are strictly related to the infant's immune system, which plays a crucial role in modulating appropriate and non-exaggerated responses to luminal antigens. This fundamental enteric function, known as "oral tolerance" is based on the interaction between the luminal content (microbiota, food antigens, and other molecules), the intestinal epithelium, and the tolerogenic dendritic cells (DCs) from mesenteric lymph nodes of the gut associated lymphoid tissue (GALT) [2], and is associated with specific cytokine patterns. It has been suggested that the early composition of the intestinal microbiota at birth can influence the correct ontogenesis of the gut barrier, and motor and immune function through a complex neuroendocrine cross-talk [3,4]. Consequences of prematurity like antibiotic usage, feeding type, and being located in neonatal intensive care unit (NICU) may cause an intestinal dysbiosis that affects the intestinal integrity and disrupts the delicate balance between intestinal microbiota and the immune system of premature infants. An aberrant microbial colonization pattern might contribute to the development of an early traumatic inflammatory insult on the gut-brain axis with short- and long-term consequences on gastrointestinal well-being [5].

Early colonization of the gastrointestinal tract with a probiotic may contribute to the neonatal tolerance, as breast-feeding does, resulting in correct gut ontogenesis [6–9]. Besides, it has been demonstrated that *L. reuteri* DSM 17938 significantly reduced intestinal mucosal levels of IL-8 and interferon (IFN)-γ when newborn rat pups were fed formula containing lipopolysaccharide (LPS) $\pm$ *L. reuteri*. *L. reuteri* DSM 17938 was able to significantly reduce the intestinal histological damage produced by LPS plus cow milk formula in the same animal model. Even cow milk formula feeding without LPS produced a mild gut inflammation, evidenced by elevated mucosal IFN-γ and IL-13 levels, and that process could be suppressed by the strain 17938 [10].

In this framework, we hypothesized that giving the probiotic strain *L. reuteri* DSM 17938 to preterm, formula-fed infants would prevent an early traumatic intestinal inflammatory insult modulating intestinal cytokine profile and would reduce the onset of feeding intolerance acting also on gastrointestinal motility.

2. Methods

A randomized, double-blinded, clinical, and placebo-controlled trial, was conducted in two Italian neonatal intensive care units (NICUs), Brindisi and Crotone, from January 2011 to November 2012. Preterm neonates (gestational age <37 weeks), within the first 48 h of life: adequate for gestational age weight, formula fed, Apgar score at 5 min >7, <24 h of age, hemodynamically stable, with absence of congenital malformations, inborn errors of metabolism, proven sepsis, or infections at birth were included. The ethical committees of each participating institution approved the study protocol. All preterm newborns were screened at birth and the parents of eligible newborns gave signed consent. Trial registered ClinicalTrials.gov (National Institutes of Health) with the number NCT00985816.

2.1. Randomization and Interventions

Preterm newborns were randomly assigned to receive a *L. reuteri* DSM 17938 supplementation or placebo by the use of a computer-generated randomization scheme. The study personnel, health care workers, and parents were masked to the study group allocation. The active study product consisted of freeze-dried *L. reuteri* DSM 17938 suspended in a mixture of pharmaceutical grade sunflower and medium-chain triglyceride oils supplied in a dark bottle fitted with a dropper cap and an individual number indicating the randomization sequence. Five drops of the formulation, delivering a dose of 1×10^8 colony-forming units (CFUs) of *L. reuteri* DSM 17938, were administered to infants in the probiotic group each day regardless of whether enteric feeds were started and until 30 days of life. The placebo consisted of an identical formulation of oils supplied in an identical bottle and was administered following the same protocol as that described for the probiotic group. There were no differences in smell or taste between the two formulations. Analysis of total Lactobacillus counts was performed in our laboratory on three randomly selected bottles from separate batches to ensure the viability of the live bacteria. Each bottle of 10 mL, containing at least 45 dosages, was confirmed to conform with the stated content of *L. reuteri* of at least 4.5×10^9. The study products were stored refrigerated, which keeps the live content at a stable level.

L. reuteri DSM 17938 has the ability to colonize the entire human gastrointestinal tract with a blood safety profile similar to *L. reuteri* ATCC 55730 (*L. reuteri* DSM 17938 is daughter strain of *L. reuteri ATCC 55730*). Its colonization is only temporary, and genome annotation did not reveal any further gene or gene cluster known to be involved in virulence or antibiotic resistance [11].

Both the *L. reuteri* DSM 17938 and placebo were manufactured and donated by BioGaia AB (Stockholm, Sweden). The viability and purity of the packaging data was guaranteed by the certificate of analysis provided from the manufacturer for each of the batches. In order to minimize differences in feeding and nutrition practices among participating NICUs, the preterm newborns were all exclusively bottle-fed with the same preterm standard formula. Minimal Enteral Feeding was started on day 1 or 2 with small amounts of enteral feedings of formula at intakes of 10–20 mL/kg/day. The limit of tolerance for increasing formula amount (10–20 mL/kg/day) was set at 50% of previous feeds on the assessment of pre-feed gastric residual volumes. Parenteral nutrition, when needed, was started on the second day of life following a standardized protocol.

2.2. Symptoms and Data Evaluation

Anthropometrical parameters, occurrence of adverse reactions, time to regain birth weight, time taken to reach full enteral feeding, duration of antibiotic treatment, days of hospital stay, and stool frequency were recorded. In order to perform quantification of fecal cytokines and fecal calprotectin, a stool sample was obtained at the end of supplementation (30 days of life). Fecal interleukin (IL)-1β, IL-6, IL-8, IL-10, IL-17, TNFα, and fecal calprotectin were evaluated. Briefly, for measurement of fecal IL, TNF, and calprotectin, fecal samples were taken from the diaper with a sterile plastic spoon. Samples were stored in a sterile screw cap tube at 2–8 °C for a maximum of 7 days. Samples were extracted and diluted 1:50 with an incubation buffer. The homogenate was microcentrifuged for 5 min at $10{,}000\times g$, and the supernatant was stored at -20 °C until analysis. The concentrations of fecal cytokines were determined in each fecal sample photometrically with commercially available enzyme-linked immunosorbent assay (ELISA) kits (IL-1β, IL-6, IL-8, IL-10, IL-17, and TNFα (IDK® TNFα), ELISA (Immunodiagnostik, Bensheim, Germany), according to the instructions provided by the manufacturer. Calprotectin levels were measured by ELISA using the Calprotectin-MPR8/14 kit (Buhlmann, Basel, Switzerland). All of the concentrations quantified were adjusted to the wet weight of the individual fecal sample.

Scintigraphy is considered the "gold standard" among methods to evaluate gastric emptying in clinical practice [12]. Scintigraphy allows a complete and physiologic study of the motor function of the stomach. However, it is an expensive technique and specialized personnel from nuclear medicine are needed to perform a scintigraphic study. Moreover, scintigraphy induces significant radiation emission [13], and as result it has limited application in newborns and children, and does not allow repetitive measurements in a short period of time. In comparison, the study of gastric emptying time by ultrasound is a non-invasive method and can be used for research or practical purposes to evaluate gastric emptying in healthy adults, children, and newborns, and in those with gastrointestinal motility disorders. On considering these factors, an ultrasound gastric emptying examination was performed on day 30 after birth, according to a previously reported procedure [14,15]. Lastly, a cost-analysis assessment during NICU hospitalization was performed.

2.3. Outcome Measures

The primary outcome was the assessment of *L. reuteri* DSM 17938 supplementation on feeding tolerance through evaluation of cytokine fecal profile, clinical parameters, and ultrasound measurement during the first month of life. The secondary outcome was to evaluate the costs of supplementation, calculated based on duration of hospitalization.

2.4. Sample Size

To calculate the minimum sample size, we used previous published data [7] about the reduction of average time of gastric emptying; we hypothesized a reduction of 10% of the average time and we used an alpha of 0.05 and a power of 0.9. Using Stata Software, we estimated a required sample size of 20 for each group.

We repeated the sample size calculation using, as the main outcome, the reduction of the cytokine fecal profile and setting an alpha of 0.05 and a power of 0.9. In this case, the required sample was around 30. We hypothesized a drop-out rate of 20%; then, we planned to enroll 72 subjects.

2.5. Data Analysis

Clinical and functional gastrointestinal variables were considered prospectively. The mean and standard deviation of each quantitative parameter were calculated and means were compared by unpaired Student's *t*-test, after establishing the normal distribution of variables by Bartlett's test. Significance was set at $p < 0.05$. To evaluate the costs of the hospitalizations, we used the Diagnosis Related Group (DRG) rate as reported on the Official website of Italian Ministry of Health for DRG 388 (prematurity without major risks).

3. Results

A total of 72 preterm newborns were eligible. Twelve newborns were excluded from analysis because of parental refusal to participate (three neonates), withdrawal from the study (five neonates), or maternal desire to breastfeed (three neonates). The need for exclusive bottle-feeding should be considered the most important covert/clearly expressed cause of high drop-out of these infants. However, the response rate was 83.3% (60/72), higher than that expected (80%). A total of 60 preterm newborns were randomly assigned to *L. reuteri* DSM 17938 or to the placebo group. Clinical and demographic characteristics of the infants at birth are shown in Table 1. No significant differences were observed between the two groups at baseline. The newborns receiving *L. reuteri* DSM 17938 had a significant decrease in the number of days needed to reach full enteral feeding ($p < 0.01$), days of hospital stay ($p < 0.01$), and days of antibiotic treatment ($p < 0.01$) compared with those given placebo. Further, significant differences were found in time to regain birth weight, which was reduced in the *L. reuteri* DSM 17938 supplemented group ($p < 0.05$), and in body weight at the end of the study, which was lower in the placebo group ($p < 0.05$), Table 2. Multiple statistically significant differences were observed in the pattern of fecal cytokine profiles between the two groups. The anti-inflammatory cytokine IL-10, which is involved in immune tolerance, was increased in newborns receiving *L. reuteri* DSM 17938. Pro-inflammatory cytokines: IL-17, IL-8, and TNFα levels were increased in newborns given placebo. The newborns receiving *L. reuteri* DSM 17938 had a significant decrease in calprotectin level compared with the placebo group. The IL-1β was increased in the group treated with *L. reuteri* DSM 17938. IL-6 was increased in newborns receiving *L. reuteri* DSM 17938, but the difference was not statistically significant (Table 3). Regarding gastric emptying, significant differences in the half-emptying (T1/2) time and fasting antral area (FAA) were reported, confirming the improved motility pattern in the probiotic administration group (Table 4). There were no adverse events related to the trial in the *L. reuteri* DSM 17938 supplemented babies.

Table 1. Clinical and demographic data at baseline.

Total $n = 60$	*L. reuteri* DSM 17938 ($n = 30$)	Placebo ($n = 30$)	p
Gestational age	30.2 ± 1.2	30.1 ± 1.2	n.s.
Gender (M/F)	15/15	16/14	n.s.
Delivery (VD/CD)	4/26	5/25	n.s.
Birth weight (g)	1471.5 ± 455.1	1406.6 ± 536.4	n.s.

Gender: M/F = Male/Female; Delivery: vaginal delivery (VD)/cesarean delivery (CD). Non significant (n.s.)

Table 2. Clinical results at the end of the study.

Clinical Parameter	*L. reuteri* DSM 17938	Placebo	*p*
Time taken to reach full enteral feeding (day)	4.2 ± 1.1	7.5 ± 3.2	<0.01
Day of hospitalization (day)	13.4 ± 2.2	22.4 ± 3.2	<0.01
Duration of antibiotic treatment (day)	4.2 ± 4.3	12.5 ± 7.2	<0.01
Time to regain birth weight (day)	6.4 ± 1.6	7.3 ± 1.3	<0.05
Weight at the end of the study (g)	1955.3 ± 653.4	1737.6 ± 512	<0.05
Stool frequency (*n*/day on the last week)	2.5 ± 0.7	2.8 ± 0.9	<0.05

Table 3. Fecal cytokines.

Group	IL-1β pg/mL	IL-8 pg/mL	IL-10 pg/mL	IL-17 pg/mL	Calprotectin µg/g	TNFα pg/mL	IL-6 pg/mL
LR	57.4 ± 73.3	56.7 ± 72.4	6.3 ± 3.2	6.5 ± 1.9	246.6 ± 78.4	8.0 ± 3.1	3.2 ± 2.8
Placebo	17.1 ± 16.7	197.3 ± 222.1	4.2 ± 1.7	8.8 ± 3.5	323.9 ± 111.7	12.7 ± 7.7	2.9 ± 1.7
p	0.04	0.04	0.02	0.02	0.01	0.01	n.s.

LR = *L. reuteri* DSM 17938; IL = interleukin; TNF = tumor necrosis factor.

Table 4. Gastric emptying parameters at the end of the study.

Parameter	*L. reuteri* DSM 17938	Placebo	*p*
T1/2 (Half-emptying time) (min)	73.8 ± 7.5	80.4. ± 6.1	0.0004
Fasting antral area (cm^2)	0.6 ± 0.2	0.8 ± 0.3	0.009

The cost of treatment saved by the reduction of hospitalization by giving *L. reuteri* DSM 17938 amounted to 2043 Euros per infant.

4. Discussion

L. reuteri DSM 17938 supplementation in preterm newborns improves intestinal motility and changes the cytokine profile in stools. Our study underlines the potential beneficial effects of *L. reuteri* DSM 17938 supplementation on clinical and functional variables related to maturation of gastrointestinal function. In particular, it shows that oral supplementation with *L. reuteri* DSM 17938 improves feeding tolerance in preterm newborns with clinical effects on growth, hospitalization, and antibiotic treatment.

Primary colonization of the gut can be considered an important step in the development of intestinal functions and the transferal of the microbiota at birth from maternal vaginal and intestinal flora to the newborn gut is fundamental [16]. The continuous and complex cross-talk between the gut and its microbial content is a normal part of development and plays a crucial role in the ability to distinguish harmless bacterial and food antigens from potentially dangerous antigens. This function requires a sophisticated system that is responsive to a wide variety of microbial and food antigens that transit or populate the gut [17].

An imbalance of normal intestinal microbiota, or the host response to such an imbalance are thought to be involved in the pathogenesis of several intestinal diseases [18]. The beneficial effect of probiotic supplementation on feeding intolerance and immunomodulation has been reported in several studies [4]. A recent study by Rojas [19] reported feeding intolerance episodes and duration of hospitalization significantly lower in preterm infants <1500 g exposed to *L. reuteri* DSM 17938 in comparison to placebo exposed infants. Different from the study by Rojas, our newborns supplemented with probiotic reached the full enteral feeding in a shorter time.

The specific mechanism of probiotic supplementation on gastrointestinal function is not yet clear. Functional components of the human gastrointestinal tract do not evolve simultaneously and it has been shown that a reduced or an abnormal microbial colonization during the first months of life would provoke a slower postnatal maturation of epithelial cell barrier functions, of neuronal route, and of the immunomodulation system of the GALT [20]. This aberrant development of gut functions could finally lead to mucosal inflammation and play a pivotal role in the development of feeding intolerance [21] or other diseases later in life. In an animal model, *L. reuteri* DSM 17938 significantly reduced intestinal mucosal IL and interferon levels, and such reduction corresponded to a reduction in the low grade histological damage induced by cow milk formula feeding [10].

In agreement with these data, in our study, early probiotic supplementation induced a decrease in fecal pro-inflammatory cytokines, IL-17, IL-8, and TNFα, and an increase in the fecal anti-inflammatory cytokine IL-10. Our data suggest a potential anti-inflammatory effect of probiotic with a shift in the tolerogenic mechanism on naïve CD4+ T cells that suppress the expression of T effector cells (Th1 and Th2) and stimulate the expansion of regulatory T cells (Tregs). Furthermore, significant changes in IL-1β and IL-6 levels were found in preterms given probiotic compared to placebo, and previous studies in animals have shown that these two cytokines can have excitatory and neuromodulatory roles in the myenteric plexus, stimulating gastrointestinal motility [22,23]. Also, fecal calprotectin, a well-known marker of gut inflammation, was reduced in the infants supplemented with *L. reuteri* DSM 17938. The modulation of fecal calprotectin by this specific probiotic strain has been reported in the literature [24,25].

Another important aspect is the growing evidence suggesting that the intestinal microbiota may be emitting and receiving a multiplicity of signals to and from the brain, thus playing a critical role in the modulation of the gut-brain axis [26,27]. An immature ontogenesis of this bidirectional interrelationship between the enteric microbiota and the nervous system could affect the pathophysiology of feeding intolerance [28]. In this context, the strength of contemporary action on the motility and immunity of the intestine could result in a better functionality of the whole intestinal function. Our study demonstrates that gastric motility was improved in preterm infants given *L. reuteri* DSM 17398, as shown by the significantly increased gastric emptying time, and the significantly reduced FAA. The clinical counterpart of such improved gastric activity is the decreased gastric residual in preterm infants given *L. reuteri* DSM 17938 and the consequent earlier achievement of full enteral feeding and the faster regain to birth weight compared to the placebo group. This bacterial strain has already been used in a pediatric population [29], and a recent paper [30] showed that LR DSM 17938 increased both colonic migrating motor complex frequency and velocity in an animal model. The authors, based upon the effects of LR DSM 17938 on the adult mouse colon, speculated that this approach may help to screen and identify the therapeutic effect of LR DSM 17938 on constipation and, generally, to correlate the given effect of the probiotic on the enteric nervous system with the action on GI motility.

5. Conclusions

Our study demonstrates an effective role for *L. reuteri* DSM 17938 supplementation in preventing feeding intolerance and improving gut motor and immune function development in bottle-fed stable preterm newborns. The physiological mechanisms underlying these effects may involve changes in cytokine inflammatory patterns. Finally, in light of our cost-analysis assessment, another benefit from the use of this probiotic is in the form of reductions in the costs for the Health Care service.

Acknowledgments: Funding Sources The authors state that they do not receive any founding for the publication fees for this article: All phases of this study were supported by each of the institutions with which the authors are affiliated (University of Bari, IRCCS "S de Bellis" Castellana Grotte, Ospedale Perrino Brindisi, Ospedale San Giovanni di Dio Crotone). Financial Disclosure: The authors have indicated they have no financial relationships relevant to this article to disclose.

Author Contributions: Flavia Indrio: conceptualized and designed the study, interpreted the results, drafted, reviewed and revised the manuscript, and approved the final manuscript; Giuseppe Riezzo: calculated and interpreted all the gastric emptying parameters, reviewed and revised the manuscript, and approved the final manuscript; Silvio Tafuri: conducted and interpreted the statistical analyses, drafted the initial manuscript, reviewed and revised the manuscript, and approved the final manuscript; Barbara Carlucci, Maria Ficarella, and Massimo Bisceglia: participated in the clinical study, recruited the newborns, reviewed and approved the final manuscript; Lorenzo Polimeno: coordinated and supervised the laboratory analyses, interpreted the results, reviewed and revised the manuscript, and approved the final manuscript; Ruggiero Francavilla: supervised the clinical study, reviewed and approved the final manuscript.

Abbreviations

DCs	Dendritic cells
GALT	Gut associated lymphoid tissue
NICU	Neonatal intensive care unit
CFU	Colony forming unit
IL	Interleukin

References

1. Indrio, F.; Riezzo, G.; Cavallo, L.; Di Mauro, A.; Francavilla, R. Physiological basis of food intolerance in VLBW. *J. Matern. Fetal Neonatal Med.* **2011**, *24*, 64–66. [CrossRef] [PubMed]
2. Schatzmann Peron, J.P.; Ligeiro de Oliveira, A.P.; Rizzo, L.V. It takes guts for tolerance: The phenomenon of oral tolerance and the regulation of autoimmune response. *Autoimmun. Rev.* **2009**, *9*, 1–4. [CrossRef] [PubMed]
3. Isolauri, E. Development of healthy gut microbiota early in life. *J. Paediatr. Child Health* **2012**, *48*, 1–6. [CrossRef] [PubMed]
4. Deshpande, G.; Rao, S.; Patole, S.; Bulsara, M. Updated meta-analysis of probiotics for preventing necrotizing enterocolitis in preterm neonates. *Pediatrics* **2010**, *125*, 921–930. [CrossRef] [PubMed]
5. Torrazza, R.M.; Ukhanova, M.; Wang, X.; Sharma, R.; Hudak, M.L.; Neu, J.; Mai, V. Intestinal microbial ecology and environmental factors affecting necrotizing enterocolitis. *PLoS ONE* **2013**, *8*, e83304. [CrossRef] [PubMed]
6. Verhasselt, V. Neonatal tolerance under breastfeeding influence. *Curr. Opin. Immunol.* **2010**, *22*, 620–630. [CrossRef] [PubMed]
7. Indrio, F.; Riezzo, G.; Raimondi, F.; Bisceglia, M.; Cavallo, L.; Francavilla, R. The effects of probiotics on feeding tolerance, bowel habits, and gastrointestinal motility in preterm newborns. *J. Pediatr.* **2008**, *152*, 801–806. [CrossRef] [PubMed]
8. Indrio, F.; Riezzo, G.; Raimondi, F.; Francavilla, R.M.; Montagna, O.; Valenzano, M.L.; Cavallo, L.; Boehm, G. Prebiotics improve gastric motility and gastric electrical activity in preterm newborn. *J. Pediatr. Gastroenterol. Nutr.* **2009**, *49*, 258–261. [CrossRef] [PubMed]
9. Indrio, F.; Riezzo, G.; Raimondi, F.; Bisceglia, M.; Cavallo, L.; Francavilla, R. Effects of probiotic and prebiotic on gastrointestinal motility in newborns. *J. Physiol. Pharmacol.* **2009**, *60*, 27–31. [PubMed]
10. Liu, Y.; Fatheree, N.Y.; Mangalat, N.; Rhoads, J.M. Human-derived probiotic *Lactobacillus reuteri* strains differentially reduce intestinal inflammation. *Am. J. Physiol. Gastrointest. Liver Physiol.* **2010**, *299*, G1087–G1096. [CrossRef] [PubMed]
11. Rosander, A.; Connolly, E.; Roos, S. Removal of antibiotic resistance gene-carrying plasmids from *Lactobacillus reuteri* ATCC 55730 and characterization of the resulting daughter strain, *L. reuteri* DSM 17938. *Appl. Environ. Microbiol.* **2008**, *74*, 6032–6040. [CrossRef] [PubMed]
12. Griffith, G.H.; Owen, G.M.; Kirkman, S.; Shields, R. Measurement of rate of gastric emptying using chromium-51. *Lancet* **1966**, *1*, 1244–1245. [CrossRef]
13. Siegel, J.; Wu, R.; Knight, L.; Zelac, R.E.; Stern, H.S.; Malmud, L.S. Radiation dose estimates for oral agents used in upper gastrointestinal disease. *J. Nucl. Med.* **1983**, *24*, 835–837. [PubMed]
14. Riezzo, G.; Indrio, F.; Montagna, O.; Tripaldi, C.; Laforgia, N.; Chiloiro, M.; Mautone, A. Gastric electrical activity and gastric emptying in term and preterm newborns. *Neurogastroenterol. Mot.* **2000**, *12*, 223–229. [CrossRef]

15. Bolondi, L.; Bortolotti, M.; Santi, V.; Calletti, T.; Gaiani, S.; Labò, G. Measurement of gastric emptying time by real-time ultrasonography. *Gastroenterology* **1985**, *89*, 752–759. [CrossRef]
16. Hattori, M.; Taylor, T.D. The human intestinal microbiome: A new frontier of human biology. *DNA Res.* **2009**, *16*, 1–12. [CrossRef] [PubMed]
17. Nagler-Anderson, C. Man the barrier! Strategic defences in the intestinal mucosa. *Nat. Rev. Immunol.* **2001**, *1*, 59–67. [CrossRef] [PubMed]
18. Sharma, R.; Young, C.; Neu, J. Molecular modulation of intestinal epithelial barrier: Contribution of microbiota. *J. Biomed. Biotechnol.* **2010**, *2010*. [CrossRef] [PubMed]
19. Rojas, M.A.; Lozano, J.M.; Rojas, M.X.; Rodriguez, V.A.; Rondon, M.A.; Bastidas, J.A.; Perez, L.A.; Rojas, C.; Ovalle, O.; Garcia-Harker, J.E.; et al. Prophylactic probiotics to prevent death and nosocomial infection in preterm infants. *Pediatrics* **2012**, *130*, e1113–e1120. [CrossRef] [PubMed]
20. Perrier, C.; Corthésy, B. Gut permeability and food allergies. *Clin. Exp. Allergy* **2011**, *41*, 20–28. [CrossRef] [PubMed]
21. Martin, C.R.; Walker, W.A. Probiotics: Role in pathophysiology and prevention in necrotizing enterocolitis. *Semin. Perinatol.* **2008**, *32*, 127–137. [CrossRef] [PubMed]
22. Kelles, A.; Janssens, J.; Tack, J. IL-1beta and IL-6 excite neurones and suppress cholinergic neurotransmission in the myenteric plexus of the guinea pig. *Neurogastroenterol. Motil.* **2000**, *12*, 531–538. [CrossRef] [PubMed]
23. Kindt, S.; Vanden Berghe, P.; Boesmans, W.; Roosen, L. Tack, J. IL-1beta exposure alters neurotransmitter and electrically induced Ca(2+) responses in the myenteric plexus. *Neurogastroenterol. Motil.* **2010**, *22*. [CrossRef] [PubMed]
24. Moles, L.; Escribano, E.; de Andrés, J.; Montes, M.T.; Rodríguez, J.M.; Jiménez, E.; Sáenz de Pipaón, M.; Espinosa-Martos, I. Administration of *Bifidobacterium breve* PS12929 and *Lactobacillus salivarius* PS12934, two strains isolated from human milk, to very low and extremely low birth weight preterm infants: A pilot study. *J. Immunol. Res.* **2015**, *2015*. [CrossRef] [PubMed]
25. Campeotto, F.; Suau, A.; Kapel, N.; Magne, F.; Viallon, V.; Ferraris, L.; Waligora-Dupriet, A.J.; Soulaines, P.; Leroux, B.; Kalach, N.; et al. A fermented formula in pre-term infants: Clinical tolerance, gut microbiota, down-regulation of faecal calprotectin and up-regulation of faecal secretory IgA. *Br. J. Nutr.* **2011**, *105*, 1843–1851. [CrossRef] [PubMed]
26. Cryan, J.F.; O'Mahony, S.M. The microbiome-gut-brain axis: From bowel to behavior. *Neurogastroenterol. Motil.* **2011**, *23*, 187–192. [CrossRef] [PubMed]
27. Collins, S.M.; Bercik, P. The relationship between intestinal microbiota and the central nervous system in normal gastrointestinal function and disease. *Gastroenterology* **2009**, *136*, 2003–2014. [CrossRef] [PubMed]
28. Calder, P.C. Feeding the immune system. *Proc. Nutr. Soc.* **2013**, *72*, 299–309. [CrossRef] [PubMed]
29. Urbanska, M.; Szajewska, H. The efficacy of *Lactobacillus reuteri* DSM 17938 in infants and children: A review of the current evidence. *Eur. J. Pediatr.* **2014**, *173*, 1327–1337. [CrossRef] [PubMed]
30. Wu, R.Y.; Pasyk, M.; Wang, B.; Forsythe, P.; Bienenstock, J.; Mao, Y.K.; Sharma, P.; Stanisz, A.M.; Kunze, W.A. Spatiotemporal maps reveal regional differences in the effects on gut motility for *Lactobacillus reuteri* and *rhamnosus* strains. *Neurogastroenterol. Motil.* **2013**, *25*, e205–e214. [CrossRef] [PubMed]

12

Modulation of Gut Microbiota of Overweight Mice by Agavins and their Association with Body Weight Loss

Alicia Huazano-García [1,†], Hakdong Shin [2,†] and Mercedes G. López [1,*]

1 Departamento de Biotecnología y Bioquímica, Centro de Investigación y de Estudios Avanzados del IPN, Unidad Irapuato 36821, México; ahuazano@ira.cinvestav.mx

2 Faculty of Food Science and Biotechnology, College of Life Science, Sejong University, Seoul 05006, Korea; hakdong.shin@gmail.com

* Correspondence: mlopez@ira.cinvestav.mx

† These authors contributed equally to this work.

Abstract: Agavins consumption has led to accelerated body weight loss in mice. We investigated the changes on cecal microbiota and short-chain fatty acids (SCFA) associated with body weight loss in overweight mice. Firstly, mice were fed with standard (ST5) or high-fat (HF5) diet for five weeks. Secondly, overweight mice were shifted to standard diet alone (HF-ST10) or supplemented with agavins (HF-ST + A10) or oligofructose (HF-ST + O10), for five more weeks. Cecal contents were collected before and after supplementation to determine microbiota and SCFA concentrations. At the end of first phase, HF5 mice showed a significant increase of body weight, which was associated with reduction of cecal microbiota diversity (PD whole tree; non-parametric t test, $p < 0.05$), increased Firmicutes/Bacteroidetes ratio and reduced SCFA concentrations (t test, $p < 0.05$). After diet shifting, HF-ST10 normalized its microbiota, increased its diversity, and SCFA levels, whereas agavins (HF-ST + A10) or oligofructose (HF-ST + O10) led to partial microbiota restoration, with normalization of the Firmicutes/Bacteroides ratio, as well as higher SCFA levels ($p < 0.1$). Moreover, agavins noticeably enriched *Klebsiella* and *Citrobacter* (LDA > 3.0); this enrichment has not been reported previously under a prebiotic treatment. In conclusion, agavins or oligofructose modulated cecal microbiota composition, reduced the extent of diversity, and increased SCFA. Furthermore, identification of bacteria enriched by agavins opens opportunities to explore new probiotics.

Keywords: agavins; prebiotics; microbiota; overweight; body weight loss; short chain fatty acids

---

1. Introduction

Agavins are branched neo-fructans found in *Agave* plants, which contain a mixture of β(2-1) and β(2-6) linkages [1,2]. The degree of polymerization (DP) and the chemical structure of agavins become more complex as the plant ages. Plants from two to four years old have a high content of agavins with low DP and simpler chemical structures, while plants from five to seven years old contain a large proportion of high-DP agavins and highly-complex chemical structures [3].

Agavins act as prebiotics inducing benefits to host health by providing specific changes in the composition and/or activity of the gut microbiota [4]. Due to their structural complexity, endogenous gastrointestinal enzymes cannot degrade agavins during their passage through the stomach and the small intestine; so they reach both the cecum and colon, where they are fermented by saccharolytic microbiota present in these sites, producing short chain fatty acids (SCFA), mostly acetate, propionate, and butyrate. SCFA are very important because they reduce body weight gain, through G-protein-coupled receptors (GPRs), influencing the secretion of hormones involved in appetite control [5–7]. In addition, SCFA increment through agavins fermentation in both cecum and gut induces a pH drop; which might change the intestinal microbiota structure [8,9].

On the other hand, earlier investigations showed that mice fed with standard or high-fat diets with agavins of low DP led to body weight loss [10–12]. However, the microbial mechanisms remain unclear [12,13]. New molecular techniques that enable analysis of non-cultivable bacteria are starting to be applied in studies investigating the impact of prebiotics on the cecal microbiota. For example, investigations examined the effects of oligofructose (linear fructans) on cecal microbiota using the 16S rRNA gene sequencing technique, showed that the intake of oligofructose in mice not only stimulated the growth of *bifidobacteria* and *lactobacilli*, but also increased other bacteria such as *Streptococcus*, *Clostridium*, *Enterococcus*, *Olsenella*, *Akkermansia*, and *Allobaculum* [14,15]. The abundance of specific taxa, such as *Bifidobacterium* spp. and *Akkermansia muciniphila* has been negatively associated with inflammation in adipose tissue, circulating glucose, leptin, triglycerides, and insulin [16], whereas the enrichment of *Allobaculum* has been associated with body weight loss in obese mice [17]. On the other hand, Firmicutes and Bacteroidetes are usually the most abundant members of the cecal microbiota; however, the ratio of these bacterial groups can change over time or by different factors, such as age, environment, or diet, and especially those with a high fat content [18–20].

In the present work we used agavins from four-year-old *Agave tequilana* plants containing a high proportion of short DP fructans, and studied the response on the microbiota of mice, continuing our previous study on prebiotic supplementation in overweight mice [21]. Here we present changes of cecal microbiota after a diet shift and agavins supplementation, and the possibility of their association with body weight loss in overweight mice. Our hypothesis was that agavins supplementation might improve the host health, through the enrichment of probiotic bacteria, in relation to the diet shift alone.

To our knowledge, this is the first report on the global effects of a diet shift and agavins supplementation on the cecal microbiota composition through a 16S rRNA analysis in overweight mice. Finally, agavins (branched fructans) effects were compared to oligofructose (linear fructans), which was used as a positive control to evaluate the cecal microbiota changes.

2. Materials and Methods

2.1. Animals and Diets

Forty-two male C57BL/6 mice (12 weeks old at the beginning of the experiment were obtained from the Universidad Autonoma Metropolitana, Mexico City, Mexico) and housed in a temperature and humidity controlled room with a 12 h light-dark cycles. Mice were maintained in individual cages since water intake containing the fructans was measured every day. The animals were subject to a two-phase trial, the first to gain weight and the second to lose weight (Supplementary Figure S1). In the first phase mice were fed with standard (n = 12; 5053 Lab Diet, St. Louis, MO, USA) or high-fat diets (n = 30; 58Y1 Test Diet, St. Louis, MO, USA) for five weeks. The standard diet (5053 Lab Diet) contained 62.4% calories from carbohydrates (28.6% starch, 3.24% sucrose, 1.34% lactose, 0.24% fructose, and 0.19% glucose), 24.5% from proteins, and 13.1% from fat. The high-fat diet (58Y1 Test Diet) had 20.3% calories from carbohydrates (16.15% maltodextrin, 8.85% sucrose, and 6.46% powdered cellulose), 18.1% from proteins, and 61.6% from fat (31.7% lard and 3.2% soybean oil). In the second phase, healthy control mice were kept with the standard diet (ST-ST10; n = 8), and the overweight mice were shifted to the standard diet alone (HF-ST10; n = 8) or supplemented with agavins (HF-ST + A10; n = 8) or oligofructose (HF-ST + O10; n = 8) for five more weeks. Food and water were provided ad libitum throughout the experiment.

Mice experiments were conducted according to the Mexican Norm NOM-062-ZOO-1999 and approved by the Institutional Care and Use of Laboratory Animals Committee from Cinvestav-Mexico (CICUAL; protocol number 0091-14).

2.2. *Agavins and Oligofructose Fructans*

Agavins from four-year-old *Agave tequilana* Weber blue variety plants were extracted and purified in our laboratory and presented an average DP of 8 [21]. Oligofructose was bought from Megafarma® (Mexico City, Mexico) and possess an average DP of 5. Agavins and oligofructose were added in the water at a concentration of 0.38 g/mouse/day [15,22].

2.3. *gDNA Extraction*

Cecal contents were collected before and after the fructans supplementation (at five and 10 weeks, respectively). At the end of first and second experimental phase, mice were anaesthetized with a 60 mg/kg intraperitoneal dose of sodium pentobarbital and the gastrointestinal tract was exposed for cecum removal. Cecal content was snap frozen in liquid nitrogen and stored at −70 °C until their use. Genomic DNA was extracted using the ZR Fungal/Bacterial DNA MiniPrep (Irvine, CA, USA), following the manufacturer's instructions. The concentration and purity of DNA were evaluated using a Nanodrop spectrophotometer. Extracted DNA was stored at −20 °C until its use.

2.4. *PCR Amplification of the V4 Region of the Bacterial 16S rRNA Gene*

To assess microbial composition, the V4 region of the bacterial 16S *rRNA* gene was amplified with barcoded fusion primers (F515/R806) [23]. PCR reactions were carried out in triplicate, 25 μL reactions with 5 μM forward and reverse primers, 2 μL template DNA, and 1X of HotMasterMix (5 PRIME, Gaithersburg, MD, USA). Thermal cycling of PCR reactions consisted of an initial denaturation at 94 °C for 3 min, followed by 35 cycles of denaturation at 94 °C for 45 s, annealing at 50 °C for 1 min, and extension at 72 °C for 90 s, with a final extension of 10 min at 72 °C.

2.5. *Amplicon Quantitation, Pooling, and Sequencing*

DNA concentration for each amplicon was measured using the Quant-iT PicoGreen dsDNA reagent and kit (Thermo Scientific, Waltham, MA, USA). Assays were carried out using 2 μL of cleaned PCR product in a total reaction volume of 200 μL in black, 96-well microtiter plates. Fluorescence was measured on a BioTek Synergy HT plate reader using the 480/520-nm excitation/emission filter pair. Following quantitation, cleaned amplicons were combined in equimolar ratios into a single tube. The final concentration of the pooled DNA was determined using the Qubit high-sensitivity dsDNA assay (Invitrogen, Carlsbad, CA, USA). Sequencing was carried out on the Illumina MiSeq platform at New York University.

2.6. *Sequence Analysis*

Sequences were processed and analyzed in the QIIME software package (Quantitative Insights Into Microbial Ecology, v1.8.0, La Jolla, CA, USA) following the pipeline described by Caporaso et al. [24]. Sequences were removed from the analysis if they were <200 or >350 nt in length, had a mean quality score < 20, contained ambiguous characters, contained an uncorrectable barcode, or did not contain the primer sequence. Remaining sequences were assigned to samples by examining the 12-nt barcode. Similar sequences were clustered into operational taxonomic units (OTUs) using the open reference method. Taxonomic assignments for each OTU were made using the Greengenes database (May 2013) with a minimum identity of 97%. Finally, an OTU table was used to generate relative abundance plots and to calculate alpha and beta diversity (alpha diversity refers to the diversity within each sample, and beta diversity refers to patterns of similarities and differences among samples). All communities were rarefied up to 6525 reads per sample to calculate the bacterial diversity.

The raw sequences supporting the results of this article are available in the NCBI Sequence Read Archive repository under accession no. SRX1532779.

2.7. LEfSe Analysis

Linear discriminant analysis effect size (LEfSe) was used to detect significant changes in relative abundance of microbial taxa between overweight mice fed with the standard diet and fructans supplements. Briefly, LEfSe is an algorithm for applying 16S *rRNA* gene datasets to detect bacterial organisms that are differentially abundant between two or more microbial environments [25]. LEfSe first identifies features that are significantly different among biological classes using the non-parametric factorial Kruskal-Wallis ran-sum test, and then LEfSe utilizes linear discriminant analysis (LDA) to estimate the effect of each differentially-abundant feature.

2.8. SCFA and pH Determinations

A weight of 0.05 g of homogenized cecal content was placed in a conic tube. The pH was measured directly in the cecal sample through insertion of a microelectrode (PHR-146, Lazar Research Laboratories Inc., Los Angeles, CA, USA) in the tube. The pH value was read when stability was achieved; after each reading, the microelectrode was removed and rinsed with distilled water. SCFA analysis was carried out in the same sample using gas chromatography and flame ionization detection (GC-FID) [26]. Briefly, 0.3 mL of Milli-Q water was added to the tube with cecal content. The solution was acidified with 0.05 mL of H_2SO_4 and SCFA were extracted by shaking with 0.6 mL of diethylether and subsequent centrifugation at 10,000× *g* for 30 s. One microliter of the ether phase was injected directly onto a Nukol™ capillary column (30 m × 0.32 mm; Supelco, Bellefonte, PA, USA) using an injector temperature of 180 °C and nitrogen as the carrier gas. The column temperature was initially 80 °C, then increased to 120 °C at 15 °C/min and kept at this temperature for 10 min, following an increment to 200 °C at 10 °C/min and remaining at this temperature for 10 min. The detector temperature was 230 °C. The identification and quantification of the SCFA were carried out using the retention times and calibration curves for each acid, respectively.

2.9. Statistical Analysis

Results are presented as mean ± SEM. Differences between ST5 and HF5 groups were assessed by Student's *t* test. Differences between the diets were determined using a one-way ANOVA followed by Bonferroni's multiple comparison tests. Differences were considered significant when $p < 0.05$. Statistical analyses were performed using GraphPad Prism (GraphPad Software, La Jolla, CA, USA).

3. Results

To assess the impact of agavins on cecal microbiota of overweight mice, we sequenced V4 amplicons of 16S rRNA genes. After trimming, assembly, and quality filtering, we obtained a total of 635,054 sequence reads from 42 samples using a MiSeq sequencing platform. The average sequence read was 15,041 ± 1561 per sample (Supplementary Table S1).

The results of present work showed that the mouse cecal microbiota was greatly dominated by three phyla (Firmicutes, Bacteroidetes, and Proteobacteria) with six other minor phyla (Tenericutes, Actinobacteria, Cyanobacteria, Defferribacteres, Verrucomicrobia, and TM7; Supplementary Figure S2).

3.1. High-Fat Diet Induced Overweight and Altered Microbial Diversity and Composition

At the end of the first phase trial, after a high-fat diet consumption for five weeks, HF5 mice showed a significant increase in body gain weight (reaching overweight levels [27]) in relation to the ST5 group (7.26 ± 0.54 g vs. 2.22 ± 0.23 g, respectively; *t* test, $p < 0.001$; Figure 1A); which was associated with a substantial loss of bacterial alpha diversity in cecum of HF5 mice, compared to the standard diet control group ST5 (438 ± 61 vs. 774 ± 75, the number of observed species, respectively; non-parametric *t* test, $p < 0.05$; Figure 1B). In addition, a clear separation of bacterial structures between mice fed with the high-fat or standard diet was observed (weighted UniFrac distances; PERMANOVA, $p < 0.05$; Figure 1C).

On the other hand, HF5 mice were characterized by the increased relative abundance in approximately 41% of Proteobacteria (Helicobacteraceae and Desulfovibrionaceae families, including the *Bilophila* genus) and decreased in about of 17% the Firmicutes (Ruminococcaceae, Lactobacillaceae, Erysipelotrichaceae, Lachnospiraceae, and Dehalobacteriaceae families, including the genera *Lactobacillus*, *Coprobacillus*, *Allobaculum*, *Roseburia*, and *Dehalobacterium*) and approximately 25% the Bacteroidetes (S24_7 and Prevotellaceae families including *Prevotella* genus) (LDA > 3.0; Figure 1D and Supplementary Figure S3), with an increase of the Firmicutes/Bacteroidetes ratio (1.78 vs. 1.17 for HF5 and ST5, respectively; t test, $p < 0.05$; Figure 1E).

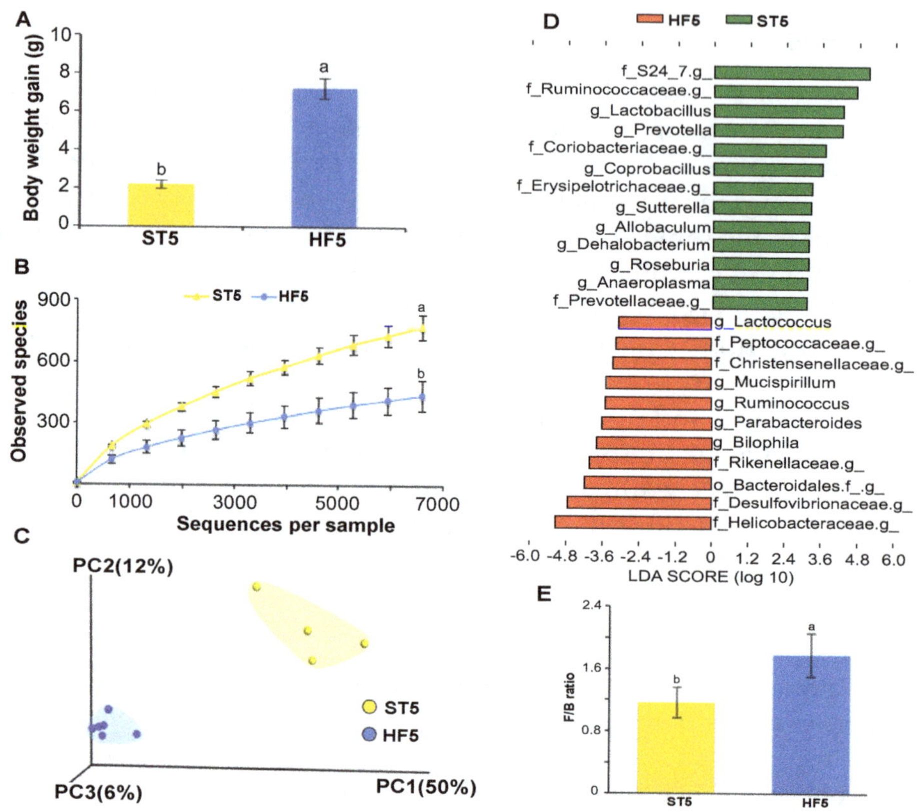

Figure 1. High-fat diet consumption for five weeks induced overweight and modified the cecal microbiota composition of mice. Body weight gain (**A**); bacterial alpha diversity in cecum according to diet (**B**); principal coordinate analysis (PCoA) plot of cecal communities (**C**); linear discriminant analysis showing the differentially-overrepresented genera between mice fed with standard and high-fat diets (**D**); and the effect of the diet on the Firmicutes/Bacteroidetes ratio (**E**). Treatments with different superscript letters indicate significant differences (t test, $p < 0.05$).

High-fat diet consumption not only induced alterations in the body weight and composition of the cecal microbiota, but also changed the biochemical environment and microbiota activity in the cecum of HF5 mice which showed a significant reduction of SCFA levels and an increment of pH in the cecal content in relation to the standard diet (ST5) group (t test, $p < 0.05$; Table 1).

Table 1. The effect of high-fat diet intake for five weeks on short-chain fatty acid concentration and pH in the cecal content of mice.

Group	Acetic Acid *	Propionic Acid *	Butyric Acid *	pH
ST5	15.13 ± 0.92^{a}	3.85 ± 0.20^{a}	4.54 ± 0.33^{a}	7.60 ± 0.12^{b}
HF5	5.43 ± 0.65^{b}	1.96 ± 0.11^{b}	1.72 ± 0.09^{b}	8.18 ± 0.06^{a}

ST5: mice fed with a standard diet; HF5: mice fed with a high-fat diet. Data are shown as mean ± SEM. Means with different letters (a,b) indicate significant differences (t test, $p < 0.05$). * μmoles/g of wet weight.

3.2. *Diet Shift Induced Body Weight Loss and Restored Altered Microbial Diversity in Overweight Mice*

At the end of the second phase, after overweight mice were switched for five weeks to the standard diet, HF-ST10 mice exhibited a body weight loss (Figure 2A). In addition, the return to standard diet in all cases—with or without prebiotic supplementation—decreased the Firmicutes/Bacteroidetes ratio from 1.78, observed in HF5, to 1.64, 1.52, and 0.75 for HF-ST10, HF-ST10 + A, and HF-ST + O, respectively (Bonferroni's test, $p < 0.05$; Figure 2B), as well as the relative abundance of Proteobacteria in approximately 34% (Helicobacteraceae and Desulfovibrionaceae families; Figure 2C).

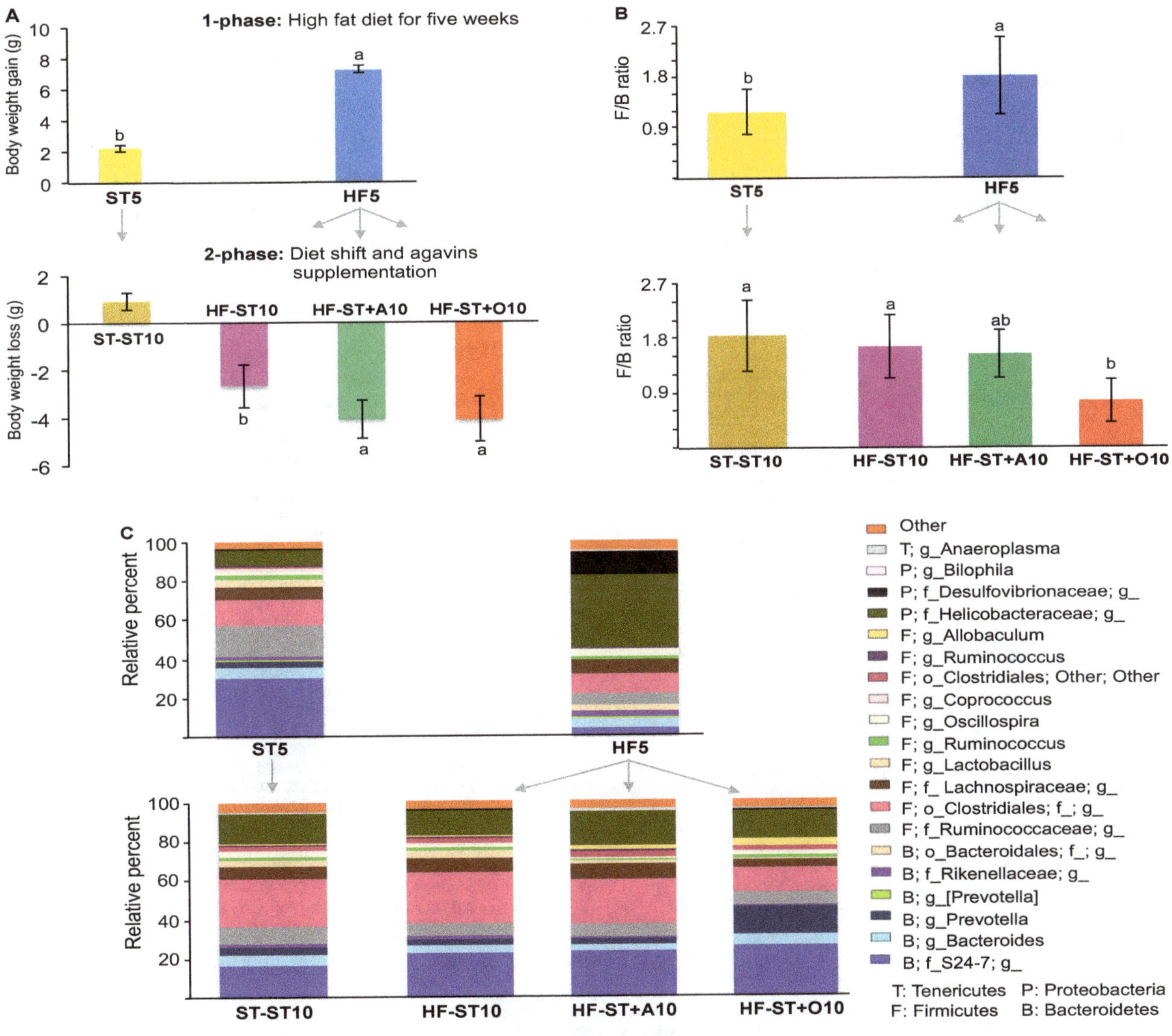

Figure 2. The effect of the diet shift and prebiotic supplementation on body weight loss and cecal microbiota composition in overweight mice. Body weight loss (**A**); Firmicutes/Bacteroidetes (F/B) ratio after the switch to a standard diet alone, or supplemented with agavins or oligofructose (**B**); differences in relative abundance of bacterial taxa in cecum according to diet group (**C**). Each taxon representing >1% of the average relative abundance in study groups is indicated by a different color.

HF-ST10 mice were characterized by a complete restoration of bacterial alpha diversity in relation to the HF5 group (771 ± 115 vs. 438 ± 61, the number of observed species, respectively; non-parametric *t* test, $p > 0.05$; Figure 3A), as well as the bacterial community structures in cecum, compared to the standard diet (ST-ST10) group (weighted UniFrac distances; PERMANOVA, $p > 0.05$; Figure 3B).

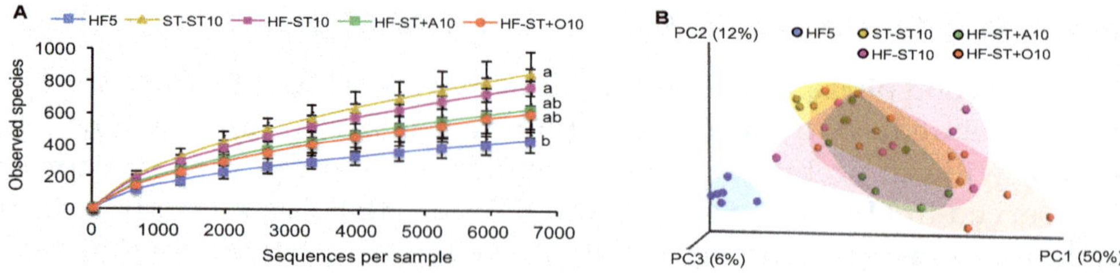

Figure 3. The effect of the diet shift and prebiotic supplementation on the cecal microbiota composition of overweight mice. Bacterial alpha diversity in cecum according to diet group (**A**); treatments with different superscript letters indicate significant differences (Bonferroni's test, $p < 0.05$). Principal coordinate analysis (PCoA) plot of cecal communities (**B**). Weighted UniFrac distances were used to evaluate beta diversity.

Furthermore, the HF-ST10 group showed a drastic change on the cecal microbiota composition in relation to the HF5 group, increasing the abundance of the genera *Lactobacillus, Prevotella, Allobaculum, Anaeroplasma, Blautia, Coprobacillus, Dehalobacterium, Candidatus Arthromitus, Sutterella,* and *Adlercreutzia* and decreased *Lactococcus, Acinetobacter, Anaerotruncus, AF12, Mucispirillum, Parabacteroides,* and *Bilophila* (LDA > 3.0; Figures 2C and 4A).

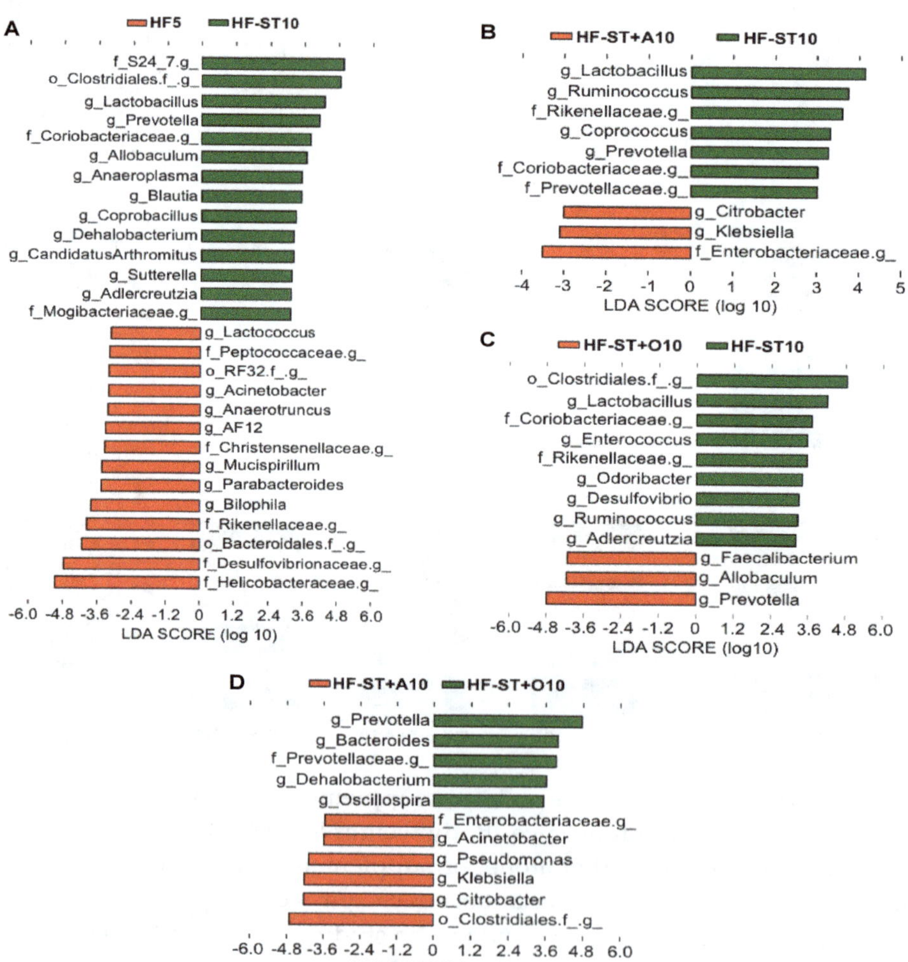

Figure 4. Linear discriminant analysis showing the differentially-overrepresented genera between overweight mice fed with: a high-fat diet and the diet shift (**A**); the diet shift and agavins supplement (**B**); the diet shift and oligofructose supplement (**C**); and agavins and oligofructose supplements (**D**). LDA effect size (3.0-fold) was used to determine the significant biomarkers.

Moreover, the diet shift led HF-ST10 mice to recover the biochemical environment and microbiota activity in the cecum, displaying similar SCFA concentration and pH values in relation to the standard diet (ST-ST10) group (t test, $p > 0.05$; Table 2).

Table 2. The effect of the diet shift and agavins supplementation on short-chain fatty acid concentration and pH in the cecal content of overweight mice.

Group	Acetic Acid *	Propionic Acid *	Butyric Acid *	pH
ST-ST10	20.73 ± 2.07^{c}	$6.07 \pm 0.60^{a,b}$	$6.53 \pm 0.60^{a,b}$	7.65 ± 0.07^{a}
HF-ST10	26.68 ± 0.69^{b}	6.48 ± 0.26^{b}	6.16 ± 0.39^{b}	7.26 ± 0.08^{a}
HF-ST + A10	34.27 ± 1.77^{a}	7.16 ± 0.44^{a}	7.51 ± 0.46^{a}	6.92 ± 0.03^{b}
HF-ST + O10	34.89 ± 1.85^{a}	7.73 ± 0.29^{a}	6.95 ± 0.40^{a}	6.79 ± 0.06^{a}

ST-ST10: healthy mice fed with the standard diet for ten weeks. HF-ST10: overweight mice switched for five weeks to the standard diet alone; or supplemented with agavins (HF-ST + A10) or oligofructose (HF-ST + O10). Data are shown as mean ± SEM. Means with different letters (a,b,c) indicate significant differences (Bonferroni's test, $p < 0.1$).
* μmoles/g of wet weight.

3.3. *Effects of Prebiotic Supplementation on Cecal Microbiota in Overweight Mice*

In contrast, to standard diet alone, overweight mice that were shifted to the standard diet and received any prebiotic treatments (agavins or oligofructose) exhibited an accelerated body weight loss (Figure 2A), as well as a partial restoration of the cecal diversity in relation to the HF5 group (635 ± 177 and 607 ± 117, the number of observed species for HF-ST + A and HF-ST + O, respectively, vs. 438 ± 75, the number of observed species; non-parametric t test, $p < 0.05$; Figure 3A). Alpha bacterial diversity was not significantly different between mice fed agavins (branched fructans) or oligofructose (linear fructans). Interestingly, bacterial community structures from the agavins and oligofructose supplementation were not different to those from the unsupplemented standard diet (non-parametric t test, $p < 0.001$; Figure 3B and Supplementary Figure S4A). Noticeably, the HF-ST + O10 group showed the highest dispersion along the PC1 axis in relation to HF-ST + A10 and ST-ST10 groups (non-parametric t test, $p < 0.01$; Figure 3B and Supplementary Figure S4B). In addition, the cecal microbiota of the agavins-supplemented diet group (HF-ST + A10) was more similar to the standard diet groups (ST-ST10 or HF-ST10) compared to the oligofructose (HF-ST + O10) (weighted UniFrac distance; t test, $p < 0.05$; Supplementary Figure S4C,D).

On the other hand, the supplementation of agavins (HF-ST + A10) or oligofructose (HF-ST + O10) was associated with different communities: in relation to HF-ST10 group, agavins increased two genera (*Citrobacter* and *Klebsiella*) and decreased four genera (*Lactobacillus*, *Ruminococcus*, *Prevotella*, and *Coprococcus*), while oligofructose increased three genera (*Prevotella*, *Faecalibacterium* and *Allobaculum*) and decreased six genera (*Lactobacillus*, *Enterococcus*, *Odoribacter*, *Adlercreutzia*, *Desulfovibrio*, and *Ruminococcus*). In relation to oligofructose, agavins increased *Citrobacter*, *Klebsiella*, *Pseudomonas*, and *Acinetobacter*, and decreased *Prevotella*, *Bacteroides*, *Dehalobacterium*, and *Oscillospira* (LDA > 3.0; Figures 2C and 4B–D).

In the same way as the diet shift alone, prebiotic (agavins or oligofructose) supplementation modified not only the cecal microbiota composition, but also the microbiota activity. However, supplementation with agavins (HF-ST + A10) or oligofructose (HF-ST + O10) significantly increased the concentration of acetic, propionic, and butyric acids with a noticeable reduction of pH in the cecal content in relation to non-supplemented controls (ST-ST10 and HF-ST10; Bonferroni's test, $p < 0.1$; Table 2).

4. Discussion

We previously reported that agavins supplementation to a standard diet reverted the metabolic syndrome (including body weight loss) induced by high-fat diet consumption [21]. However, we do not know that the changes originated with agavins consumption on the gut microbiota, which could be associated with this effect. Therefore, the present study describes the changes in the cecal microbiota, SCFA production, and pH values associated with body weight loss in overweight mice.

High-fat diet consumption for five weeks significantly increased the body weight gain of mice, and also led to a substantial decrease of bacterial diversity in the cecal microbiota (Figures 2A and 3A); which is consistent with the effects of fat in reducing diversity, as previously reported [28–30].

Firmicutes and Bacteroidetes are the most abundant members of the cecal microbiota, however, the ratio of these bacterial groups can change over time or by different factors, such environment and diet (especially those with a high fat content) [18–20]. An increase of the ratio of Firmicutes/Bacteroidetes was seen in overweight mice, which has been associated with obesity [18,20].

We found that a high-fat diet enriched *Bilophila*, a genus that include some opportunistic pathogens (for example *B. wadsworthia* [31]). Microbial changes under a high fat diet reduced cecal SCFA concentrations and increased pH, which is consistent with altered microbial metabolic activity, as previously reported [32].

Supplementation with agavins or oligofructose showed an accelerated body weight loss with partially restored the cecal microbiota diversity (Figures 2A and 3A), as well as an increase in the SCFA concentrations and acidic pH (Table 2). This might be mediated by selected supplement addition for specific bacterial taxa that tolerate a more acidic pH [33], since the direct effect of probiotic supplements on the microbiota have not been demonstrated [9,14,34]. Moreover, acetic acid suppresses appetite [35] and propionate and butyrate acids modulate hormones, such as GLP-1 and PYY, involved in satiety [5–7], and this mechanism might also contribute to body weight loss.

Weight loss was associated with a decrease in the Firmicutes/Bacteroidetes ratio, as in previous reports [18,36], and the effect is due, in part, to a reduction of caloric intake in fructans-supplemented mice [21]. Taxa associated with greater body weight loss included *Klebsiella* and *Citrobacter* (Enterobacteriaceae; Figure 4B). Enterobacteriaceae have also been reported to increase during weight loss in obese mice [37] and humans [38,39]. Other bacteria enriched by supplementation with oligofructose included *Prevotella*, *Allobaculum*, and *Faecalibacterium* genera (Figure 4C). Similarly, a previous study has reported an association between *Allobaculum* and a reduction of body weight in obese mice [17].

Interestingly, agavins and oligofructose supplementation led to the highest cecum SCFA, despite of structural differences between these fructans. However, fructan structure and the degree of polymerization were associated with differences in the bacteria genera enriched by agavins (branched) or oligofructose (linear). In relation to supplementation with oligofructose, agavins supplementation enriched *Citrobacter*, *Klebsiella*, *Pseudomonas*, and *Acinetobacter*, and decreased *Prevotella*, *Bacteroides*, *Dehalobacterium*, and *Oscillospira* (Figure 4D). Nevertheless, both supplements shared the physiological response of accelerating body weight loss perhaps due to functional redundancy of the gut microbiota [40].

5. Conclusions

In conclusion, diet supplementation of agavins restored microbiota diversity depleted by a high-fat diet, reduced the Firmicutes/Bacteroidetes ratio, enriched members of the Enterobacteriaceae, and increased the SCFA concentration in cecum, which could induce an accelerated weight loss in mice. These results could provide novel insight to develop a new supplementary strategy using agavins to modulate gut microbiota in overweight or obese individuals, which might have positive consequences on body weight loss. Furthermore, the enrichment of members of Enterobacteriaceae has not been reported previously under a prebiotic supplement, which opens opportunities to explore new probiotics.

Acknowledgments: The authors would like to thank Maria Gloria Dominguez-Bello for her advice on the microbiota analyses.

Author Contributions: A.H.-G. and M.G.L. had the idea, designed the study, and performed the mouse experiments. H.S. and A.H.-G. performed the analysis of microbiota sequence data. A.H.-G., H.S., and M.G.L. contributed to the discussion of the data and wrote the manuscript. All authors read and approved the final manuscript.

References

1. López, M.G.; Mancilla-Margalli, N.A.; Mendoza-Diaz, G. Molecular structures of fructans from *Agave tequilana* Weber var. azul. *J. Agric. Food Chem.* **2003**, *51*, 7835–7840. [CrossRef] [PubMed]
2. Mancilla-Margalli, N.A.; López, M.G. Water-soluble carbohydrates and fructan structure patterns from *Agave* and *Dasylirion* species. *J. Agric. Food Chem.* **2006**, *54*, 7832–7839. [CrossRef] [PubMed]
3. Mellado-Mojica, E.; López, M.G. Fructan metabolism in *A.* tequilana Weber blue variety along its developmental cycle in the field. *J. Agric. Food Chem.* **2012**, *60*, 11704–11713. [CrossRef] [PubMed]
4. Gibson, G.R.; Scott, K.P.; Rastall, R.A.; Tuohy, K.M.; Hotchkiss, A.; Dubert-Ferrandon, A.; Gareau, M.; Murphy, E.F.; Saulnier, D.; Loh, G.; et al. Dietary prebiotics: Current status and new definition. *Food Sci. Technol. Bull. Funct. Foods* **2010**, *7*, 1–19. [CrossRef]
5. Psichas, A.; Sleeth, M.L.; Murphy, K.G.; Brooks, L.; Bewick, G.A.; Hanyaloglu, A.C.; Ghatei, M.A.; Bloom, S.R.; Frost, G. The short chain fatty acid propionate stimulates GLP-1 and PYY secretion via free fatty acid receptor 2 in rodents. *Int. J. Obes.* **2015**, *39*, 424–429. [CrossRef] [PubMed]
6. Tolhurst, G.; Heffron, H.; Lam, Y.S.; Parker, H.E.; Habib, A.M.; Diakogiannaki, E.; Cameron, J.; Grosse, J.; Reimann, F.; Gribble, F.M. Short-chain fatty acids stimulate glucagon-like peptide-1 secretion via the G-protein-couples receptor FFAR2. *Diabetes* **2012**, *61*, 364–371. [CrossRef] [PubMed]
7. Lin, H.V.; Frassetto, A.; Kowalik, E.J., Jr.; Nawrocki, A.R.; Lu, M.M.; Kosinski, J.R.; Hubert, J.A.; Szeto, D.; Yao, X.; Forrest, G.; et al. Butyrate and propionate protect against diet-induced obesity and regulate gut hormones via free fatty acids receptor 3-independent mechanisms. *PLoS ONE* **2012**, *7*, e35240. [CrossRef] [PubMed]
8. Duncan, S.H.; Louis, P.; Thomson, J.M.; Flint, H.J. The role of pH in determining the species composition on the human colonic microbiota. *Environ. Microbiol.* **2009**, *11*, 2112–2122. [CrossRef] [PubMed]
9. Chung, W.S.; Walker, A.W.; Louis, P.; Parkhill, J.; Vermeiren, J.; Bosscher, D.; Duncan, S.H.; Flint, H.J. Modulation of the human gut microbiota by dietary fibres occurs at the species level. *BMC Biol.* **2016**, *14*, 3. [CrossRef] [PubMed]
10. Santiago-García, P.A.; López, M.G. Agavins from *Agave angustifolia* and *Agave potatorum* affect food intake, body weight gain and satiety-related hormones (GLP-1 and ghrelin) in mice. *Food Funct.* **2014**, *5*, 3311–3319. [CrossRef] [PubMed]
11. Márquez-Aguirre, A.L.; Camacho-Ruíz, R.M.; Gutiérrez-Mercado, Y.K.; Padilla-Camberos, E.; González-Ávila, M.; Gálvez-Gastélum, F.J.; Díaz-Martínez, N.E.; Ortuño-Sahagún, D. Fructans from *Agave tequilana* with a lower degree of polymerization prevent weight gain, hyperglycemia and liver steatosis in high-fat diet-induced obese mice. *Plant Foods Hum. Nutr.* **2016**, *71*, 416–421. [CrossRef] [PubMed]
12. Márquez-Aguirre, A.L.; Camacho-Ruiz, R.M.; Arriaga-Alba, M.; Padilla-Camberos, E.; Kirchmayr, M.R.; Blasco, J.L.; González-Avila, M. Effects of *Agave tequilana* fructans with different degree of polymerization profiles on the body weight, blood lipids and count of fecal *Lactobacilli/Bifidobacteria* in obese mice. *Food Funct.* **2013**, *4*, 1237–1244. [CrossRef] [PubMed]
13. Rendón-Huerta, J.A.; Juárez-Flores, B.; Pinos-Rodríguez, J.M.; Aguirre-Rivera, J.; Delgado-Portales, R.E. Effects of different sources of fructans on body weight, blood metabolites and fecal bacteria in normal and obese non-diabetic and diabetic rats. *Plant Foods Hum. Nutr.* **2012**, *67*, 64–70. [CrossRef] [PubMed]
14. Mao, B.; Li, D.; Zhao, J.; Liu, X.; Gu, Z.; Chen, Y.Q.; Zhang, H.; Chen, W. Metagenomic insight into the effects of fructo-oligosaccharides (FOS) on the composition of fecal microbiota in mice. *J. Agric. Food Chem.* **2015**, *63*, 856–863. [CrossRef] [PubMed]

15. Everard, A.; Lazarevic, V.; Gaïa, N.; Johansson, M.; Ståhlman, M.; Backhed, F.; Delzenne, N.M.; Schrenzel, J.; François, P.; Cani, P.D. Microbiome of prebiotic-treated mice reveals novel targets involved in host response during obesity. *ISME J.* **2014**, *8*, 2116–2130. [CrossRef] [PubMed]
16. Schneeberger, M.; Everard, A.; Gómez-Valadés, A.G.; Matamoros, S.; Ramírez, S.; Delzenne, N.M.; Gomis, R.; Claret, M.; Cani, P.D. *Akkermansia muciniphila* inversely correlates with the onset of inflammation, altered adipose tissue metabolism and metabolic disorders during obesity in mice. *Sci. Rep.* **2015**, *5*, 16643. [CrossRef] [PubMed]
17. Ravussin, Y.; Koren, O.; Spor, A.; LeDuc, C.; Gutman, R.; Stombaugh, J.; Knight, R.; Ley, R.E.; Libel, R.L. Responses of gut microbiota to diet composition and weight loss in lean and obese mice. *Obesity* **2012**, *20*, 738–747. [CrossRef] [PubMed]
18. Zhang, C.; Zhang, M.; Pang, X.; Zhao, Y.; Wang, L.; Zhao, L. Structural resilience of the gut microbiota in adult mice under high-fat dietary perturbations. *ISME J.* **2012**, *6*, 1848–1857. [CrossRef] [PubMed]
19. Murphy, E.F.; Cotter, P.D.; Healy, S.; Marques, T.M.; O'Sullivan, O.; Fouhy, F.; Clarke, S.F.; O'Toole, P.W.; Quigley, E.M.; Stanton, C.; et al. Composition and energy harvesting capacity of the gut microbiota: Relationship to diet, obesity and time in mouse models. *Gut* **2010**, *59*, 1635–1642. [CrossRef] [PubMed]
20. Ley, R.E.; Bäckhed, F.; Turnbaugh, P.; Lozupone, C.A.; Knight, R.D.; Gordon, J.I. Obesity alters gut microbial ecology. *Proc. Natl. Acad. Sci. USA* **2005**, *102*, 11070–11075. [CrossRef] [PubMed]
21. Huazano-García, A.; López, M.G. Agavins reverse the metabolic disorders in overweight mice through the increment of short chain fatty acids and hormones. *Food Funct.* **2015**, *6*, 3720–3727. [CrossRef] [PubMed]
22. Everard, A.; Belzer, C.; Geurts, L.; Ouwerkerk, J.P.; Druart, C.; Bindels, L.B.; Guiot, Y.; Derrien, M.; Muccioli, G.G.; Delzenne, N.M.; et al. Cross-talk between *Akkermansia muciniphila* and intestinal epithelium controls diet-induced obesity. *Proc. Natl. Acad. Sci. USA* **2013**, *110*, 9066–9071. [CrossRef] [PubMed]
23. Caporaso, J.G.; Lauber, C.L.; Walters, W.A.; Berg-Lyons, D.; Huntley, J.; Fierer, N.; Owens, S.M.; Betley, J.; Fraser, L.; Bauer, M.; et al. Ultra-high-throughput microbial community analysis on the Illumina HiSeq and MiSeq platforms. *ISME J.* **2012**, *6*, 1621–1624. [CrossRef] [PubMed]
24. Caporaso, J.G.; Kuczynski, J.; Stombaugh, J.; Bittinger, K.; Bushman, F.D.; Costello, E.K.; Fierer, N.; Peña, A.G.; Goodrich, J.K.; Gordon, J.I.; et al. QIIME allows analysis of high-throughput community sequencing data. *Nat. Methods* **2010**, *7*, 335–336. [CrossRef] [PubMed]
25. Segata, N.; Izard, J.; Waldron, L.; Gevers, D.; Miropolsky, L.; Garrett, W.S.; Huttenhower, C. Metagenomic biomarker discovery and explanation. *Genome Biol.* **2011**, *12*, R60. [CrossRef] [PubMed]
26. Femia, A.P.; Luceri, C.; Dolara, P.; Giannini, A.; Biggeri, A.; Salvadori, M.; Clune, Y.; Collins, K.J.; Paglierani, M.; Caderni, G. Antitumorigenic activity of the prebiotic inulin enriched with oligofructose in combination with the probiotics *Lactobacillus rhamnosus* and *Bifidobacterium lactis* on azoxymethane-induced colon carcinogenesis in rats. *Carcinogenesis* **2002**, *23*, 1953–1960. [CrossRef] [PubMed]
27. Long, R.T.; Zeng, W.S.; Chen, L.Y. *Bifidobacterium* as an oral delivery carrier of oxyntomodulin for obesity therapy: Inhibitory effects on food intake and body weight in overweight mice. *Int. J. Obes.* **2010**, *34*, 712–719. [CrossRef] [PubMed]
28. Hannelore, D.; Moghaddas Gholami, A.; Berry, D.; Desmarchelier, C.; Hahne, H.; Loh, G.; Mondot, S.; Lepage, P.; Rothballer, M.; Walker, A.; et al. High-fat diet alters gut microbiota physiology in mice. *ISME J.* **2014**, *8*, 295–308.
29. Hildebrandt, M.A.; Hoffmann, C.; Sherrill-Mix, S.A.; Keilbaugh, S.A.; Hamady, M.; Chen, Y.Y.; Knight, R.; Ahima, R.S.; Bushman, F.; Wu, G.D. High-fat diet determines the composition of the murine gut microbiome independently of obesity. *Gastroenterology* **2009**, *137*, 1716–1724. [CrossRef] [PubMed]
30. Turnbaugh, P.J.; Bäckhed, F.; Fulton, L.; Gordon, J.I. Diet-induced obesity is linked to marked but reversible alterations in the mouse distal gut microbiome. *Cell Host Microbe* **2008**, *3*, 213–223. [CrossRef] [PubMed]
31. Devkota, S.; Wang, Y.; Musch, M.W.; Leone, V.; Fehlner-Peach, H.; Nadimpalli, A.; Antonopoulos, D.A.; Jabri, B.; Chang, E.B. Dietary-fat-induced taurocholic acid promotes pathobiont expansion and colitis in *Il10*$^{-/-}$ mice. *Nature* **2012**, *487*, 104–108. [CrossRef] [PubMed]
32. Lawrence, A.D.; Maurice, C.F.; Carmody, R.N.; Gootenberg, D.B.; Button, J.E.; Wolfe, B.E.; Ling, A.V.; Devlin, A.S.; Varma, Y.; Fischbach, M.A.; et al. Diet rapidly and reproducibly alters the human gut microbiome. *Nature* **2014**, *505*, 559–563.
33. Flint, H.J.; Duncan, S.H.; Scott, K.P.; Louis, P. Links between diet, gut microbiota composition and gut metabolism. *Proc. Nutr. Soc.* **2015**, *74*, 13–22. [CrossRef] [PubMed]

34. Bindels, L.B.; Neyrinck, A.M.; Salazar, N.; Taminiau, B.; Druart, C.; Muccioli, G.G.; François, E.; Blecker, C.; Richel, A.; Daube, G.; et al. Non digestible oligosaccharides modulate the gut microbiota to control the development of leukemia and associated cachexia in mice. *PLoS ONE* **2015**, *10*, e0131009. [CrossRef] [PubMed]
35. Frost, G.; Sleeth, M.L.; Sahuri-Arisoylu, M.; Lizarbe, B.; Cerdan, S.; Brody, L.; Anastasovska, J.; Ghourab, S.; Hankir, M.; Zhang, S.; et al. The short-chain fatty acid acetate reduces appetite via a central homeostatic mechanism. *Nat. Commun.* **2014**, *5*, 3611. [CrossRef] [PubMed]
36. Chang, C.J.; Lin, C.S.; Lu, C.C.; Martel, J.; Ko, Y.F.; Ojcius, D.M.; Tseng, S.F.; Wu, T.R.; Chen, Y.Y.; Young, J.D.; et al. *Ganoderma lucidum* reduces obesity in mice by modulating the composition of the gut microbiota. *Nat. Commun.* **2015**, *6*, 7489. [CrossRef] [PubMed]
37. Liou, A.P.; Paziuk, M.; Luevano, J.M., Jr.; Machineni, S.; Turnbaugh, P.J.; Kaplan, L.M. Conserved shifts in the gut microbiota due to gastric bypass reduce host weight and adiposity. *Sci. Transl. Med.* **2013**, *5*, 178ra41. [CrossRef] [PubMed]
38. Tremaroli, V.; Karlsson, F.; Werling, M.; Ståhlman, M.; Kovatcheva-Datchary, P.; Olbers, T.; Fändriks, L.; le Roux, C.W.; Nielsen, J.; Bäckhed, F. Roux-en-Y gastric bypass and vertical banded gastroplasty induce long-term changes on the human gut microbiome contribution to fat mass regulation. *Cell Metal.* **2015**, *22*, 228–238. [CrossRef] [PubMed]
39. Zhang, H.; DiBaise, J.K.; Zuccolo, A.; Kudrna, D.; Braidotti, M.; Yu, Y.; Parameswaran, P.; Crowell, M.D.; Wing, R.; Rittmann, B.E.; et al. Human gut microbiota in obesity and after gastric bypass. *Proc. Natl. Acad. Sci. USA* **2009**, *106*, 2365–2370. [CrossRef] [PubMed]
40. Mahowald, M.A.; Rey, F.E.; Seedorf, H.; Turnbaugh, P.J.; Fulton, R.S.; Wollan, A.; Shah, N.; Wang, C.; Magrini, V.; Wilson, R.K.; et al. Characterizing a model human gut microbiota composed of members of its two dominant bacterial phyla. *Proc. Natl. Acad. Sci. USA* **2009**, *106*, 5859–5864. [CrossRef] [PubMed]

13

The Efficacy of *Bifidobacterium longum* BORI and *Lactobacillus acidophilus* AD031 Probiotic Treatment in Infants with Rotavirus Infection

Myeong Soo Park [1], Bin Kwon [2], Seockmo Ku [3] and Geun Eog Ji [2,4,*]

1. Department of Hotel Culinary Arts, Yeonsung University, Anyang 430-749, Korea; mspark@yeonsung.ac.kr
2. Research Center, BIFIDO Co. Ltd., Hongcheon 250-804, Korea; 531083@hanmail.net
3. Fermentation Science Program, School of Agribusiness and Agriscience, College of Basic and Applied Sciences, Middle Tennessee State University, Murfreesboro, TN 37132, USA; Seockmo.Ku@mtsu.edu
4. Department of Food and Nutrition, Research Institute of Human Ecology, Seoul National University, Seoul 151-742, Korea

* Correspondence: geji@snu.ac.kr

Abstract: A total of 57 infants hospitalized with rotavirus disease were included in this study. The children were randomly divided into the study's two treatment groups: three days of the oral administration of (i) a probiotics formula containing both *Bifidobacterium longum* BORI and *Lactobacillus acidophilus* AD031 ($N = 28$); or (ii) a placebo (probiotic-free skim milk, $N = 29$) and the standard therapy for diarrhea. There were no differences in age, sex, or blood characteristics between the two groups. When the 57 cases completed the protocol, the duration of the patients' diarrhea was significantly shorter in the probiotics group (4.38 ± 1.29, $N = 28$) than the placebo group (5.61 ± 1.23, $N = 29$), with a p-value of 0.001. Symptoms such as duration of fever ($p = 0.119$), frequency of diarrhea ($p = 0.119$), and frequency of vomiting ($p = 0.331$) tended to be ameliorated by the probiotic treatment; however, differences were not statistically significant between the two groups. There were no serious, adverse events and no differences in the frequency of adverse events in both groups.

Keywords: probiotics; rotavirus; *Bifidobacterium*; *Lactobacillus*

1. Introduction

Diarrhea-associated deaths in children under five years old in developing countries have been a major cause of childhood mortality [1]. These illnesses are caused by multiple factors, including infections by pathogenic microorganisms, viruses, and parasites [2]. Among the many acute diarrheal diseases, infections caused by rotavirus may be more fatal in infants than in adults [3]. Global reports show that most babies and toddlers are infected with rotavirus by the age of five [4]. This causes serious problems in developing and/or low-income countries (e.g., South Asian and sub-Saharan African countries), and hundreds of thousands of babies are killed by rotavirus annually [5]. Recently, the developments of rotavirus vaccines (e.g., RotaTeg and Rotarix) have dramatically reduced the number of outbreaks in many countries and were proven safe; however, concerns remain regarding the cost of the rotavirus vaccines and their limited effectiveness in some cases [6]. Accordingly, supported therapeutic methods that are compatible with common rotavirus medical treatments and effectively relieve its symptoms should be developed.

A number of studies have identified the effect of several probiotic species (e.g., *Bifidobacterium*, *Enterococcus*, *Lactobacillus*, *Lactococcus*, *Propionibacterium*, *Saccharomyces* and *Streptococcus*) in the treatment and prevention of intestinal infections [7]. These probiotic bacteria have been shown to inhibit intestinal disease [8–11]. *Bifidobacterium* and *Lactobacillus* spp. are the most common bacteria and are considered the most beneficial probiotic organisms [12].

Although multiple probiotic microorganisms could be utilized in rotavirus treatments, some studies have not identified any significant therapeutic effects; therefore, the underlying mechanisms of the therapeutic effects of probiotics in humans are still unclear [13]. Studies have shown that some probiotic bacteria have little or no statistically significant effect on rotavirus [14,15]. Moreover, we can deduce that the effect of probiotics may vary based on the type of microorganism administered to the host. We aim to determine the efficacy of a commercially available probiotic product containing two probiotic cell types, i.e., *Bifidobacterium longum* BORI and *Lactobacillus acidophilus* AD031, in infants and/or toddlers with rotavirus-associated symthoms.

2. Materials and Methods

Design: All participants' guardians completed written, informed consent forms prior to the clinical experiment. All patients were recruited and classified from the inpatient Department of Pediatrics at Yonsei University Hospital in Seoul, Korea. This double-blind, randomized, and placebo-controlled clinical study tests the efficacy of probiotics formula to ameliorate the pathological symptoms in children hospitalized with rotavirus infections. The criteria applied to the experimental subjects are as follows: nine- to 16-month-old male and female infants were diagnosed as infected with rotavirus via a latex agglutination test. A total of 57 infants hospitalized with rotavirus infection were enrolled in this study. 28 patients were assigned to the probiotics treatment group, and the remaining 29 patients were assigned to the placebo group. The probiotics group was fed probiotic formula containing *B. longum* BORI and *L. acidophilus* AD031.

Diet and probiotic microorganisms: The probiotic powder contained two lyophilized probiotic species. Each probiotic packet contained 20 billion CFU/g of *B. longum* BORI and two billion CFU/g of *L. acidophilus* AD031 in powder form. The probiotics-free skim milk powder (placebo packet) was not visually distinguishable from the composite probiotic packet. Both the probiotic and placebo packets were supplied by BIFIDO Co., Ltd. (Hongchun, Korea). Each participant consumed the packets (i) twice a day (ii) for a total of three days (iii) within 10 min of each meal.

Statistical analysis: Paired *t*-tests were performed to assess the quantitative changes in the symptoms of rotavirus infection: duration of fever, frequency of diarrhea, frequency of vomiting, and duration of diarrhea before and after the study period in both groups. Results were considered statistically significant when the p-values were < 0.05.

3. Results and Discussion

A total of 57 infants hospitalized with rotavirus infection were enrolled in this study. Twenty-eight patients were randomly assigned to the probiotics group and 29 to the placebo group. The probiotics group was fed a probiotic formula containing *B. longum* BORI and *L. acidophilus* AD031. There were no differences in the age, sex, or blood characteristics of the two groups. The experimental outcomes are summarized in Table 1. The probiotics group showed a slightly reduced duration of fever ($p = 0.119$), frequency of diarrhea ($p = 0.119$), and frequency of vomiting ($p = 0.331$) compared to the placebo group; however, these differences were not significant. By contrast, the duration of diarrhea during the three-day treatment showed a significant difference between the probiotics group (4.38 ± 1.29) and the placebo group (5.61 ± 1.23) with a p-value of 0.001 (Table 1). There were no serious, adverse events and no difference in the frequency of adverse events in both groups.

Table 1. Duration and frequency of rotavirus-associated symptoms in patients treated with probiotics and placebo.

Symptoms		Condition		p-Value
Category	**Parameter**	**Placebo (N = 29)**	**Probiotics (N = 28)**	
Duration	Fever	4.32 ± 1.94	3.66 ± 1.14	0.119
(Days)	*Diarrhea*	*5.61 ± 1.23*	*4.38 ± 1.29*	*0.001*
Frequency	Vomiting	1.82 ± 0.94	1.55 ± 1.12	0.119
(Times/Day)	Diarrhea	2.64 ± 0.73	2.38 ± 0.49	0.331

The probiotic formula containing *B. longum* BORI and *L. acidophilus* AD031 utilized in this work is likely be an effective adjuvant to relieve acute diarrhea caused by rotavirus. Several studies showed that various strains of probiotic bacteria, such as *L. reuteri* and *L. rhamnosus*, were effective in managing acute diarrhea caused by rotavirus in toddlers. In the present experiment, the efficacy of *B. longum* BORI and *L. acidophilus* AD031 probiotic products was tested. Our rationale for the *L. acidophilus* and *B. longum* combination was based on the general microbial composition, which shows a predominance of *Lactobacillus* sp. in the small intestine and *Bifidobacterium* sp. in the large intestine (among a variety of beneficial bacteria present in healthy human subjects). Eighteen of 23 clinical trials of probiotic formulas resulted in mitigating acute diarrhea, and the reduction of the duration of diarrhea in the studies' probiotics treatment group was reported to be 0.5 to 1.5 days [16]. The duration of diarrhea may vary depending on a child's health status, diet, and prescribed medication. Our study demonstrated a statistically significant diarrhea reduction of 1.2 days. The efficacy of probiotics is strain-specific, so this may be due to the use of different strains in different studies. Basu et al. [17] conducted a clinical study with 10^7 CFU/day LGG and concluded that it was not effective, but when they performed the same study again [18] with 10^{10} and 10^{12} CFU/day LGG, they concluded that a higher concentration of LGG administration in acute diarrhea patients was effective in reducing the diarrhea frequency, diarrhea period, and hospitalization period. Fang et al. [19] reported a dose-dependent effect of *Lb. rhamnosus* on fecal rotavirus concentration and suggested 6×10^8 CFU/day as the minimal effective dose, which was similar to the data of Guanidalin [20], who concluded that at least 10 billion cells/day was necessary. Dubay [21] also applied the commercially available probiotic formula (VSL#3, CD Pharma India, New Delhi, India) to mitigate acute diarrhea, which showed a more rapid recovery compared to the control group and decreased the necessity of electrolyte treatments. In contrast to the positive results mentioned above, a probiotic formula containing 10^9 CFU/day of *B. lactis* and 10^8 CFU/day of *S. thermophilus* failed to decrease the duration of rotavirus diarrhea [22]. These contrasting results suggest that further clinical experiments are necessary in order to understand the scientific basis of the efficacy of probiotics and its relation to a number of criteria the strain of probiotics, the type of rotavirus, the severity of the symptoms, the ages and races of the children, etc. Further study using animal models also should be considered since the experimental conditions in this model can be better controlled [23–27].

4. Conclusions

The results of the present study demonstrated that a probiotic formula containing *Bifidobacterium longum* BORI and *Lactobacillus acidophilus* AD031 reduced the duration of rotavirus diarrhea in young Korean children.

Acknowledgments: This work was supported by Health and Welfare (03-PJI-PG11-VN01-SV04-0018), Republic of Korea and the Promoting Regional specialized Industry (R0004140), the Ministry of Trade, Industry and Energy (MOTIE) and Korea Institute for Advancement of Technology (KIAT), Republic of Korea. The authors wish to thank Lauren B. Mallet at Purdue University for her review and feedback.

Author Contributions: Myeong Soo Park and Bin Kwon designed the experiment under the supervision of Geun Eog Ji. Myeong Soo Park and Bin Kwon performed the research. Myeong Soo Park, Seockmo Ku and Geun Eog Ji analyzed the data and wrote the manuscript. All authors were involved in the revision and editing of this work.

References

1. Lanata, C.; Fischer-Walker, C.; Olascoaga, A.; Torres, C.; Aryee, M.; Black, R. Global Causes of Diarrheal Disease Mortality in Children <5 Years Of Age: A Systematic Review. *PLoS ONE* **2013**, *8*, e72788. [PubMed]
2. Youssef, M.; Shurman, A.; Bougnoux, M.; Rawashdeh, M.; Bretagne, S.; Strockbine, N. Bacterial, Viral and Parasitic Enteric Pathogens Associated with Acute Diarrhea in Hospitalized Children from Northern Jordan. *FEMS Immunol. Med. Microbiol.* **2000**, *28*, 257–263. [CrossRef] [PubMed]
3. Vaccine Information Statement | Rotavirus | VIS | CDC. Available online: https://www.cdc.gov/vaccines/hcp/vis/vis-statements/rotavirus.html (accessed on 26 June 2017).
4. Bernstein, D. Rotavirus Overview. *Pediatr. Infect. Dis. J.* **2009**, *28*, S50–S53. [CrossRef] [PubMed]
5. Rotavirus. Available online: http://www.who.int/immunization/diseases/rotavirus/en/ (accessed on 26 June 2017).
6. Kirkwood, C.; Steele, A. Rotavirus Vaccine Will Have an Impact in Asia. *PLoS Med.* **2017**, *14*, e1002298. [CrossRef] [PubMed]
7. Fung, W.Y.; Lye, H.S.; Lim, T.J.; Kuan, C.Y.; Liong, M.T. Roles of Probiotic on Gut Health. In *Probiotics*; Liong, M.T., Ed.; Springer: Berlin/Heidelberg, Germany, 2011; pp. 139–165.
8. Lee, A.; Lee, Y.; Yoo, H.; Kim, M.; Chang, Y.; Lee, D.; Lee, J. Consumption of Dairy Yogurt Containing *Lactobacillus paracasei* ssp. *paracasei*, *Bifidobacterium animalis* ssp. *lactis* and Heat-Treated *Lactobacillus plantarum* Improves Immune Function Including Natural Killer Cell Activity. *Nutrients* **2017**, *9*, 558. [CrossRef] [PubMed]
9. Plaza-Díaz, J.; Ruiz-Ojeda, F.; Vilchez-Padial, L.; Gil, A. Evidence of the Anti-Inflammatory Effects of Probiotics and Synbiotics in Intestinal Chronic Diseases. *Nutrients* **2017**, *9*, 555. [CrossRef] [PubMed]
10. Ku, S.; You, H.J.; Ji, G.E. Enhancement of anti-tumorigenic polysaccharide production, adhesion, and branch formation of Bifidobacterium bifidum BGN4 by phytic acid. *Food Sci. Biotechnol.* **2009**, *18*, 749–754.
11. Ku, S.; Park, M.; Ji, G.; You, H. Review on Bifidobacterium bifidum BGN4: Functionality and Nutraceutical Applications as a Probiotic Microorganism. *Int. J. Mol. Sci.* **2016**, *17*, 1544. [CrossRef] [PubMed]
12. Matur, E.; Eraslan, E. *The Impact of Probiotics on the Gastrointestinal Physiology, New Advances in the Basic and Clinical Gastroenterology*; InTech: Rijeka, Croatia, 2012.
13. Ahmadi, E.; Alizadeh-Navaei, R.; Rezai, M.S. Efficacy of probiotic use in acute rotavirus diarrhea in children: A systematic review and meta-analysis. *Casp. J. Intern. Med.* **2015**, *6*, 187.
14. Costa-Ribeiro, H.; Ribeiro, T.; Mattos, A.; Valois, S.; Neri, D.; Almeida, P.; Cerqueira, C.; Ramos, E.; Young, R.; Vanderhoof, J. Limitations of Probiotic Therapy in Acute, Severe Dehydrating Diarrhea. *J. Pediatr. Gastroenterol. Nutr.* **2003**, *36*, 112–115. [CrossRef] [PubMed]
15. Abbaskhanian, A.; Rezai, M.S.; Karami, H.; Hasanpour, A. The Effect of Fermented Yogurt on Rotavirus Diarrhea in Children. *Health Med.* **2012**, *6*, 1600–1604.
16. Lee, Y.K.; Salminen, S. *Handbook of Probiotics and Prebiotics*, 2nd ed.; John Wiley & Sons, Inc.: Hoboken, NJ, USA, 2009; pp. 272–275.
17. Basu, S.; Chatterjee, M.; Ganguly, S.; Chandra, P.K. Efficacy of Lactobacillus rhamnosus GG in Acute Watery diarrhoea of Indian children: A randomized controlled trial. *J. Paediatr. Child Health* **2007**, *43*, 837–842. [CrossRef] [PubMed]
18. Basu, S.; Paul, D.K.; Ganguly, S.; Chatterjee, M.; Chandra, P.K. Efficacy of High-dose Lactobacillus rhamnosus GG in Controlling Acute Watery Diarrhea in Indian Children: A Randomized Controlled Trial. *J. Clin. Gastroenterol.* **2009**, *43*, 208–213. [CrossRef] [PubMed]
19. Fang, S.B.; Lee, H.C.; Hu, J.J.; Hou, S.Y.; Liu, H.L.; Fang, H.W. Dose-Dependent Effect of Lactobacillus rhamnosus on Quantitative Reduction of Faecal Rotavirus Shedding in Children. *J. Trop. Pediatr.* **2009**, *55*, 297–301. [CrossRef] [PubMed]
20. Guandalini, S. Probiotics for children with diarrhea: An update. *J. Clin. Gastroenterol.* **2008**, *42*, S53–S57. [CrossRef] [PubMed]

21. Dubey, A.P.; Rajeshwari, K.; Chakravarty, A.; Famularo, G. Use of VSL#3 in the Treatment of Rotavirus Diarrhea in Children: Preliminary Results. *J. Clin. Gastroenterol.* **2008**, *42*, S126–S129. [PubMed]
22. Mao, M.; Yu, T.; Xiong, Y.; Wang, Z.; Liu, H.; Gotteland, M.; Brunser, O. Effect of a lactose-free milk formula supplemented with bifidobacteria and streptococci on the recovery from acute diarrhoea. *Asia Pac. J. Clin. Nutr.* **2008**, *17*, 30–34. [PubMed]
23. Kandasamy, S.; Chattha, K.S.; Vlasova, A.N.; Rajashekara, G.; Saif, L.J. Lactobacilli and Bifidobacteria enhance mucosal B cell responses and differentially modulate systemic antibody responses to an oral human rotavirus vaccine in a neonatal gnotobiotic pig disease model. *Gut Microbes* **2014**, *5*, 639–651. [CrossRef] [PubMed]
24. Liu, F.; Li, G.; Wen, K.; Wu, S.; Zhang, Y.; Bui, T.; Yang, X.; Kocher, J.; Sun, J.; Jortner, B.; Yuan, L. Lactobacillus rhamnosus GG on rotavirus-induced injury of ileal epithelium in gnotobiotic pigs. *J. Pediatr. Gastroenterol. Nutr.* **2013**, *57*, 750–758. [CrossRef] [PubMed]
25. Vlasova, A.N.; Chattha, K.S.; Kandasamy, S.; Liu, Z.; Esseili, M.; Shao, L. Lactobacilli and Bifidobacteria promote immune homeostasis by modulating innate immune responses to human rotavirus in neonatal Gnotobiotic pigs. *PLoS ONE* **2013**, *8*, e76962. [CrossRef] [PubMed]
26. Laycock, G.; Sait, L.; Inman, C.; Lewis, M.; Smidt, H.; van Diemen, P.; Jorgensen, F.; Stevens, M.; Bailey, M. A defined intestinal colonization microbiota for gnotobiotic pigs. *Vet. Immunol. Immunopathol.* **2012**, *15*, 216–224. [CrossRef] [PubMed]
27. Zhang, W.; Azevedo, M.S.; Wen, K.; Gonzalez, A.; Saif, L.J.; Li, G.; Yousef, A.E.; Yuan, L. Probiotic Lactobacillus acidophilus enhances the immunogenicity of an oral rotavirus vaccine in gnotobiotic pigs. *Vaccine* **2008**, *4*, 3655–3661. [CrossRef] [PubMed]

14

Live *Faecalibacterium prausnitzii* does not Enhance Epithelial Barrier Integrity in an Apical Anaerobic Co-Culture Model of the Large Intestine

Eva Maier [1,2,*], Rachel C. Anderson [1,2] and Nicole C. Roy [1,2,3]

1 Food Nutrition & Health Team, Food & Bio-Based Products Group, AgResearch Grasslands, Palmerston North 4442, New Zealand; rachel.anderson@agresearch.co.nz (R.C.A.); nicole.roy@agresearch.co.nz (N.C.R.)
2 Riddet Institute, Massey University, Palmerston North 4442, New Zealand
3 High-Value Nutrition National Science Challenge, Auckland 1142, New Zealand
* Correspondence: eva.maier@agresearch.co.nz

Abstract: Appropriate intestinal barrier maturation during infancy largely depends on colonization with commensal bacteria. *Faecalibacterium prausnitzii* is an abundant obligate anaerobe that colonizes during weaning and is thought to maintain colonic health throughout life. We previously showed that *F. prausnitzii* induced Toll-like receptor 2 (TLR2) activation, which is linked to enhanced tight junction formation. Therefore, we hypothesized that *F. prausnitzii* enhances barrier integrity, an important factor in appropriate intestinal barrier maturation. In order to test metabolically active bacteria, we used a novel apical anaerobic co-culture system that allows the survival of both obligate anaerobic bacteria and oxygen-requiring intestinal epithelial cells (Caco-2). The first aim was to optimize the culture medium to enable growth and active metabolism of *F. prausnitzii* while maintaining the viability and barrier integrity, as measured by trans-epithelial electrical resistance (TEER), of the Caco-2 cells. This was achieved by supplementing the apical cell culture medium with bacterial culture medium. The second aim was to test the effect of *F. prausnitzii* on TEER across Caco-2 cell layers. Live *F. prausnitzii* did not improve TEER, which indicates that its benefits are not via altering tight junction integrity. The optimization of the novel dual-environment co-culturing system performed in this research will enable the investigation of new probiotics originating from indigenous beneficial bacteria.

Keywords: intestinal barrier maturation; intestinal microbiota; obligate anaerobic bacteria; tight junctions

1. Introduction

Faecalibacterium prausnitzii is one of the most abundant bacterial species in the colon of healthy human adults [1,2]. This bacterium is thought to be critical for maintaining colonic health because its abundance is reduced in people with gastrointestinal diseases [3–10]. Therefore, increasing the abundance of *F. prausnitzii* in the colonic microbiota has become the target of much research, either by directly delivering the bacterium as a probiotic [11] or by using food ingredients that preferentially stimulate the growth of endogenous *F. prausnitzii* [12]. Despite this, little is known about the role of *F. prausnitzii* in appropriate development of the intestinal barrier during infancy and whether it has the potential to be a probiotic during early life.

Intestinal maturation, including the development of the intestinal barrier integrity and immune function as well as the establishment and stabilization of the microbiota, occurs throughout the first two years of life. Much of this process is regulated by diet (e.g., breast milk versus infant formula), which in turn influences the colonization patterns of the early microbiota and their interactions with the host [13]. *F. prausnitzii* colonizes the large intestine between six and 12 months of life [14–16], so it is likely to have an impact on intestinal maturation during weaning.

One key area of intestinal maturation is the education of the immune system by the resident bacteria. *F. prausnitzii* has been associated with anti-inflammatory effects in adult gnotobiotic rodents colonized with *Escherichia coli* [17] or *Bacteroides thetaiotaomicron* [18]. However, *F. prausnitzii* is unable to mono-colonize gnotobiotic rodents [17], which means that targeted in vivo studies are not possible. An alternative is to use in vitro techniques to investigate the specific immune-modulatory effects of *F. prausnitzii* on host cells. Such studies have been limited due to the difficulty of co-culturing obligate anaerobes and human oxygen-requiring cells using conventional culturing systems. Using a novel dual-environment co-culturing system we previously showed that live *F. prausnitzii* induced TLR2 activation in transfected human embryonic kidney cells (HEK293) [19], which has been implicated in maintaining homeostasis between immunity and tolerance in the intestinal epithelium [20].

Another key to appropriate intestinal maturation is development of the barrier integrity, which is crucial not only for nutrient absorption but also to prevent the entry of bacteria and food antigens from the lumen into underlying tissues [21]. *F. prausnitzii* improved barrier integrity in mice with DSS-induced colitis [22]. However, our previous study using Caco-2 cell monolayers as a model of the large intestinal epithelium showed that *F. prausnitzii* did not alter ion permeability, as measured by the trans-epithelial electrical resistance (TEER) assay, and increased small molecule permeability, as measured by the ^{3}H-mannitol flux assay, which could be considered detrimental [23]. In the study described above using the dual-environment co-culturing system the viability of *F. prausnitzii* in apical anaerobic conditions was improved compared to when cultured in the presence of oxygen, but the bacterium was not actively growing. The discrepancy between the in vivo and in vitro results may be due to this lack of growth, especially since mammalian cells have been shown to respond differently to the same bacterium depending on its growth phases [24].

Therefore, the specific hypothesis of this research was that actively growing *F. prausnitzii* improves intestinal barrier integrity, as measured by the TEER across Caco-2 cells, indicating that it has potential to be a probiotic to improve intestinal barrier maturation during early life. In order to test the hypothesis the first aim of this study was to optimize the apical medium to suit the requirements of both the bacterium and the intestinal epithelial cells, and in particular to encourage growth and active metabolism of *F. prausnitzii*. The second aim was then to test the effects of three *F. prausnitzii* strains, A2-165, American Type Culture Collection (ATCC) 27768, and HTF-F, on TEER across Caco-2 cells to ensure that our results were not limited to one strain.

2. Materials and Methods

2.1. *F. prausnitzii* Culturing Conditions

The three *F. prausnitzii* strains A2-165 (DSM 17677), ATCC 27768, and HTF-F (DSM 26943) were kindly provided by Hermie J. M. Harmsen (Department of Medical Microbiology, University of Groningen, Groningen, The Netherlands). Bacteria were cultured anaerobically in Brain Heart Infusion (BHI) broth containing 3.7% (*w/v*) BHI powder (Becton Dickinson, Auckland, New Zealand) supplemented with 0.5% (*w/v*) yeast extract, 0.0005% (*w/v*) hemin, 0.0005% vitamin K and 0.2% L-cysteine (Sigma-Aldrich, Auckland, New Zealand) in an atmosphere of 10% CO_2, 10% H_2 in N_2 at 37 °C (Concept Plus Anaerobic Workstation, Ruskinn Technology Ltd., Bridgend, UK) as previously described [19].

2.2. Caco-2 Cell Culturing Conditions

Caco-2 cells (HTB37) were obtained from the ATCC and used in experiments between passage 25 and 35. Caco-2 cells were maintained in cell culture flasks (Corning, New York, NY, USA) in Medium 199 (M199) cell culture medium supplemented with 10% fetal bovine serum (FBS),

1% non-essential amino acids (NEAA; 100× solution), and 1% penicillin-streptomycin (10,000 units/mL penicillin, and 10 mg/mL streptomycin (Life Technologies, Auckland, New Zealand), referred to as M199 Standard medium (M199 Std) and incubated at 37 °C in 5% CO_2. Medium was replaced twice a week. For co-culture experiments Caco-2 cells were seeded on semi-permeable polyester membranes (Transwell inserts, 6.5 mm diameter, 0.4 μm pore size, Corning, New York, NY, USA) at a density of 8×10^4 cells per insert and cultured for 16–18 days to attain differentiated cell monolayers (TEER over 400 $\Omega \cdot cm^2$).

2.3. Apical Anaerobic Co-Culture Model

The apical anaerobic co-culture model utilized an in-house designed and built dual-environment co-culture chamber inside an anaerobic workstation (Figure 1). The Caco-2 cells received oxygen through the semi-permeable membrane from the oxygenated medium in the basal compartment and the bacterial cells were maintained in the apical anaerobic medium. The chamber was sterilized and consumables and solutions were made anaerobic before each experiment as previously described [19].

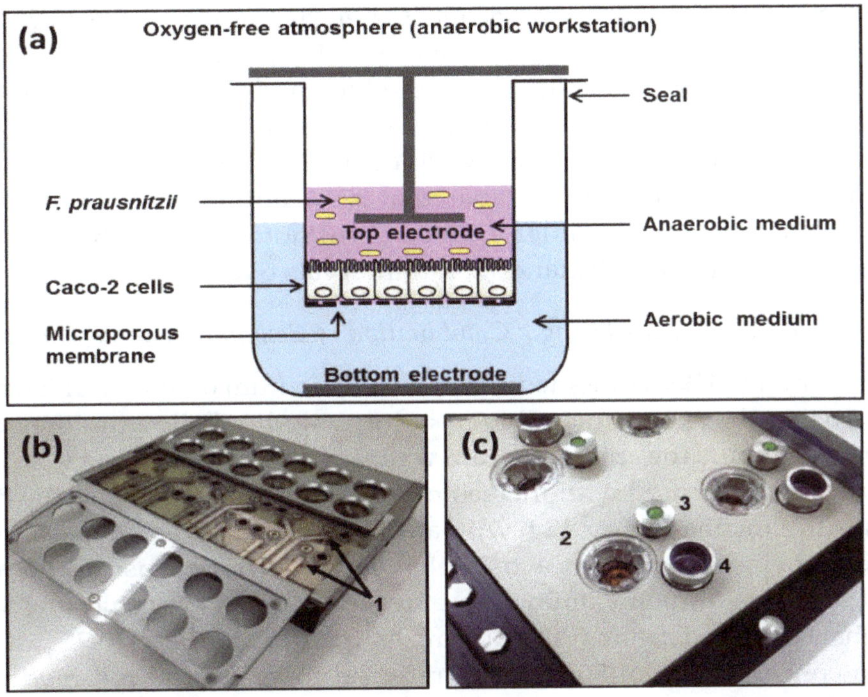

Figure 1. Apical anaerobic co-culture model. (**a**) Schematic diagram of a single well of the apical anaerobic co-culture model used for the co-culture of Caco-2 cell monolayers with anaerobic *F. prausnitzii*. The top and bottom electrodes enable the determination of the effect of *F. prausnitzii* on TEER across the Caco-2 cell monolayers; (**b**,**c**) Photographs of the co-culture chamber including details of the components. 1: Top electrodes; 2: Transwell insert containing Caco-2 cell monolayer; 3: Septum for basal media sampling; 4: One-way pressure relief valve.

2.4. TEER Experiment Protocol

Twenty-four hours before the experiments, the apical and basal M199 Std was removed from the Caco-2 cell monolayers grown on Transwell inserts and replaced with M199 supplemented only with 10% FBS and 1% NEAAs, referred to as M199 TEER, in order to remove the antibiotics before co-culturing the cells with bacteria. On the day of the experiment, the basal wells of the co-culture chamber were filled with 3 mL of M199 TEER. The Transwell inserts containing the cell monolayers were carefully inserted into the co-culture chamber using a twisting motion. The co-culture chamber was transferred into the interlock chamber of the anaerobic workstation, purged with nitrogen and after finishing the interlock cycle moved into the anaerobic workstation. The co-culture chamber was connected to the commercially available CellZscope automated TEER monitoring system (CellZscope controller and CellZscope software version 2.2.3; nanoAnalytics, Münster, Germany). The TEER across each Caco-2 cell monolayer was measured twice and the second reading (after 1 h adaptation to the environment) was used as a baseline reading. The apical aerobic medium was removed and replaced with 260 μL of anaerobic medium or treatments. The TEER measurements were resumed and recorded hourly over 12 h. Since the initial TEER for each insert was different, the effect on TEER over time was expressed as the change in TEER compared to the initial TEER for each insert using the following Equation (1):

$$\text{Change in TEER } (\%) = \frac{(\text{TEER}_{\text{current}} - \text{TEER}_{\text{initial}})}{\text{TEER}_{\text{initial}}} \times 100. \quad (1)$$

2.5. *Survival of F. prausnitzii in Anaerobic Cell Culture Media*

The three *F. prausnitzii* strains were incubated in M199 TEER medium to monitor their survival. Secondary bacterial cultures in stationary phase were pelleted by centrifugation at 2500× *g* for 6 min (11180/13190 rotor, Sigma 3-18K centrifuge, Osterode am Harz, Germany) and resuspended in anaerobic media inside the anaerobic workstation. Bacterial number was estimated using a Petroff-Hauser counting chamber and solutions diluted to yield a concentration of 2.4×10^7 bacterial cells/mL. This bacterial density was chosen so that when used in the co-culture experiments described below it resulted in a multiplicity of infection (MOI) of 100 bacterial cells per intestinal epithelial cell. Triplicates of the bacterial solutions were incubated at 37 °C and the optical density at a wavelength of 600 nm (OD_{600nm}) was recorded (Implen OD600 DiluPhotometer with DC10 DiluCell cuvettes; Total Lab Solutions, Auckland, New Zealand) at 2-h intervals over 24 h.

2.6. *TEER and Viability of Caco-2 Cells Using a Combination of Cell and Bacterial Culture Media*

The effect of combining M199 TEER medium and BHI medium on the TEER and viability of Caco-2 cells was examined using the apical anaerobic co-culture model. Following the measurement of the initial resistance after two hours the apical medium was removed and replaced with 260 μL of anaerobic M199 TEER medium supplemented with increasing concentrations of anaerobic BHI (0%, 25%, 50%, 75%, or 100% BHI). After incubation for 12 h with automated hourly TEER measurements, the inserts were removed and the viability of the Caco-2 cells was determined using the neutral red uptake assay. Neutral red (3-amino-7-dimethylamino-2-methyl-phenazine hydrochloride; Sigma-Aldrich) was dissolved in phosphate-buffered saline (PBS) at 5 mg/mL, filter sterilized (0.22 μm filter), and diluted with M199 Std to a concentration of 50 μg/mL (referred to as neutral red medium). The medium was removed from all the Caco-2 cell monolayers and replenished with 200 μL neutral red medium. After incubation for 2 h at 37 °C in a CO_2 incubator, the neutral red medium was removed and cell monolayers washed twice with PBS. The dye was extracted from viable cells by adding 200 μL solubilization solution (1% acetic acid–50% ethanol) and incubating at room temperature on a plate shaker at 200 rpm for 7 min. 150 μL of extract was transferred to a 96-well plate and the absorbance of neutral red was determined on a microplate reader at 540 nm (FlexStation 3, Molecular Devices, Sunnyvale, CA, USA). The background absorbance of the 96-well plate was measured at 690 nm and subtracted from the 540 nm measurement. The experiment was completed in five blocks with four replicates per treatment group in each block.

2.7. *Viability of the F. prausnitzii Strains in the Apical Anaerobic Co-Culture Model Using a Combination of Cell and Bacterial Culture Media*

Combinations of anaerobic M199 TEER medium and BHI medium were used for co-culturing Caco-2 cells and the three *F. prausnitzii* strains in the apical anaerobic co-culture model and it was determined if the bacteria were growing in these adapted conditions. The media compositions chosen were anaerobic M199 TEER supplemented with 25% or 50% of anaerobic BHI (referred to as 25% and

50% BHI). This adapted medium was only used for the apical compartment of the co-culture chamber; the basal compartments had aerobic M199 TEER medium. The bacterial suspensions were diluted with 25% and 50% BHI to a concentration of 2.4×10^7 bacterial cells/mL as described previously. The viability of the *F. prausnitzii* strains in the co-culture model was assessed by determining the viable colony forming units (CFU) of the bacteria at 0 h and 12 h after co-culture with the Caco-2 cells in both the cell supernatant and cell lysate. Duplicate ten-fold serial dilutions of the bacterial solutions were made in 96-well plates for each sample. Three 20-μL spots of each dilution were pipetted onto anaerobic BHI agar, allowed to dry, and then incubated anaerobically for 48 h at 37 °C. Spots with between 10 and 100 colonies were counted and the CFU were calculated. This experiment was done in five blocks, with three replicates per treatment group per block.

2.8. TEER Assay Using F. prausnitzii in Different Apical Media

To assess the effects of *F. prausnitzii* on TEER, each of the strains (A2-165, ATCC 27768, or HTF-F) was co-cultured with differentiated Caco-2 monolayers in the apical anaerobic co-culture model using 25% or 50% BHI as apical medium. There were eight treatment groups: the two control media (25% and 50% BHI) and the three *F. prausnitzii* strains diluted with the two different media. The TEER was recorded hourly for 12 h. The experiment was done in five blocks, with three replicates per treatment in each block.

2.9. TEER Assay Using Live and UV-Killed F. prausnitzii

The effect of both live and UV-killed *F. prausnitzii* on TEER across Caco-2 monolayers in the apical anaerobic co-culture model was determined using 50% BHI as the apical medium. The bacterial suspensions of the three *F. prausnitzii* strains were prepared for the co-culture experiments as follows. A 2-mL aliquot was removed from each bacterial suspension, and transferred to wells of a six-well plate. With the lid removed, the plate was placed on ice and the bacterial suspension treated with a UV lamp (UVP 3UV-38, Bio-Strategy Ltd., Auckland, New Zealand). The bacteria were exposed for 15 min to UVC light. The UV-treated bacteria were plated on anaerobic BHI agar plates and incubated anaerobically for 48 h at 37 °C to confirm that the bacteria were dead. For the TEER experiment there were seven treatment groups: the control medium (50% BHI), the three live *F. prausnitzii* strains and the three UV-killed *F. prausnitzii* strains. The experiment was done in three blocks, with three replicates per treatment per block.

2.10. Statistical Analysis

The statistical analyses were performed using SAS (SAS/STAT version 9.3; SAS Institute Inc., Cary, NC, USA). An analysis of repeated measures was conducted to test the effect of the treatment and time and their interaction on the response variables (change in TEER or change in OD_{600nm}). The most appropriate covariance structure of the mixed model for each response variable was selected after fitting the models by restricted maximum likelihood method and comparing them using the log-likelihood ratio test. When an interaction was not significant it was removed from the model. An analysis of variance (ANOVA) was also conducted to test the effect of the BHI concentration on the viability of Caco-2 cells in apical anaerobic conditions. When the F-value of the analyses were significant ($p < 0.05$), the means were compared using Tukey tests. A two independent samples t-test procedure was performed to compare the viability of the three *F. prausnitzii* strains before and after the co-culture with Caco-2 cells in the apical anaerobic co-culture model. Additionally, a paired t-test was conducted to compare the viability of the three *F. prausnitzii* strains before and after the incubation in 50% BHI. For all the analyses the model assumptions (e.g., normal distribution and the homogeneity of variance) was evaluated using the Output Delivery System (ODS) graphics in SAS. When the response variable did not fulfil these assumptions a $\log_{10}$ transformation was performed to reach these assumptions.

3. Results and Discussion

3.1. *F. prausnitzii Did Not Grow in an Anaerobic Cell Culture Medium*

For bacterial–mammalian cell co-culture experiments, it is common to harvest bacterial cells by centrifugation and then resuspend the bacteria in mammalian cell culture media [23,25,26]. Studies have shown that there was no difference in the viability for strains of *Escherichia coli*, *Salmonella typhimurium*, and *Lactobacillus fructosus* in mammalian and bacterial culture medium [25]. In contrast to this, our results showed that the three *F. prausnitzii* strains did not grow in the anaerobic cell culture medium over the period of 24 h of incubation at 37 °C, as shown in the change in the OD_{600nm} graph (Figure 2). There were no significant differences in the change of the OD_{600nm} until 8 h of incubation for each of the three strains. However, after 24 h of incubation, all three strains showed a decrease in the OD_{600nm} compared to the previous time points (0 to 8 h; $p < 0.05$). Therefore, it concluded it was necessary to supplement the cell culture medium to stimulate the growth and metabolic activity of *F. prausnitzii*.

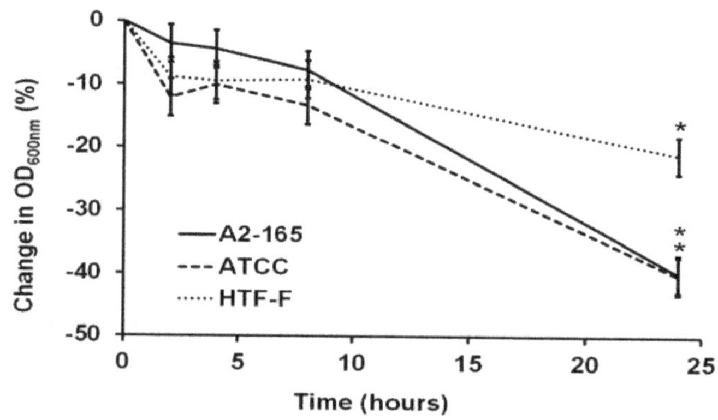

Figure 2. Normalized change in OD_{600nm} (%) of the three *F. prausnitzii* strains in an anaerobic cell culture medium. The three *F. prausnitzii* strains (A2-165, ATCC 27768, and HTF-F) in stationary phase were resuspended in anaerobic M199 TEER, incubated at 37 °C, and the OD_{600nm} was measured over 24 h. The graph shows the mean values (±SEM; $n = 3$) after normalizing by the OD_{600nm} at time 0 h for each of the three *F. prausnitzii* strains over 24 h. * Change in OD_{600nm} different compared to previous time point for the same strain ($p < 0.05$).

When considering which supplements should be added to the medium first the nutrient composition of M199 TEER was investigated. Iron and vitamin K_1 were identified as nutrients that may be lacking in this medium. Bacterial culture media often contain hemin as the iron source [1,23,27], whereas ferric nitrate is the only iron source in the M199 cell culture medium. This may not be optimum for *F. prausnitzii* since bacteria have developed heme acquisition systems to obtain iron from host heme-sequestering proteins [28]. Similarly, bacterial culture media often contain vitamin K_1 [27,29], which bacteria convert into the vitamin K_2 required for electron transport processes during anaerobic respiration [30]; whereas M199 only contains vitamin K_3 (menadione), a synthetic type of vitamin K, which is a provitamin that requires conversion to menaquinone-4 in order to be active [23,31]. The bioavailability of vitamin K_3 may therefore be lower for *F. prausnitzii* compared to other vitamin K sources.

Further investigation in the literature indicated that *F. prausnitzii* likely requires a complex medium to grow. A recent study used a combined approach of computational modeling, in vitro experiments, metabolomic analysis and genomic analysis to identify the metabolic capabilities of *F. prausnitzii* A2-165 and to develop a chemically defined medium, CDM1, for this bacterium [32]. However, CDM1 did not enable growth of *F. prausnitzii* A2-165, and even when enriched with additional vitamins, amino acids, and bases, *F. prausnitzii* A2-165 growth was still less than on the bacterial medium YCFAG [32]. Therefore, it was decided to supplement cell culture medium with a complex bacterial culture medium.

3.2. Bacterial Medium Did Not Affect Caco-2 Viability, but Reduced TEER at High Concentrations

As our previous experience indicated that bacterial medium can be detrimental to mammalian cells, initially the effect of the bacterial medium on the Caco-2 cell monolayers was investigated. The viability of the Caco-2 cells treated with anaerobic M199 TEER mixed with anaerobic BHI in different ratios (0%, 25%, 50%, 75%, or 100% BHI) in apical anaerobic conditions (co-culture chamber inside the anaerobic workstation) over 12 h was determined using the neutral red viability assay (Figure 3a). There was no significant difference ($p = 0.07$) between the viability of Caco-2 cell monolayers treated with 0%, 25%, 50%, 75%, or 100% BHI in the apical anaerobic co-culture model.

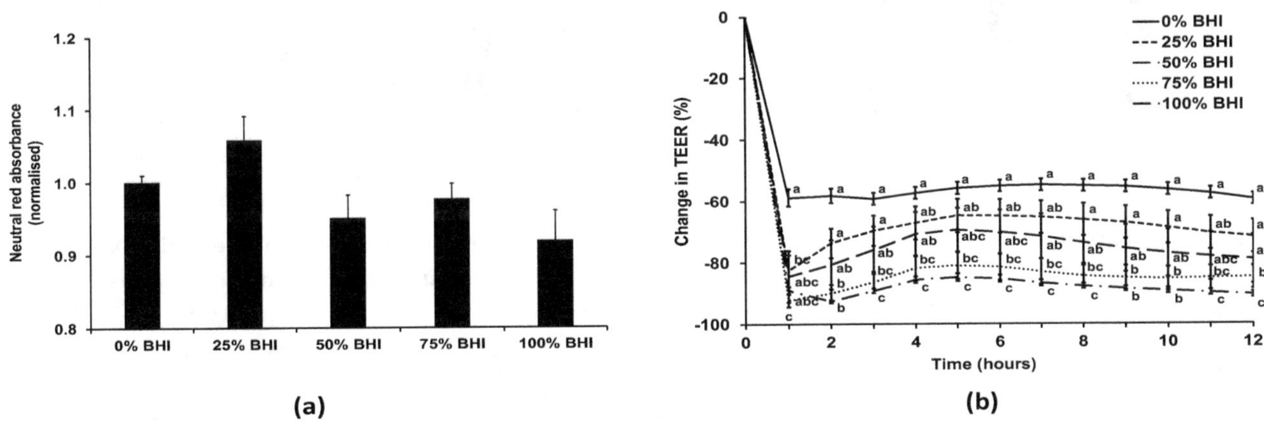

Figure 3. Effect of combining cell and bacterial culture medium on the viability and TEER of Caco-2 cells in the apical anaerobic co-culture model. The apical compartment of Caco-2 cell monolayers were exposed to non-supplemented anaerobic M199 TEER medium (0% BHI), or M199 TEER medium supplemented with increasing concentrations of anaerobic BHI medium (25%, 50%, 75%, or 100% BHI). (**a**) Viability (mean ± SEM; $n = 20$) of Caco-2 cells after 12 h incubation. Neutral red absorbance was normalized by adjusting the 0% BHI exposed cells to 1. Viability of the Caco-2 cells was unchanged as a consequence of differing culture medium composition ($p = 0.07$). (**b**) Mean (±SEM; $n = 20$) change in TEER as a percentage of initial TEER across Caco-2 cell monolayers over 12 h for each medium. There was a significant interaction between the time and the BHI concentration on the change in TEER ($p < 0.01$). Treatments that do not share the same letters are significantly different ($p < 0.05$).

The effect of the different M199 TEER-BHI media combinations on TEER across Caco-2 monolayers in apical anaerobic conditions was tested over 12 h (Figure 3b). There was a significant interaction between the time and the BHI concentration on the change in TEER ($p < 0.01$). When treated with 25% BHI, the normalized TEER across Caco-2 cell monolayers was significantly lower at one hour after adding the treatments compared to 0% BHI, however after that time point onwards there was no difference between 0% and 25% BHI. Caco-2 cell monolayers treated with 50% BHI showed no difference in TEER to Caco-2 cells treated with 0% BHI across all time points. In contrast, when 75% or 100% BHI were added to the apical side of Caco-2 cell monolayers, the normalized TEER values were significantly lower compared to cells treated with 0% BHI across all time points ($p < 0.05$).

The TEER of the Caco-2 cells treated with 50% BHI reached a plateau of approximately 300 $\Omega \cdot cm^2$ following the initial drop in TEER, whereas those with cell culture medium had TEER values that plateaued at approximately 600 $\Omega \cdot cm^2$. The Caco-2 cell monolayers treated with this combination of bacterial and cell culture medium had TEER values that were more comparable to those reported for human colon tissues (100 to 300 $\Omega \cdot cm^2$) [33,34].

3.3. Two *F. prausnitzii* Strains Grew in 50% Bacterial Medium When Co-Cultured with Caco-2 Cells

Based on the results above, the viability of the *F. prausnitzii* strains was tested using the anaerobic M199 TEER: BHI ratio (1:1), which was referred to as 50% BHI. The CFUs of the three *F. prausnitzii* strains were determined before and after their incubation in 50% BHI over 12 h (Figure 4a). The number of CFU of *F. prausnitzii* A2-165 increased by 1.7 log ($p < 0.001$), while the other two strains showed no significant differences between the CFU before and after 12 h of incubation in 50% BHI.

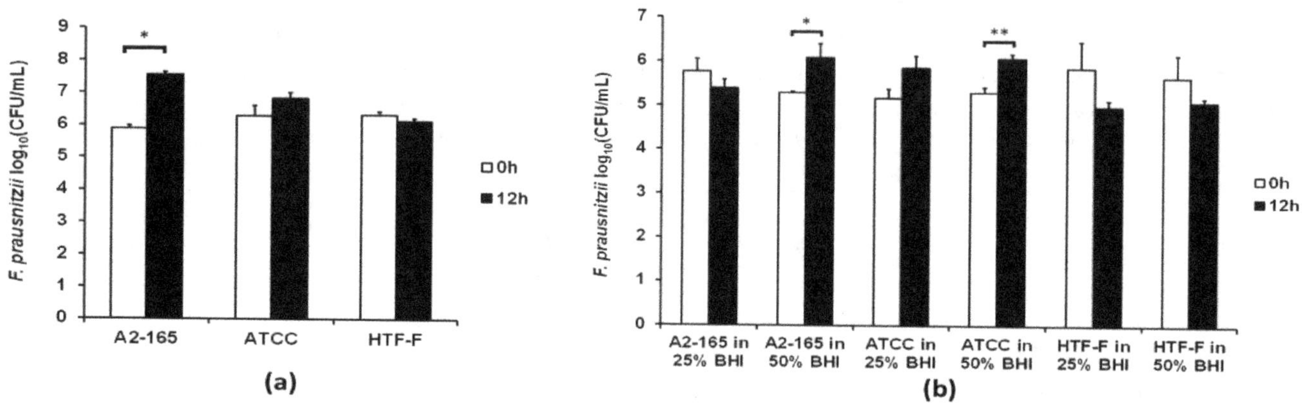

Figure 4. Viability of the three *F. prausnitzii* strains in a cell culture medium supplemented with bacterial culture medium. (**a**) In Hungate culture tubes. The three *F. prausnitzii* strains in stationary phase were resuspended in anaerobic M199 TEER: BHI (1:1) (referred to as 50% BHI) and incubated anaerobically at 37 °C. The graph shows the mean (±SEM; $n = 3$) $\log_{10}$(CFU/mL) of the three *F. prausnitzii* strains before and after 12 h of incubation in 50% BHI. * Mean $\log_{10}$(CFU/mL) differ between 0 and 12 h at $p < 0.05$. (**b**) In the apical anaerobic co-culture model with Caco-2 cells. The three *F. prausnitzii* strains were co-cultured with Caco-2 cells using two different media on the apical side of the Caco-2 cell monolayer (25% and 50% BHI). The graph shows the mean (±SEM; $n = 4$ and 8 for time 0 and 12 h, respectively) $\log_{10}$(CFU/mL) of the bacteria at 0 and 12 h of incubation with Caco-2 cells in the co-culture model. Mean $\log_{10}$(CFU/mL) differ between 0 and 12 h at * $p < 0.05$ and ** $p < 0.01$.

It was proposed that the *F. prausnitzii* strains may grow better in the presence of intestinal epithelial cells. Therefore the three strains were co-cultured with differentiated Caco-2 cell monolayers in the apical anaerobic co-culture model using M199 TEER supplemented with 25% or 50% BHI medium on the apical side of the cell monolayers. These medium compositions were chosen as they did not compromise the TEER and viability of the Caco-2 cell monolayers. The viability of the bacterial strains was determined by comparing the CFU before and after 12 h of co-culture with Caco-2 cells. No bacteria were able to be cultured from the Caco-2 cell lysate, therefore indicating that none of the three strains adhered to the Caco-2 cells. When 25% BHI was used at the apical side of the Caco-2 cell monolayer none of the three *F. prausnitzii* strains had an increase in CFU (Figure 4b). The number of CFU of both *F. prausnitzii* A2-165 and *F. prausnitzii* ATCC 27768 increased by 0.8 log after the 12 h of incubation ($p < 0.05$) when 50% BHI was used as the apical culture medium. However, there was no significant difference in CFU of *F. prausnitzii* HTF-F at 0 and 12 h of co-culture with Caco-2 cells when 50% BHI was used as the apical culture medium.

In agreement with published results using a simple dual-environment co-culture model [35], the presence of the Caco-2 cells improved the growth of the *F. prausnitzii* strains. This may be due to the presence of mucins. Though Caco-2 cells do not express mucin-2, the predominant mucin in the gastrointestinal tract, they express mucins 3 and 5A/C [36,37]. Furthermore, *F. prausnitzii* may benefit from the oxygen gradient close to the Caco-2 cell monolayer. *F. prausnitzii* uses an extracellular electron shuttle of flavins and thiols to transfer electrons to oxygen [38]. Small amounts of oxygen may diffuse from the aerobic basal compartment of the apical anaerobic co-culture model through the Caco-2 cell monolayer to the apical side. The *F. prausnitzii* strains may be able to use riboflavin (vitamin B_2), one component of M199, for its extracellular electron transfer, which may benefit growth at this oxic–anoxic interphase [39].

3.4. *Live F. prausnitzii Did Not Alter TEER across Caco-2 Cells*

To determine whether live *F. prausnitzii* was able to improve TEER, differentiated Caco-2 monolayers were co-cultured with the three *F. prausnitzii* strains (A2-165, ATCC 27768, or HTF-F) in the apical anaerobic co-culture model using 25% or 50% BHI as apical medium. These apical media were chosen as one of them enabled growth of *F. prausnitzii* A2-165 and ATCC 27768 in co-culture with Caco-2 cells (50% BHI), whereas the other medium did not enable growth of any of the three strains (25% BHI) in the previous experiment. It could therefore be determined if change in TEER over time across Caco-2 monolayers differed when co-cultured with growing or non-growing bacteria. The interaction between the bacterial treatment and time was significant for both media (Figure 5; $p < 0.001$). However, there were no differences between the TEER of Caco-2 cells treated with either the 25% or 50% BHI medium or the three *F. prausnitzii* strains in the respective medium for each time point ($p > 0.05$).

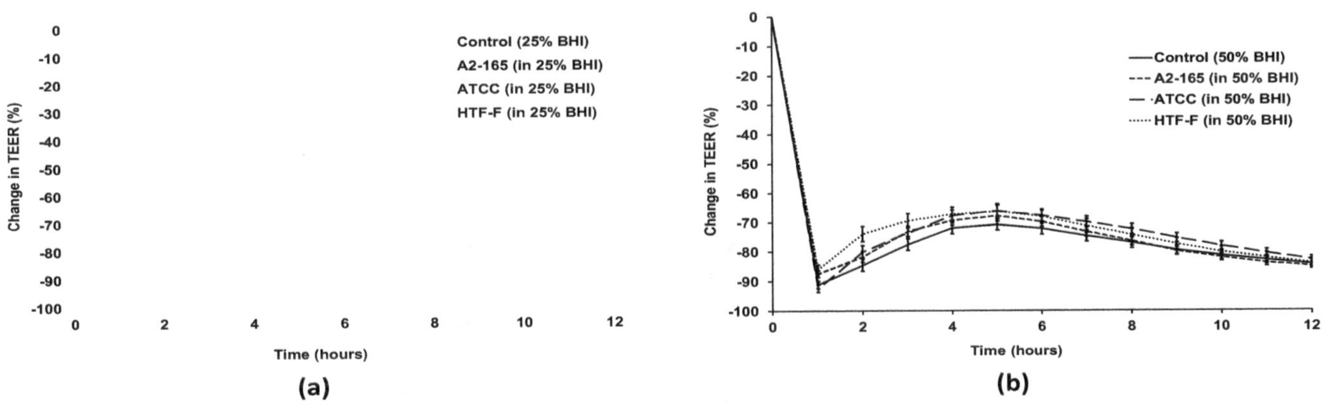

Figure 5. Change in TEER across Caco-2 monolayers co-cultured with live *F. prausnitzii* using 25% and 50% BHI as apical medium. Differentiated Caco-2 monolayers were co-cultured with the three *F. prausnitzii* strains for 12 h in the apical anaerobic co-culture model using 25% or 50% BHI as apical medium. The interaction between the treatment and time was significant for the change in TEER ($p < 0.001$). The graphs show the mean ($\pm$SEM; $n = 12$) change in TEER across Caco-2 monolayers when using (**a**) 25% BHI and (**b**) 50% BHI as apical medium. No differences were determined between the two control media and the three *F. prausnitzii* strains in the respective medium at any time point ($p > 0.05$).

Based on these results, it is likely that the maintenance of colonic health by *F. prausnitzii* is not mediated through enhancement of epithelial barrier integrity. Instead, the beneficial effects of *F. prausnitzii* may be due to it supporting immune homeostasis, as previously shown [19]. However, it is possible that metabolites secreted by live *F. prausnitzii* may require an increased treatment time than that undertaken here to exert their effects on intestinal barrier integrity. Specific probiotics and commensal bacteria influence intestinal barrier integrity through secreted metabolites [40–42], for example butyrate, a short chain fatty acid produced during bacterial fermentation, enhanced the barrier integrity through the regulation of tight junction assembly [43]. However, the barrier enhancing properties of butyrate occurred only after 24 h of incubation and TEER values reached maximum levels between 48 to 72 h [43]. In order to determine the effects of *F. prausnitzii* on TEER over a prolonged incubation time in this model, further validation studies would be necessary to ensure survival of the Caco-2 cells since the initial validation studies were performed for 12 h [23]. In addition, although *F. prausnitzii* is known as one of the major butyrate producers in the colon [1], it is unknown whether it produced butyrate when using 50% BHI as apical medium; therefore, further studies could analyze the composition of the apical medium after the co-culture of *F. prausnitzii* with Caco-2 cells.

3.5. UV-Killed *F. prausnitzii* Decreased TEER

Caco-2 cells in the apical anaerobic co-culture model were co-cultured with live or UV-killed *F. prausnitzii* (strains A2-165, ATCC 27768, or HTF-F) in 50% BHI for 12 h (Figure 6). The interaction between the treatment and time was not significant, so it was removed from the statistical analysis. There was a significant treatment effect ($p = 0.002$), so between-treatment comparisons were warranted. No differences were observed between the TEER across Caco-2 monolayers exposed to the bacterial treatments and the untreated controls ($p > 0.05$). However, the TEER across Caco-2 monolayers co-cultured with live or UV-killed *F. prausnitzii* HTF-F was significantly different ($p < 0.05$) with higher TEER values recorded for cells treated with live bacteria. It is likely that this detrimental effect of the UV-killed bacteria is due to bacteria surface proteins interacting with the host cells. It is also possible that this negative effect is mitigated by metabolites produced by the live bacterium. Live *F. prausnitzii* may also maintain barrier integrity of Caco-2 monolayers through the activation of innate signaling. For example, commensal induced TLR2 signaling was shown to enhance intestinal barrier function and thereby limit mucosal inflammation [44,45]. We have previously shown that live *F. prausnitzii* induced higher TLR2 activation compared to dead *F. prausnitzii* [19], which may cause the barrier-protecting properties.

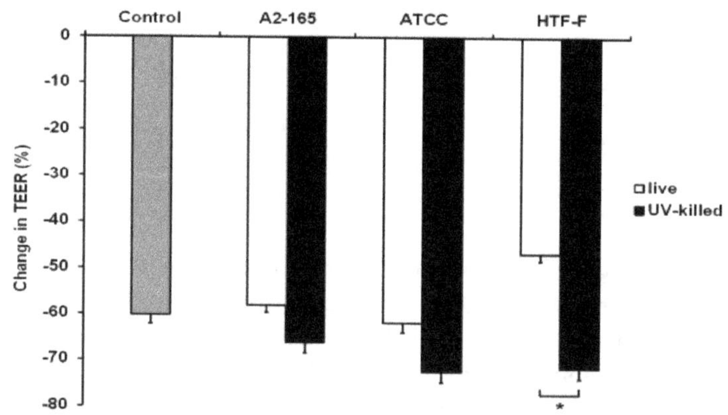

Figure 6. Change in TEER across Caco-2 monolayers co-cultured with live or UV-killed *F. prausnitzii* using 50% BHI as apical medium. Caco-2 monolayers were co-cultured with live or UV-killed *F. prausnitzii* (strains A2-165, ATCC 27768, or HTF-F). The TEER across the Caco-2 monolayers was recorded hourly over 12 h. The interaction between the treatment and time was not significant and so was removed from the statistical model. There was a significant treatment effect on the change in TEER ($p = 0.002$). The graph shows the mean (±SEM; $n = 9$) change in TEER across Caco-2 monolayers co-cultured with live or UV-killed *F. prausnitzii*. * indicates significant difference in TEER ($p < 0.05$).

4. Conclusions

In conclusion, this research resulted in further optimization of the novel dual-environment co-culturing system, which will enable the investigation of new probiotics originating from indigenous beneficial bacteria. Contrary to our hypothesis, actively growing *F. prausnitzii* (strains A2-165, ATCC 27768, or HTF-F) did not improve intestinal barrier integrity, as measured by the TEER of Caco-2 cells. This result indicates that the benefits of *F. prausnitzii* are likely not due to it altering intracellular tight junction integrity.

Acknowledgments: This research was funded by the Marsden Fund, administered by the Royal Society of New Zealand (Grant AGR1102) and the New Zealand Ministry of Business, Innovation and Employment (Grant C10X1003 Dairy-based solutions for improved intestinal function). Eva Maier was supported by a Ph.D. stipend from the Riddet Institute, a New Zealand Centre of Research Excellence, funded by the Tertiary Education Commission. The authors also acknowledge the statistical advice of Carlos Montoya.

Author Contributions: Eva Maier, Rachel C. Anderson and Nicole C. Roy conceived and designed the experiments; Eva Maier performed the experiments and analyzed the data; Eva Maier and Rachel C. Anderson wrote the paper. All authors commented, edited, approved and are responsible for the final version of the paper.

References

1. Duncan, S.H.; Hold, G.L.; Harmsen, H.J.M.; Stewart, C.S.; Flint, H.J. Growth requirements and fermentation products of *Fusobacterium prausnitzii*, and a proposal to reclassify it as *Faecalibacterium prausnitzii* gen. nov., comb. nov. *Int. J. Syst. Evol. Microbiol.* **2002**, *52*, 2141–2146. [PubMed]
2. Hold, G.L.; Schwiertz, A.; Aminov, R.I.; Blaut, M.; Flint, H.J. Oligonucleotide probes that detect quantitatively significant groups of butyrate-producing bacteria in human feces. *Appl. Environ. Microbiol.* **2003**, *69*, 4320–4324. [CrossRef] [PubMed]
3. Swidsinski, A.; Loening-Baucke, V.; Vaneechoutte, M.; Doerffel, Y. Active Crohn's disease and ulcerative colitis can be specifically diagnosed and monitored based on the biostructure of the fecal flora. *Inflamm. Bowel Dis.* **2008**, *14*, 147–161. [CrossRef] [PubMed]
4. Sokol, H.; Seksik, P.; Furet, J.P.; Firmesse, O.; Nion-Larmurier, I.; Beaugerie, L.; Cosnes, J.; Corthier, G.; Marteau, P.; Doraé, J. Low counts of *Faecalibacterium prausnitzii* in colitis microbiota. *Inflamm. Bowel Dis.* **2009**, *15*, 1183–1189. [CrossRef] [PubMed]
5. Mondot, S.; Kang, S.; Furet, J.P.; Aguirre De Carcer, D.; McSweeney, C.; Morrison, M.; Marteau, P.; Doré, J.; Leclerc, M. Highlighting new phylogenetic specificities of Crohn's disease microbiota. *Inflamm. Bowel Dis.* **2011**, *17*, 185–192. [CrossRef] [PubMed]
6. Kabeerdoss, J.; Sankaran, V.; Pugazhendhi, S.; Ramakrishna, B.S. *Clostridium leptum* group bacteria abundance and diversity in the fecal microbiota of patients with inflammatory bowel disease: A case-control study in India. *BMC Gastroenterol.* **2013**, *13*, 20. [CrossRef] [PubMed]
7. Fujimoto, T.; Imaeda, H.; Takahashi, K.; Kasumi, E.; Bamba, S.; Fujiyama, Y.; Andoh, A. Decreased abundance of *Faecalibacterium prausnitzii* in the gut microbiota of Crohn's disease. *J. Gastroenterol. Hepatol.* **2013**, *28*, 613–619. [CrossRef] [PubMed]
8. Rajilic-Stojanovic, M.; Biagi, E.; Heilig, H.G.; Kajander, K.; Kekkonen, R.A.; Tims, S.; de Vos, W.M. Global and deep molecular analysis of microbiota signatures in fecal samples from patients with irritable bowel syndrome. *Gastroenterology* **2011**, *141*, 1792–1801. [CrossRef] [PubMed]
9. Balamurugan, R.; Rajendiran, E.; George, S.; Samuel, G.V.; Ramakrishna, B.S. Real-time polymerase chain reaction quantification of specific butyrate-producing bacteria, *Desulfovibrio* and *Enterococcus faecalis* in the feces of patients with colorectal cancer. *J. Gastroenterol. Hepatol.* **2008**, *23*, 1298–1303. [CrossRef] [PubMed]
10. De Palma, G.; Nadal, I.; Medina, M.; Donat, E.; Ribes-Koninckx, C.; Calabuig, M.; Sanz, Y. Intestinal dysbiosis and reduced immunoglobulin-coated bacteria associated with coeliac disease in children. *BMC Microbiol.* **2010**, *10*, 63. [CrossRef] [PubMed]
11. Martín, R.; Miquel, S.; Benevides, L.; Bridonneau, C.; Robert, V.; Hudault, S.; Chain, F.; Berteau, O.; Azevedo, V.; Chatel, J.M.; et al. Functional characterization of novel *Faecalibacterium prausnitzii* strains isolated from healthy volunteers: A step forward in the use of *F. prausnitzii* as a next-generation probiotic. *Front. Microbiol.* **2017**, *8*, 1226. [CrossRef] [PubMed]
12. Blatchford, P.; Stoklosinski, H.; Walton, G.; Swann, J.; Gibson, G.; Gearry, R.; Ansell, J. Kiwifruit fermentation drives positive gut microbial and metabolic changes irrespective of initial microbiota composition. *Bioact. Carbohydr. Diet. Fibre* **2015**, *6*, 37–45. [CrossRef]
13. Neu, J. Gastrointestinal maturation and implications for infant feeding. *Early Hum. Dev.* **2007**, *83*, 767–775. [CrossRef] [PubMed]
14. Talarico, S.T.; Santos, F.E.; Brandt, K.G.; Martinez, M.B.; Taddei, C.R. Anaerobic bacteria in the intestinal microbiota of Brazilian children. *Clinics (Sao Paulo)* **2017**, *72*, 154–160. [CrossRef]

15. Hopkins, M.J.; Macfarlane, G.T.; Furrie, E.; Fite, A.; Macfarlane, S. Characterisation of intestinal bacteria in infant stools using real-time PCR and northern hybridisation analyses. *FEMS Microbiol. Ecol.* **2005**, *54*, 77–85. [CrossRef] [PubMed]
16. Pop, M.; Walker, A.W.; Paulson, J.; Lindsay, B.; Antonio, M.; Hossain, M.A.; Oundo, J.; Tamboura, B.; Mai, V.; Astrovskaya, I.; et al. Diarrhea in young children from low-income countries leads to large-scale alterations in intestinal microbiota composition. *Genome Biol.* **2014**, *15*, R76. [CrossRef] [PubMed]
17. Miquel, S.; Leclerc, M.; Martin, R.; Chain, F.; Lenoir, M.; Raguideau, S.; Hudault, S.; Bridonneau, C.; Northen, T.; Bowen, B.; et al. Identification of metabolic signatures linked to anti-inflammatory effects of *Faecalibacterium prausnitzii*. *MBio* **2015**, *6*, e00300-15. [CrossRef] [PubMed]
18. Wrzosek, L.; Miquel, S.; Noordine, M.-L.; Bouet, S.; Chevalier-Curt, M.J.; Robert, V.; Philippe, C.; Bridonneau, C.; Cherbuy, C.; Robbe-Masselot, C.; et al. *Bacteroides thetaiotaomicron* and *Faecalibacterium prausnitzii* influence the production of mucus glycans and the development of goblet cells in the colonic epithelium of a gnotobiotic model rodent. *BMC Biol.* **2013**, *11*, 61. [CrossRef] [PubMed]
19. Maier, E.; Anderson, R.C.; Altermann, E.; Roy, N.C. Live *Faecalibacterium prausnitzii* induces greater TLR2 and TLR2/6 activation than the dead bacterium in an apical anaerobic co-culture system. *Cell. Microbiol.* **2017**, e12805. [CrossRef] [PubMed]
20. Wells, J.M.; Loonen, L.M.; Karczewski, J.M. The role of innate signaling in the homeostasis of tolerance and immunity in the intestine. *Int. J. Med. Microbiol.* **2010**, *300*, 41–48. [CrossRef] [PubMed]
21. Groschwitz, K.R.; Hogan, S.P. Intestinal barrier function: Molecular regulation and disease pathogenesis. *J. Allergy Clin. Immunol.* **2009**, *124*, 3–20. [CrossRef] [PubMed]
22. Carlsson, A.H.; Yakymenko, O.; Olivier, I.; Håkansson, F.; Postma, E.; Keita, Å.V.; Söderholm, J.D. *Faecalibacterium prausnitzii* supernatant improves intestinal barrier function in mice DSS colitis. *Scand. J. Gastroenterol.* **2013**, *48*, 1136–1144. [CrossRef] [PubMed]
23. Ulluwishewa, D.; Anderson, R.C.; Young, W.; McNabb, W.C.; van Baarlen, P.; Moughan, P.J.; Wells, J.M.; Roy, N.C. Live *Faecalibacterium prausnitzii* in an apical anaerobic model of the intestinal epithelial barrier. *Cell. Microbiol.* **2015**, *17*, 226–240. [CrossRef] [PubMed]
24. Haller, D.; Bode, C.; Hammes, W.P. Cytokine secretion by stimulated monocytes depends on the growth phase and heat treatment of bacteria: A comparative study between lactic acid bacteria and invasive pathogens. *Microbiol. Immunol.* **1999**, *43*, 925–935. [CrossRef] [PubMed]
25. Yu, Q.; Yuan, L.; Deng, J.; Yang, Q. *Lactobacillus* protects the integrity of intestinal epithelial barrier damaged by pathogenic bacteria. *Front. Cell. Infect. Microbiol.* **2015**, *5*, 26. [CrossRef] [PubMed]
26. Anderson, R.C.; Young, W.; Clerens, S.; Cookson, A.L.; McCann, M.J.; Armstrong, K.M.; Roy, N.C. Human oral isolate *Lactobacillus fermentum* AGR1487 reduces intestinal barrier integrity by increasing the turnover of microtubules in Caco-2 cells. *PLoS ONE* **2013**, *8*, e78774. [CrossRef] [PubMed]
27. Wilkins, T.D.; Chalgren, S. Medium for use in antibiotic susceptibility testing of anaerobic bacteria. *Antimicrob. Agents Chemother.* **1976**, *10*, 926–928. [CrossRef] [PubMed]
28. Wandersman, C.; Delepelaire, P. Bacterial iron sources: From siderophores to hemophores. *Annu. Rev. Microbiol.* **2004**, *58*, 611–647. [CrossRef] [PubMed]
29. Bentley, R.; Meganathan, R. Biosynthesis of vitamin K (menaquinone) in bacteria. *Microbiol. Rev.* **1982**, *46*, 241–280. [PubMed]
30. Kurosu, M.; Begari, E. Vitamin K_2 in electron transport system: Are enzymes involved in vitamin K_2 biosynthesis promising drug targets? *Molecules* **2010**, *15*, 1531. [CrossRef] [PubMed]
31. Nakagawa, K.; Hirota, Y.; Sawada, N.; Yuge, N.; Watanabe, M.; Uchino, Y.; Okuda, N.; Shimomura, Y.; Suhara, Y.; Okano, T. Identification of UBIAD1 as a novel human menaquinone-4 biosynthetic enzyme. *Nature* **2010**, *468*, 117–121. [CrossRef] [PubMed]
32. Heinken, A.; Khan, M.T.; Paglia, G.; Rodionov, D.A.; Harmsen, H.J.M.; Thiele, I. Functional metabolic map of *Faecalibacterium prausnitzii*, a beneficial human gut microbe. *J. Bacteriol.* **2014**, *196*, 3289–3302. [CrossRef] [PubMed]
33. Miyakawa, M.F.; Creydt, V.P.; Uzal, F.; McClane, B.; Ibarra, C. *Clostridium perfringens* enterotoxin damages the human intestine in vitro. *Infect. Immun.* **2005**, *73*, 8407–8410. [CrossRef] [PubMed]
34. Soler, A.P.; Miller, R.D.; Laughlin, K.V.; Carp, N.Z.; Klurfeld, D.M.; Mullin, J.M. Increased tight junctional permeability is associated with the development of colon cancer. *Carcinogenesis* **1999**, *20*, 1425–1432. [CrossRef] [PubMed]

35. Sadaghian Sadabad, M.; von Martels, J.Z.H.; Khan, M.T.; Blokzijl, T.; Paglia, G.; Dijkstra, G.; Harmsen, H.J.M.; Faber, K.N. A simple coculture system shows mutualism between anaerobic faecalibacteria and epithelial Caco-2 cells. *Sci. Rep.* **2015**, *5*, 17906. [CrossRef] [PubMed]
36. Shekels, L.L.; Lyftogt, C.T.; Ho, S.B. Bile acid-induced alterations of mucin production in differentiated human colon cancer cell lines. *Int. J. Biochem. Cell Biol.* **1996**, *28*, 193–201. [CrossRef]
37. Klinken, B.J.-W.; Oussoren, E.; Weenink, J.-J.; Strous, G.J.; Büller, H.A.; Dekker, J.; Einerhand, A.W.C. The human intestinal cell lines Caco-2 and LS174T as models to study cell-type specific mucin expression. *Glycoconj. J.* **1996**, *13*, 757–768. [CrossRef] [PubMed]
38. Khan, M.T.; Duncan, S.H.; Stams, A.J.M.; van Dijl, J.M.; Flint, H.J.; Harmsen, H.J.M. The gut anaerobe *Faecalibacterium prausnitzii* uses an extracellular electron shuttle to grow at oxic-anoxic interphases. *ISME J.* **2012**, *6*, 1578–1585. [CrossRef] [PubMed]
39. Khan, M.T.; Browne, W.R.; Van Dijl, J.M.; Harmsen, H.J.M. How can *Faecalibacterium prausnitzii* employ riboflavin for extracellular electron transfer? *Antioxid. Redox Signal.* **2012**, *17*, 1433–1440. [CrossRef] [PubMed]
40. Ewaschuk, J.B.; Diaz, H.; Meddings, L.; Diederichs, B.; Dmytrash, A.; Backer, J.; Looijer-van Langen, M.; Madsen, K.L. Secreted bioactive factors from *Bifidobacterium infantis* enhance epithelial cell barrier function. *Am. J. Physiol. Gastrointest. Liver Physiol.* **2008**, *295*, G1025–G1034. [CrossRef] [PubMed]
41. Segawa, S.; Fujiya, M.; Konishi, H.; Ueno, N.; Kobayashi, N.; Shigyo, T.; Kohgo, Y. Probiotic-derived polyphosphate enhances the epithelial barrier function and maintains intestinal homeostasis through integrin–p38 MAPK pathway. *PLoS ONE* **2011**, *6*, e23278. [CrossRef] [PubMed]
42. Otte, J.-M.; Podolsky, D.K. Functional modulation of enterocytes by gram-positive and gram-negative microorganisms. *Am. J. Physiol. Gastrointest. Liver Physiol.* **2004**, *286*, G613–G626. [CrossRef] [PubMed]
43. Peng, L.; Li, Z.-R.; Green, R.S.; Holzman, I.R.; Lin, J. Butyrate enhances the intestinal barrier by facilitating tight junction assembly via activation of AMP-activated protein kinase in Caco-2 cell monolayers. *J. Nutr.* **2009**, *139*, 1619–1625. [CrossRef] [PubMed]
44. Karczewski, J.; Troost, F.J.; Konings, I.; Dekker, J.; Kleerebezem, M.; Brummer, R.-J.M.; Wells, J.M. Regulation of human epithelial tight junction proteins by *Lactobacillus plantarum* in vivo and protective effects on the epithelial barrier. *Am. J. Physiol. Gastrointest. Liver Physiol.* **2010**, *298*, G851–G859. [CrossRef] [PubMed]
45. Cario, E.; Gerken, G.; Podolsky, D.K. Toll-like receptor 2 controls mucosal inflammation by regulating epithelial barrier function. *Gastroenterology* **2007**, *132*, 1359–1374. [CrossRef] [PubMed]

In Vitro and In Vivo Evaluation of *Lactobacillus delbrueckii* subsp. *bulgaricus* KLDS1.0207 for the Alleviative Effect on Lead Toxicity

Bailiang Li [1,†], Da Jin [1,†], Shangfu Yu [1], Smith Etareri Evivie [1,2], Zafarullah Muhammad [1], Guicheng Huo [1,3,*] and Fei Liu [1,*]

1 Key Laboratory of Dairy Science, Ministry of Education, Northeast Agricultural University, Harbin 150030, China; 15846092362@163.com (B.L.); 18846420263@163.com (D.J.); yushangf@163.com (S.Y.); besta_intercom@yahoo.com (S.E.E.); zaf_wahla@hotmail.com (Z.M.)

2 Food Science and Nutrition Unit, Department of Animal Science, Faculty of Agriculture, University of Benin, PMB 1154 Benin City, Nigeria

3 Food College, Northeast Agricultural University, Harbin 150030, China

* Correspondence: gchuo@neau.edu.cn (G.H.); wangyt@neau.edu.cn (F.L.); Tel.: +86-451-55191807 (G.H.)

† These authors contributed equally to this work.

Abstract: Lead (Pb) is a toxic contaminating heavy metal that can cause a variety of hazardous effects to both humans and animals. In the present study, *Lactobacillus delbrueckii* subsp. *bulgaricus* KLDS1.0207 (*L. bulgaricus* KLDS1.0207), which has a remarkable Pb binding capacity and Pb tolerance, was selected for further study. It was observed that the thermodynamic and kinetic model of *L. bulgaricus* KLDS1.0207 Pb binding respectively fit with the Langmuir–Freundlich model and the pseudo second-order kinetic model. Scanning electron microscopy and energy dispersive spectroscopy analysis disclosed that the cell surfaces were covered with Pb and that carbon and oxygen elements were chiefly involved in Pb binding. Combined with Fourier transform infrared spectroscopy analysis, it was revealed that the carboxyl, phosphoryl, hydroxyl, amino and amide groups were the main functional groups involved in the Pb adsorption. The protective effects of *L. bulgaricus* KLDS1.0207 against acute Pb toxicity in mice was evaluated by prevention and therapy groups, the results in vivo showed that *L. bulgaricus* KLDS1.0207 treatment could reduce mortality rates, effectively increase Pb levels in the feces, alleviate tissue Pb enrichment, improve the antioxidant index in the liver and kidney, and relieve renal pathological damage. Our findings show that *L. bulgaricus* KLDS1.0207 can be used as a potential probiotic against acute Pb toxicity.

Keywords: *Lactobacillus delbrueckii* subsp. *bulgaricus*; lead toxicity; adsorption; antioxidative activity

1. Introduction

Lead (Pb) is a toxic contaminating heavy metal, with no constructive biological role, that remains a public health concern. The key sources of Pb in the human environment are diet, cosmetics, Pb-based paint, soil and dust from Pb-contaminated paint, gasoline, mining, and industrial activity [1–3]. Pb can be inhaled, as it can enter the atmosphere through industrial burning, smelting, and the emissions of vehicles with leaded gasoline. Pb can also enter drinking water through water supply pipes. Consumption of contaminated food and water are also potent sources of Pb exposure and toxicity. Pb is immensely toxic even at low concentrations, and mainly accumulates in bones, the brain [4,5], the liver, kidneys [6] and muscles causing several serious disorders, such as oxidative stress [6,7], carcinogenesis [8], disruption of calcium homeostasis, degenerative changes, nervous disorders [9,10], and sickness and tissue diseases, predominantly in children [11]. The half-life of Pb in blood plasma is 27 days, in blood is 35 days, in the brain it is about two years, and in bone it may persist for decades [12,13]. Oxidative stress is an imbalance between reactive oxygen species (ROS) and cellular antioxidant systems. Many studies propose oxidative stress as one of the significant mechanisms of the toxic effects of Pb [5,14,15].

The standard treatment for heavy metal poisoning is chelation therapy with the most commonly used chelating agents being $CaNa_2EDTA$ and Meso-2,3-dimercaptosuccinic acid (DMSA). However, adverse effects, including renal injury, malaise, nausea, vomiting, skin reactions [16,17] and progressive deficiencies of copper, zinc and other essential trace nutrients, which are an indispensable part of the body's antioxidant defenses [18]. Therefore, nontoxic natural alternatives of chelating agents have been studied in recent years.

It has been reported that some lactic acid bacteria (LAB) strains, including *L. rhamnosus*, *L. plantarum*, and *Leuconostoc mesenteroides*, are capable of binding and removing heavy metals, such as silver, cadmium and lead in vitro [19–21]. Furthermore, various recent studies have revealed that LAB can effectively protect against metal-induced oxidative stress through antioxidation in vivo [22–24]. Based on this, LAB may serve as a candidate to relieve the symptoms of heavy metal toxicity and their fermented products can be used as dietary fortification against heavy metal poisoning.

The aim of the present study was to select a novel probiotic LAB strain with high Pb-binding capacity and investigate different possible doses to treat acute Pb-induced tissue damage through biochemical enzyme analyses and histopathological studies. This study provides useful information on the utilization of LAB to aid recovery from Pb poisoning.

2. Materials and Methods

2.1. Chemicals and Reagents

Kits used to measure the levels of malondialdehyde (MDA; Njjcbio A003-1 kit), total superoxide dismutase (T-SOD; Njjcbio A001-1 kit), glutathione (GSH; Njjcbio A006-2kit), GSH peroxidase (GSH-PX; Njjcbio A005 kit), aspartate aminotransferase (AST; Njjcbio C010-2 kit), alanine aminotransferase (ALT; Njjcbio C009-2 kit) and a protein quantification kit, rapid (Njjcbio A045-2,) were procured from the Nanjing Jiancheng Bioengineering Institute (Nanjing, China). Lead dinitrate, lead acetate and other analytical reagents were purchased from the Tianli Chemical Reagent Company (Tianjin, China).

2.2. Bacterial Strain and Culture

L. rhamnosus KLDS1.0205, KLDS1.0911 and KLDS1.0912, *L. bulgaricus* KLDS1.0207 and KLDS1.9201, *L. plantarum* KLDS1.0386 and KLDS1.0344, *L. acidophilus* KLDS1.1003, *L. helveticus* KLDS1.0903 and *L. casei* KLDS1.0351 were isolated from traditional dairy products in Sinkiang Province, China and identified by API 50CH strips and 16S rRNA gene similarity analysis. These LAB strains were stored at the Key Laboratory of Dairy Science (KLDS), Ministry of Education, China. All strains were anaerobically incubated in De Man, Rogosa and Sharpe (MRS) broth (Hopebio Company, Qingdao, China) at 37 °C for 18 h and were sub-cultured twice prior to the experiment.

2.3. Estimation of Pb Binding and Pb Tolerance

The Pb binding ability of 10 strains was analyzed as previously described with little modification [25]. All strains were incubated for 18 h and the cultured biomass was centrifuged at 8000 rpm for 20 m. The centrifuged mass was washed twice with ultrapure water to obtain cell pellets. The bacterial concentration was adjusted to 1 g/L (wet weight) using ultrapure water containing 50 mg/L lead dinitrate and samples were then incubated at 37 °C for 24 h (pH 6.0). The samples were centrifuged at 8000 rpm for 20 m and the residual Pb concentrations of the supernatants were measured by flame atomic absorption spectrophotometry (Spectra AA 220; Varian, Palo Alto, CA, USA). The metal removal efficiency based on mass balance was calculated using the following equation:

$$\text{Removal}(\%) = \frac{C_i - C_e}{C_i} \times 100\%$$

where, C_i and C_e are the initial Pb concentration and residual Pb concentration after removal, respectively.

The Pb tolerance of each strain was determined by the minimum inhibitory concentration (MIC) approach [26]. MRS agar medium containing 50 to 1000 mg/L lead dinitrate solution was prepared, and 10 μL of cultured LAB strain was spotted on the MRS agar medium at an inoculum level of 1×10^9 CFU/mL. LAB growth was recorded after cultivation at 37 °C for 48 h. The minimum concentration of Pb that completely inhibited LAB growth was considered as the MIC in this study.

2.4. Equilibrium Isotherm and Kinetic Study

The equilibrium isotherm was performed as previously reported [27], and the harvested cell pellets were suspended in ultrapure water containing 5 to 75 mg/L lead dinitrate to give a final bacterial concentration of 1 g/L (dry weight). The Pb binding assay was then conducted with an initial pH of 6.0 and the equilibrium content of Pb bound by the bacterium was expressed as follows:

$$q_e(\text{mg metal/g biosorbent}) = \frac{C_i - C_e}{m/V} \quad (1)$$

where, C_i and C_e are the initial Pb concentration and residual Pb concentration after removal, respectively; and $m/V = 1$ g/L.

The Langmuir, Freundlich and Langmuir–Freundlich models were used to determine the sorption equilibrium between the biosorbent and metal ions. Isotherm constants for the three models were obtained by non-linear regression methods [28,29].

The kinetic study was conducted as previously described [27], the harvested cell pellets were suspended in ultrapure water containing 50 mg/L lead dinitrate to give a final bacterial concentration of 1 g/L (dry weight). The Pb binding assay was then conducted with an initial pH of 6.0 and the concentration of Pb in the supernatant was detected at different time intervals up to 240 m.

The pseudo first and second-order rate equations were used in the kinetic model of Pb biosorption with the integrated form of the pseudo first-order model as follows:

$$\lg \frac{q_e}{q_e - q_t} = \frac{k_1}{2.303} t$$

where q_t is adsorption capacity; and time t and k_1 are first-order rate constants. k_1 can be determined from the slope of the plot of $\lg \frac{q_e}{q_e - q_t}$ vs. t.

The pseudo second-order integrate equation is expressed as:

$$\frac{t}{q_t} = \frac{1}{k_2 q_e^2} + \frac{1}{q_e} t$$

where k_2 can be determined from the interception of the linearized plot of t/q_t vs. t.

2.5. Scanning Electron Microscopy (SEM) Analysis

The samples for SEM observation were prepared as described earlier [30]. The untreated harvested cell pellets and those treated with Pb (50 mg/L) were fixed by 2.5% glutaraldehyde (*v*/*v*) at 4 °C for 1.5 h, and washed thrice with phosphate buffer solution. Supernatants were discarded and the cell pellets treated with different concentrations (50%, 70%, 90% and 100%) of alcohol as well as a mixture of alcohol and t-butanol (1:1) to wash cells successively. Finally, the cell pellets were eluted with plain t-butanol. The specimens were then put in a freeze-drier for 4 h and sputter-coated with gold. The scanning and photography were performed using SEM with an energy dispersive spectrometer (EDS).

2.6. Fourier Transform Infrared Spectroscopy (FT-IR) Analysis

The untreated harvested cell pellets and those treated with Pb (50 mg/L) were lyophilized and mixed with KBr powder as KBr discs. Discs containing 2% (*w*/*w*) of finely ground powder of each sample were prepared. The FT-IR technique was employed to characterize the changes in the functional groups on the untreated cell pellets and those treated with Pb.

2.7. In Vivo Protective Potential of *L. bulgaricus* KLDS1.0207 Against Acute Pb Toxicity

2.7.1. Animals and Experimental Design

A total of 72 female BALB/c mice (6–7 weeks old, weighing 16 to 20 g) were purchased from the Vital River Laboratory Animal Technology Company (Beijing, China) and housed in a room under controlled environmental conditions at 25 °C and with a 12-h light/dark cycle. All the mice were put into plastic cages for one week before the begin of the experiments. The experimental protocol was approved by the Institutional Animal Care and Use Committee of the Northeast Agricultural University under the approved protocol number Specific pathogen free rodent management (SRM)-06.

Mice were fed with standard commercial pellets and water ad libitum and were randomly divided into two major groups. The prevention and therapy groups were divided into three subgroups and six subgroups, respectively. Each subgroup had a total of eight BALB/c mice. The details of the administration are shown in Table 1. On the basis of Azar's studies [31], the oral dose of lead acetate [$(CH_3COO)_2Pb{\cdot}3H_2O$] was 100 mg/kg body weight. The dose of DMSA used in this study was 50 mg/kg/day [17,32].

Table 1. Experimental design of the prevention and therapy groups.

Groups	Treatment on the Indicated Day(s) for the Following:	
Prevention groups	1–14 days	15 day
Pre-control (n = 8)	SM	PW
Pre-Pb (n = 8)	SM	Pb
Pre-LAB (n = 8)	SM + LAB	Pb
Therapy groups	1 day	2–15 days
Control (n = 8)	PW	SM
Pb (n = 8)	Pb	SM
High dose (n = 8)	Pb	SM + LAB
Medial dose (n = 8)	Pb	SM + LAB
Low dose (n = 8)	Pb	SM + LAB
Drug (n = 8)	Pb	DMSA(50 mg/kg/day)

PW, 0.4 mL plain water. SM, 0.4 mL skim milk. Pb, [$(CH_3COO)_2Pb{\cdot}3H_2O$] at 2 mg in 0.4 mL plain water. SM + LAB, in the Pre-LAB group, 1×10^9 CFU/mL *L. bulgaricus* KLDS1.0207 in 0.4 mL skim milk. SM + LAB in the high, medial and low dose group, 1×10^{10}, 1×10^9 and 1×10^8 CFU/mL *L. bulgaricus* KLDS1.0207 in 0.4 mL skim milk, respectively. Meso-2,3-dimercaptosuccinic acid (DMSA), DMSA at 1 g in 0.4 mL 5% sodium bicarbonate solution. All modes of administration were oral.

All of the therapy groups had their feces collected every week to determine Pb concentration. The animals were then sacrificed under ether anesthesia, and blood samples were collected with Pb-free needles, and all tissue samples were obtained and kept at −80 °C for biochemical assays and estimation of the Pb concentration. Some kidney samples were put into 10% neutral formalin to analyze their pathology.

2.7.2. Determination of Pb in Blood, Feces and Tissue

Samples were digested in concentrated HNO_3 by using a microwave digestion system. Pb concentration in the livers, kidneys, blood, and feces was determined by a graphite furnace atomic absorption spectrophotometer.

2.7.3. Biochemical Assays

The levels of MDA and GSH and the activities of T-SOD and GSH-Px in the mouse kidneys and livers, and the activities of ALT and AST in the mouse serum were measured by using the assay kit in accordance with the recommendations of the manufacturer.

2.7.4. Histopathological Studies

The kidneys were fixed in 10% neutral formalin for 48 h. Samples were then embedded in paraffin, sliced into 5 μm thickness and stained with hematoxylin-eosin (H&E) for examination by light microscopy.

2.8. Statistical Analysis

All values are expressed as the mean ± standard deviation (SD). A minimum of three independent experiments were carried out for each assay. The statistical significance of data comparisons was determined using one-way analysis of variance (ANOVA), followed by Duncan's multiple range test. Values of $p < 0.05$ were considered to be statistically significant.

3. Results

3.1. Pb Biosorption and Pb Tolerance of LAB Strains

The Pb-binding abilities of the 10 strains are presented in Figure 1. While the initial Pb concentration was 50 mg/L, the range of Pb removal by the tested strains was from 22.47% to 79.18%. *L. bulgaricus* KLDS1.0207 showed the best binding ability among the 10 strains. Moreover, *L. bulgaricus* KLDS1.0207 had the highest MIC value (>1000 mg/L) (Table 2). Based on these characteristics, *L. bulgaricus* KLDS1.0207 was selected as a candidate for the further study of its biosorption mechanism and in vivo assays.

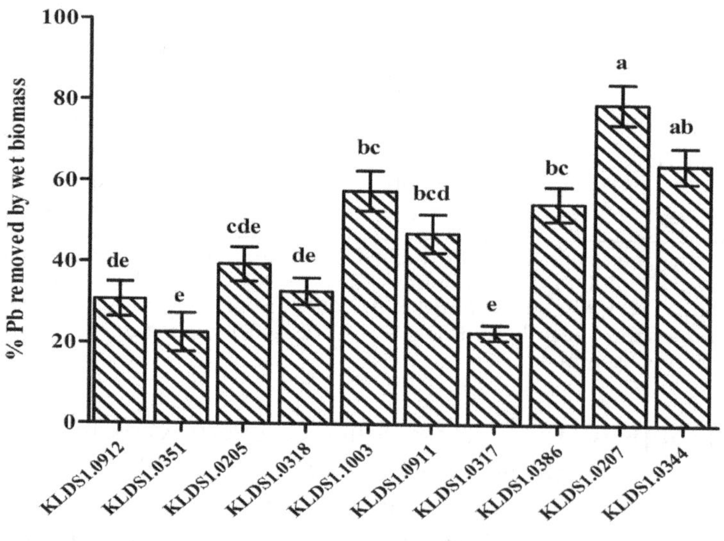

Figure 1. The Pb-binding ability of the tested lactic acid bacteria (LAB) strains when incubated with an initial Pb concentration of 50 mg/L. Values are mean ± SD of three determinations. Significant differences ($p < 0.05$) among the strains are indicated with different letters above the graphical bars. KLDS1.0205, KLDS1.0911 and KLDS1.0912 are *L. rhamnosus*. KLDS1.0207 and KLDS1.9201 are *L. bulgaricus*. KLDS1.0386 and KLDS1.0344 are *L. plantarum*. KLDS1.1003 is *L. acidophilus*. KLDS1.0903 is *L. helveticus*. KLDS1.0351 is *L. casei*.

Table 2. Pb tolerance of the tested LAB strains.

Strains	Minimum Inhibitory Concentration for Pb (mg/L)
L. bulgaricus KLDS1.0207	>1000
L. bulgaricus KLDS1.9201	200
L. helveticus KLDS1.0903	350
L. acidophilus KLDS1.1003	300
L. plantarum KLDS1.0386	150
L. plantarum KLDS1.0344	450
L. rhamnosus KLDS1.0205	100
L. rhamnosus KLDS1.0911	50
L. rhamnosus KLDS1.0912	400
L. casei KLDS1.0351	200

3.2. Biosorption Isotherms and Kinetic Models

As indicated in Figure 2, the Pb concentration in the solution was positively correlated with the Pb-binding ability of *L. bulgaricus* KLDS1.0207. The data of different isotherm models, including Langmuir, Freundnlich and Langmuir–Freundlich, are listed in Table S1, respectively. The values of the coefficients of correlation (R^2) illustrated that the Langmuir–Freundlich model ($R^2 = 0.9820$) best suited our experimental data.

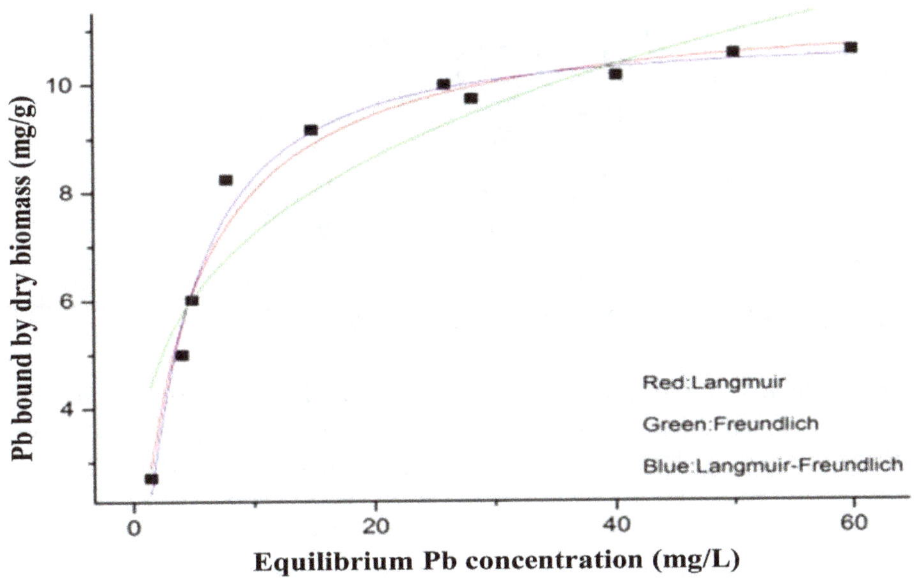

Figure 2. Adsorption isotherm of Pb binding by *L. bulgaricus* KLDS1.0207.

As shown in Figure 3, the biosorption of Pb onto *L. bulgaricus* KLDS1.0207 was efficient, because the binding process was nearly completed in 60 m. The rate kinetics of the reaction adopted pseudo first-order kinetic model ($R^2 = 0.9665$) for first 15 m (Figure S1A). Further analysis showed that the pseudo second-order kinetic model ($R^2 = 0.9916$) was far better at explaining the biosorption of Pb on the surface of *L. bulgaricus* KLDS1.0207 for the complete process (Figure S1B).

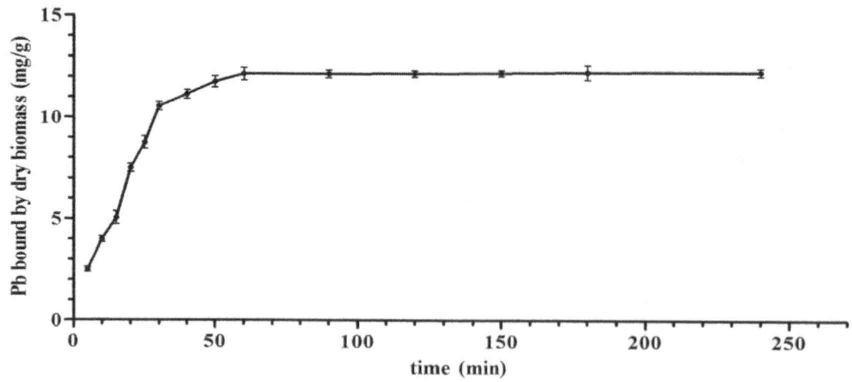

Figure 3. Pb binding of *L. bulgaricus* KLDS1.0207 at different time points. Values are mean ± standard deviation (SD) of three determinations.

3.3. Electron Microscopy Analysis

The SEM micrographs of *L. bulgaricus* KLDS1.0207 after the treatment with Pb indicated that many light clusters of metal precipitates were localized but did not cover the cell surface evenly (Figure 4B). However, no light precipitates were found on the surface of untreated cell pellets (Figure 4A). The EDS analysis confirmed that the presence of Pb resulted in the light precipitates (Figure 4C, Table S2).

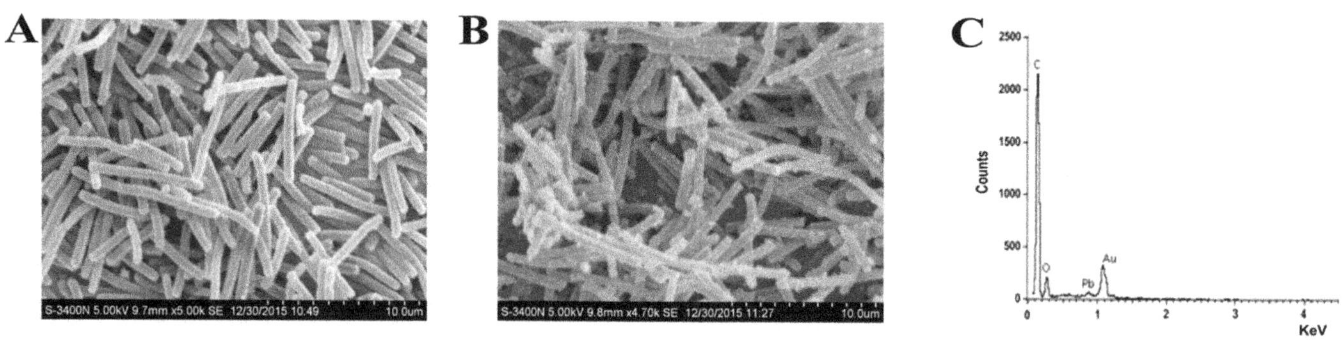

Figure 4. Scanning electron micrographs of *L. bulgaricus* KLDS1.0207 untreated and treated with Pb (50 mg/L): (**A**) Untreated biomass; (**B**) Biomass after lead binding; and (**C**) Energy dispersive spectrometer (EDS) analysis of biomass after Pb binding. Scale bar = 10.0 µm.

3.4. FT-IR Analysis

The FT-IR spectrums of untreated *L. bulgaricus* KLDS1.0207 and that treated with Pb (50 mg/L) are shown in Figure 5. The marked shift to a strong wave number at 3500–3200 cm^{-1} may be due to the interaction of the –NH group of amide and –OH group of alcohol-phenol with Pb. In the 1720–1700 cm^{-1} region, a C=O stretching vibration of carboxylic acid was observed. The amine II band (1400–1410 cm^{-1}) is related to a combination of the NH in-plane bending mode with the stretching of the C–N peptide bond. The disappearance of the peak at 1250–1150 cm^{-1} indicated that the P=O and O–H or C–O stretching vibrations of polysaccharides could play a role in Pb biosorption. These constituents can be combined with Pb by the main functional carboxyl, phosphoryl, hydroxyl, amino, and amide groups.

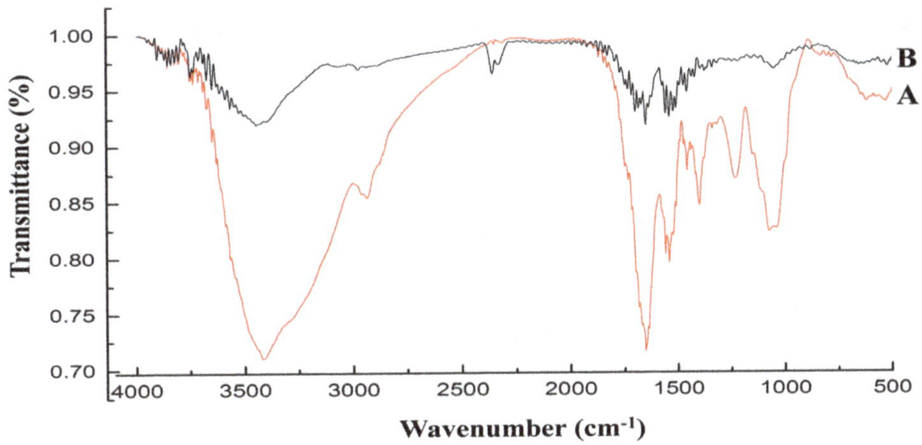

Figure 5. Fourier transform infrared spectrums of *L. bulgaricus* KLDS1.0207 untreated and treated with Pb (50 mg/L): (**A**) Untreated biomass; and (**B**) Biomass after Pb binding.

3.5. Mortality and Viscera Index Analysis

The survival rates of BALB/c mice are presented in Table 3. No mortality was recorded in the pre-control group and the mortality of pre-LAB group (1/8) was lower than the pre-Pb group (2/8). The mortality in the low dose and medial dose group were 1/8, no death was recorded in the high dose and drug group, indicating that the high dose group played a role in mitigating Pb toxicity.

In the viscera indices, the pre-Pb group was significantly different ($p < 0.05$) from the pre-control group, suggesting that some pathological changes may be present in the pre-Pb group. There was no significant difference between the pre-LAB group and the pre-control group, which may be due in part to the presence of *L. bulgaricus* KLDS1.0207. The high dose and Pb group were significantly different in the liver body ratio ($p < 0.05$), but no significant difference in the kidney body ratio was found between the high dose and control group. This was dissimilar from the low dose, medial dose and drug group, which may imply that the high dose group had a better protection against Pb exposure than the drug group as the long-term intake DMSA may have resulted in some damage to the liver and kidneys.

Table 3. The mortality and the viscera indices of different groups.

Groups	Mortality	Liver Body Ratio	Kidney Body Ratio
Pre-control	0/8	3.80 ± 0.25^{b}	1.17 ± 0.03^{bc}
Pre-Pb	2/8	3.28 ± 0.22^{a}	1.06 ± 0.04^{a}
Pre-LAB	1/8	3.65 ± 0.23^{ab}	1.16 ± 0.05^{bc}
Control	0/8	4.95 ± 0.31^{d}	1.42 ± 0.06^{d}
Pb	2/8	3.33 ± 0.14^{a}	1.11 ± 0.04^{ab}
High dose	0/8	4.47 ± 0.27^{c}	1.40 ± 0.03^{d}
Medial dose	1/8	3.43 ± 0.19^{ab}	1.31 ± 0.03^{c}
Low dose	1/8	3.37 ± 0.28^{ab}	1.21 ± 0.04^{c}
Drug	0/8	3.39 ± 0.15^{ab}	1.23 ± 0.07^{c}

Values are mean ± SD. Significant differences ($p < 0.05$) among different groups are indicated with different superscript letters.

3.6. Pb Levels in Feces and Tissues

The changes in the Pb levels in the feces of the mice in the therapy groups are presented in Table 4. In the first week, in comparison to the Pb group, the fecal Pb levels of all treated groups increased significantly ($p < 0.05$). No dose–response relationship by the administration of *L. bulgaricus* KLDS1.0207 was observed. During the second week, the excretion amounts of Pb in the Pb group and treated groups were lower than the first week, indicating that *L. bulgaricus* KLDS1.0207 and DMSA were effective against acute Pb toxicity in the first week.

Table 4. Effects of *L. bulgaricus* KLDS1.0207 on Pb level in feces under different time.

Groups	Pb (μg/g)	
	First Week	Second Week
Control	0.16 ± 0.03^{a}	0.13 ± 0.04^{a}
Pb	23.15 ± 1.35^{b}	0.40 ± 0.13^{b}
High dose	31.15 ± 2.32^{c}	0.65 ± 0.14^{bc}
Medial dose	29.48 ± 1.12^{c}	0.52 ± 0.10^{bc}
Low dose	28.81 ± 1.87^{c}	0.41 ± 0.18^{b}
Drug	42.81 ± 2.43^{d}	0.70 ± 0.16^{c}

Values are mean ± SD. Significant differences ($p < 0.05$) among different groups are indicated with different superscript letters.

The Pb concentrations of the blood, liver and kidneys in the pre-LAB group were significantly lower than the pre-Pb group ($p < 0.05$). In the blood and kidneys, the decreasing Pb levels in all dose groups were significantly different from the values obtained for the Pb group ($p < 0.05$), whereas no significant differences were observed in the liver. This implies that *L. bulgaricus* KLDS1.0207 is more efficient in the kidney than in the liver (Table 5).

Table 5. Effects of *L. bulgaricus* KLDS1.0207 on Pb levels in the blood and tissue of mice.

Groups	Blood (μg/L)	Liver (μg/g)	Kidney (μg/g)
Pre-control	0.32 ± 0.02^{a}	0.15 ± 0.02^{a}	0.17 ± 0.03^{a}
Pre-Pb	383.30 ± 23.12^{f}	1.51 ± 0.04^{e}	1.72 ± 0.07^{g}
Pre-LAB	344.03 ± 24.32^{e}	1.13 ± 0.09^{d}	1.25 ± 0.06^{f}
Control	0.43 ± 0.05^{a}	0.12 ± 0.04^{a}	0.16 ± 0.04^{a}
Pb	302.20 ± 25.32^{d}	0.46 ± 0.08^{c}	0.66 ± 0.08^{e}
High dose	234.12 ± 10.18^{c}	0.35 ± 0.07^{bc}	0.45 ± 0.06^{bc}
Medial dose	248.01 ± 7.54^{c}	0.39 ± 0.05^{c}	0.54 ± 0.04^{cd}
Low dose	258.33 ± 8.13^{c}	0.43 ± 0.07^{c}	0.63 ± 0.05^{de}
Drug	176.14 ± 6.17^{b}	0.27 ± 0.06^{b}	0.36 ± 0.08^{b}

Values are mean ± SD. Significant differences ($p < 0.05$) among different groups are indicated with different superscript letters.

3.7. Activity of Antioxidant Enzymes

The levels of antioxidant capacity in the liver and kidney of mice are shown in Figure 6. In both prevention and therapy groups, acute Pb exposure induced a remarkable increase in the levels of MDA and a marked decrease in the levels of GSH, GSH-PX and T-SOD in the liver. All *L. bulgaricus* KLDS1.0207 administrations had significant protective effects on the antioxidant capacity ($p < 0.05$). Particularly, the high dose group was significantly different with the low dose, medial dose and drug group, indicating that the high dose of *L. bulgaricus* KLDS1.0207 could more efficiently relieve oxidative stress in the liver. Generally, in the kidney, there were significant differences in MDA, GSH and GSH-PX levels in all dose group ($p < 0.05$), however, a significant increase in T-SOD levels was only observed in the high dose group. The MDA levels of the pre-LAB group showed non-significant decrease trends compared with the pre-Pb group. There was a decreasing pattern in the MDA level of all dose groups ($p < 0.05$). In contrast, the drug group was significantly higher than the Pb group in the MDA level ($p < 0.05$), indicating that the drug group had a significantly adverse effect on the kidney. In all, the high dose of *L. bulgaricus* KLDS1.0207 could serve as an effective antioxidant in the liver and kidney.

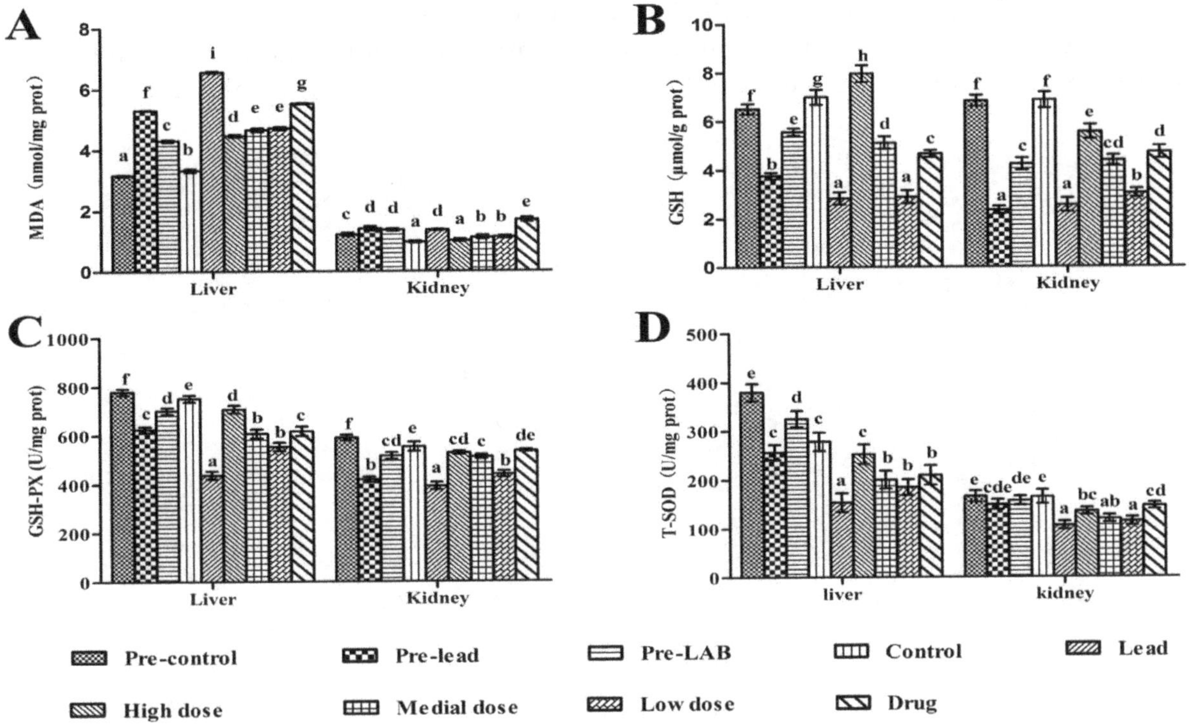

Figure 6. Effects of *L. bulgaricus* KLDS1.0207 on Pb-induced variations of antioxidant capacity in the liver and kidney of mice: (**A**): Malondialdehyde (MDA); (**B**): Glutathione (GSH); (**C**): Glutathione peroxidase (GSH-PX); and (**D**): Total superoxide dismutase (T-SOD). Values are mean ± SD. Significant differences ($p < 0.05$) among the groups are indicated with different letters above the graphical bars.

The activities of marker enzymes in the serum of mice are shown in Table 6. Although no significant difference in the activity of ALT was observed in the prevention group, a significant decrease ($p < 0.05$) in the AST/ALT ratio between the pre-LAB group and the pre-Pb group was noticed. In the therapy group, the AST/ALT ratio in all treated groups was significantly reduced ($p < 0.05$), especially the high dose group showed the lowest AST/ALT ratio.

Table 6. Effects of *L. bulgaricus* KLDS1.0207 on Pb-induced variations in the activity of marker enzymes in the serum of mice.

Groups	ALT (U/L)	AST (U/L)	AST/ALT
Pre-control	33.56 ± 2.13^{a}	55.87 ± 3.01^{a}	1.67 ± 0.02^{a}
Pre-Pb	40.74 ± 1.76^{c}	84.23 ± 3.32^{c}	2.07 ± 0.01^{b}
Pre-LAB	38.67 ± 2.38^{bc}	65.89 ± 4.21^{b}	1.70 ± 0.00^{a}
Control	35.39 ± 3.01^{ab}	100.23 ± 4.54^{d}	2.84 ± 0.11^{c}
Pb	46.19 ± 2.88^{d}	228.12 ± 5.65^{h}	4.95 ± 0.19^{g}
High dose	34.23 ± 1.47^{a}	123.33 ± 4.25^{e}	3.60 ± 0.03^{d}
Medial dose	37.87 ± 2.13^{abc}	153.33 ± 4.02^{f}	4.05 ± 0.12^{e}
Low dose	40.02 ± 2.42^{c}	167.88 ± 5.23^{g}	4.20 ± 0.12^{ef}
Drug	33.87 ± 2.12^{a}	146.46 ± 4.37^{f}	4.33 ± 0.14^{f}

Values are mean ± SD. Significant differences ($p < 0.05$) among different groups are indicated with different superscript letters. AST, aspartate aminotransferase; and ALT, alanine aminotransferase.

3.8. Histopathology

In the control groups (Figure 7A,D), normal kidney histomorphology was apparent. In the pre-Pb group (Figure 7B), glomeruli were hyperemic, the glomerular volume became significantly bigger and few glomeruli were missed, some renal tubular epithelial cells showed swelling, which was alleviated in the pre-LAB group (Figure 7C). The symptoms of all treated groups (Figure 7F–I) including inflammatory cells, swelled tubular epithelial cells and granular degeneration and glomerular hyperemic were ameliorated to some extent when compared to the Pb group (Figure 7E).

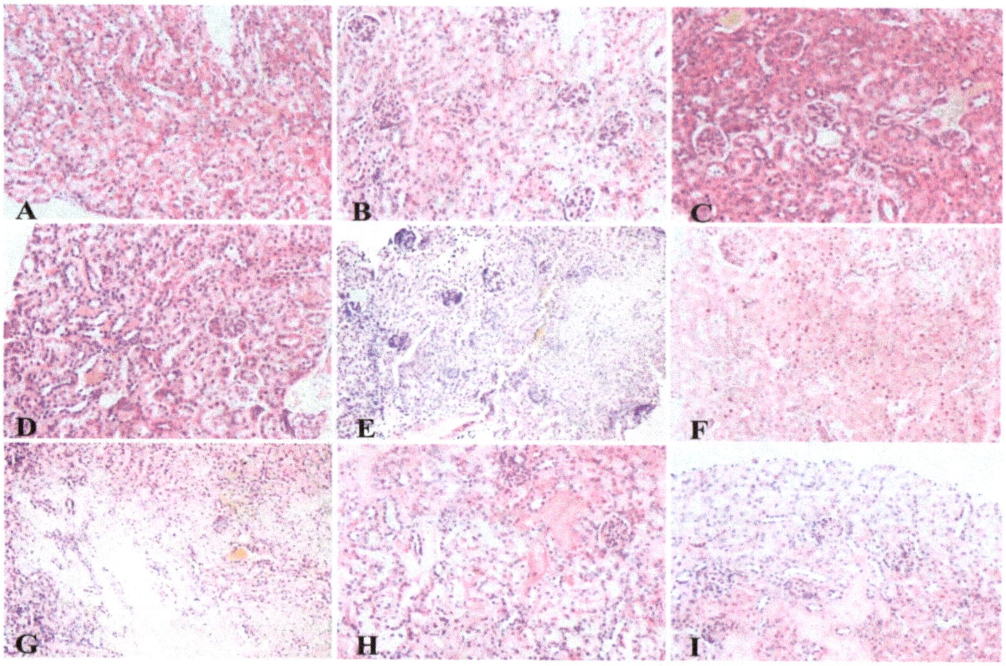

Figure 7. Representative photomicrographs of renal tissue of mice (hematoxylin-eosin (H&E) staining; magnification ×400): (**A**) Normal appearance of the renal tissue of mice in the control prevention group; (**B**) Renal tissue of mice in the pre-lead group; (**C**) Renal tissue of mice in the pre-LAB group; (**A**) Renal tissue of mice in the control therapy group; (**B**) Renal tissue of mice in the lead-only therapy group; (**C**) Renal tissue of mice in the high-dose therapy group; (**D**) Renal tissue of mice in the medial-dose group; (**E**) Renal tissue of mice in the low-dose group; and (**F**) Renal tissue of mice in the drug group.

4. Discussion

Pb is a prevalent environmental pollutant with no beneficial biological role. It adversely induces oxidative stress damage to the host. Many researches have reported that LAB can not only sequester Pb, but also relieve the oxidative damage [1,2]. Screening LAB strains against Pb toxicity should take a number of properties into consideration. First, LAB strains must show high Pb-binding ability, enabling them to bind Pb before the intestinal absorption of Pb by the host. Second, LAB strains should exhibit high resistance to Pb to avoid it being poisoned. Furthermore, to perform Pb removal in the gastrointestinal tract, it is necessary for the screened strains to remain viable in high concentrations of bile and stomach acids. In the present study, *L. bulgaricus* KLDS1.0207 showed the best binding aptitude among 10 strains (Figure 1) and had a remarkable tolerance to Pb (Table 2). In addition, *L. bulgaricus* KLDS1.0207 showed good resistance to simulated gastrointestinal tract conditions (data not shown). Based on these properties, *L. bulgaricus* KLDS1.0207 was selected as a potential strain for the further study of its Pb biosorption mechanism and in vivo assays.

Various mechanisms of metal biosorption, including adsorption, ion exchange, complexation, chelation and microprecipitation have been proposed because of differences in the bacterial structures among the species [33]. The cell walls of the gram-positive bacteria consist of peptidoglycans, teichoic acids, proteins and polysaccharides [34,35]. These contents also contain negatively charged functional groups, which serve as the primary sites of metal ion sorption on a bacterium surface [36]. The phosphate and carboxyl group present in peptidoglycans and teichoic acids are the primary sites of metal ion binding on the surface of the bacterial cell [37]. SEM micrographs and EDS analysis

(Figure 4) confirmed that the added toxic Pb metal was localized on the cell surface evenly. A previous study has reported a similar phenomenon in *L. mesenteroides* after Pb binding [21], this phenomenon may be related to the passive physicochemical adsorption mechanism.

By analyzing the FT-IR spectrum (Figure 5), it was able to be speculated that the functional groups (carboxyl, phosphoryl, hydroxyl, amino and amide) of biological macromolecules (fatty acids, polysaccharides, S-layer proteins and teichoic acid) bind Pb through complexation, ion exchange and physical adsorption (electrostatic attraction). These predictions were consistent with the previous assertion that the carboxyl, hydroxyl and amide groups were involved in Pb uptake [38–40]. It may be necessary in future studies to elucidate the effects of the specific groups in this mechanism.

The thermodynamic and kinetic models of *L. bulgaricus* KLDS1.0207 binding Pb fit with the Langmuir–Freundlich model and pseudo second-order kinetic model, respectively (Figure 2 and Figure S1), this is in line with the cadmium binding characterization of an acidophilic bacterium [27], indicating that adsorption (physical and chemical) is a complex process.

As *L. bulgaricus* KLDS1.0207 had an excellent Pb-binding capacity, the protective effects of it against acute Pb toxicity in mice was evaluated using prevention and therapy groups. In the present study, mice were orally given a lead acetate solution of 100 mg/kg bodyweight to stimulate acute Pb toxicity, followed by treatment with different concentrations of *L. bulgaricus* KLDS1.0207 for two weeks. Our study showed that the high dose therapy group had a higher ability to increase fecal excretion of Pb than low dose groups (Table 4). Similar results were observed for the other *Lactobacillus* strains, which could modulate intestinal heavy metal absorption in mice by increasing fecal heavy metal excretion [22,23,41].

The high concentration of Pb in different tissues was associated with increased oxidative reaction, which might be responsible, at least in part, for Pb-induced toxic effects [42]. Several studies have reported a possible link between oxidative stress and the disruption of metal ion homeostasis [43–45]. Our results showed that *L. bulgaricus* KLDS1.0207 lowered Pb-induced oxidative stress and facilitated a protective role in reducing the lipid peroxide by decreasing MDA concentration and improving other antioxidants, such as T-SOD, GSH and GSH-Px in the liver and kidneys (Figure 6).

Changes in the ALT and AST levels are often used for liver pathological examination, and AST/ALT is an important biochemical indicator [46,47]. ALT mainly exists in the liver cell plasma. When liver cell damage is lower, changes in liver-cell-membrane permeability elevate ALT levels in the blood. On the other hand, increased AST blood levels are a result of severely damaged liver cells. It thus follows that higher AST/ALT ratios imply more severe liver cell damage. The treatment of *L. bulgaricus* KLDS1.0207 could improve the ALT and AST levels (Table 6).

Compared with the dose groups, the drug group was able to increase Pb excretion. Nonetheless, the drug DMSA has been shown in a previous study to have some adverse effects, including depletion of zinc and copper in the body [17]. In all, the results from the present study have shown that the most effective dose in the therapy groups was 1×10^{10} CFU/mL of *L. bulgaricus* KLDS1.0207 in 0.4 mL skim milk. This was similar to the findings of earlier studies that 2×10^{10} CFU/mL of *L. plantarum* CCFM8246 (0.2 mL) and 1×10^9 Colony-Forming Units (CFU) of *L. plantarum* CCFM8610 (0.5 mL) were effective against copper and cadmium toxicity in mice, respectively [22,41]. These effective LAB strains can be freeze-dried or spray-dried to obtain the strain powders for the practical administration. Interestingly, LAB strains such as *L. plantarum* and *L. rhamnosus* can improve the absorption and bioavailability of several trace elements in animals [48,49]. Thus, it is very significant to exploit LAB as a heavy metal removal agent added to food or feed.

5. Conclusions

L. bulgaricus KLDS1.0207 had high Pb biosorption and Pb tolerance in vitro. The adsorption process of Pb was complex and efficient by the main functional groups, including the carboxyl, phosphoryl, hydroxyl, amino and amide groups. *L. bulgaricus* KLDS1.0207 facilitated Pb detoxication in vivo by increasing Pb levels in the feces, alleviated tissue Pb enrichment, improved the antioxidant index, and relieved renal pathological damages. Therefore, *L. bulgaricus* KLDS1.0207 may be used as a novel probiotic candidate against acute Pb toxicity.

Acknowledgments: Present research work was financially supported by the National Key Research and Development Program of China (No. 2017YFD0400303) and the National Natural Science Foundation of China (No. 31401512). We would like to thank Smith Etareri Evivie and Zafarullah Muhammad for revising the manuscript.

Author Contributions: B.L., F.L., S.Y. and G.H. conceived the study and designed the project. B.L., D.J. and S.Y. performed the experiment, analyzed the data and drafted the manuscript. S.E.E. and Z.M. helped to revise the manuscript. All authors read and approved the final manuscript.

References

1. Fewtrell, L.; Prüss-Üstün, A.; Landrigan, P.; Ayuso-Mateos, J. Estimating the global burden of disease of mild mental retardation and cardiovascular diseases from environmental lead exposure. *Environ. Res.* **2004**, *94*, 120–133. [CrossRef]
2. Okoro, K.I.; Igene, J.O.; Ebabhamiegbebho, P.A.; Evivie, S.E. Lead (Pb) and cadmium (Cd) levels in fresh and smoke-dried grasscutter (*Thryonomis swinderianus* Temminck) meat. *Afr. J. Agric. Res.* **2015**, *10*, 3116–3122.
3. Mielke, H.W. Research ethics in pediatric environmental health: Lessons from lead. *Neurotoxicol. Teratol.* **2002**, *24*, 467–469. [CrossRef]
4. Tangpong, J.; Satarug, S. Alleviation of lead poisoning in the brain with aqueous leaf extract of the *Thunbergia laurifolia* (Linn.). *Toxicol. Lett.* **2010**, *198*, 83–88. [CrossRef] [PubMed]
5. Struzyńska, L.; Dabrowska-Bouta, B.; Rafałowska, U. Acute lead toxicity and energy metabolism in rat brain synaptosomes. *Acta Neurobiol. Exp.* **1996**, *57*, 275–281.
6. Patra, R.; Swarup, D.; Dwivedi, S. Antioxidant effects of α tocopherol, ascorbic acid and L-methionine on lead induced oxidative stress to the liver, kidney and brain in rats. *Toxicology* **2001**, *162*, 81–88. [CrossRef]
7. Khordad, E.; Fazel, A.; Bideskan, A.E. The effect of ascorbic acid and garlic administration on lead-induced apoptosis in rat offspring's eye retina. *Iran. Biomed. J.* **2013**, *17*, 206. [PubMed]
8. Valverde, M.; Fortoul, T.I.; Díaz-Barriga, F.; Mejía, J.; del Castillo, E.R. Genotoxicity induced in CD-1 mice by inhaled lead: Differential organ response. *Mutagenesis* **2002**, *17*, 55–61. [CrossRef] [PubMed]
9. Sansar, W.; Bouyatas, M.M.; Ahboucha, S.; Gamrani, H. Effects of chronic lead intoxication on rat serotoninergic system and anxiety behavior. *Acta Histochem.* **2012**, *114*, 41–45. [CrossRef] [PubMed]
10. Sansar, W.; Ahboucha, S.; Gamrani, H. Chronic lead intoxication affects glial and neural systems and induces hypoactivity in adult rat. *Acta Histochem.* **2011**, *113*, 601–607. [CrossRef] [PubMed]
11. Goyer, R.A.; Clarkson, T.W. Toxic effects of metals. In *The Basic Science of Poisons*, 5th ed.; Klaassen, C., Ed.; McGraw-Hill Health Professions Division: New York, NY, USA, 2007; Volume 5, pp. 811–867.
12. Rentschler, G.; Broberg, K.; Lundh, T.; Skerfving, S. Long-term lead elimination from plasma and whole blood after poisoning. *Int. Arch. Occup. Environ. Health* **2012**, *85*, 311–316. [CrossRef] [PubMed]
13. Ahyayauch, H.; Sansar, W.; Rendón-Ramírez, A.; Goñi, F.M.; Bennouna, M.; Gamrani, H. Effects of chronic and acute lead treatments on the biophysical properties of erythrocyte membranes, and a comparison with model membranes. *FEBS Open Bio* **2013**, *3*, 212–217. [CrossRef] [PubMed]
14. Hosseini, A.; Sharifi, A.M.; Abdollahi, M.; Najafi, R.; Baeeri, M.; Rayegan, S.; Cheshmehnour, J.; Hassani, S.; Bayrami, Z.; Safa, M. Cerium and yttrium oxide nanoparticles against lead-induced oxidative stress and apoptosis in rat hippocampus. *Biol. Trace Element Res.* **2015**, *164*, 80–89. [CrossRef] [PubMed]
15. Flora, G.J.; Seth, P.K. Beneficial effects of *S*-Adenosyl-L-Methionine on aminolevulinic acid dehydratase, glutathione, and lipid peroxidation during acute lead—Ethanol administration in mice. *Alcohol* **1999**, *18*, 103–108. [CrossRef]
16. Gründlingh, J. Martindale: The complete drug reference 38th edition. *J. Forensic Legal Med.* **2014**, *28*, 54. [CrossRef]
17. Bradberry, S.; Vale, A. A comparison of sodium calcium edetate (edetate calcium disodium) and succimer (DMSA) in the treatment of inorganic lead poisoning. *Clin. Toxicol.* **2009**, *47*, 841–858. [CrossRef] [PubMed]
18. Yadav, A.; Mathur, R.; Samim, M.; Lomash, V.; Kushwaha, P.; Pathak, U.; Babbar, A.K.; Flora, S.J.S.; Mishra, A.K.; Kaushik, M.P. Nanoencapsulation of DMSA monoester for better therapeutic efficacy of the chelating agent against arsenic toxicity. *Nanomedicine* **2014**, *9*, 465–481. [CrossRef] [PubMed]

19. Zhai, Q.; Yin, R.; Yu, L.; Wang, G.; Tian, F.; Yu, R.; Zhao, J.; Liu, X.; Chen, Y.Q.; Zhang, H. Screening of lactic acid bacteria with potential protective effects against cadmium toxicity. *Food Control* **2015**, *54*, 23–30. [CrossRef]
20. Milanowski, M.; Pomastowski, P.; Railean-Plugaru, V.; Rafińska, K.; Ligor, T.; Buszewski, B. Biosorption of silver cations onto *Lactococcus lactis* and *Lactobacillus casei* isolated from dairy products. *PLoS ONE* **2017**, *12*, e0174521. [CrossRef] [PubMed]
21. Yi, Y.-J.; Lim, J.-M.; Gu, S.; Lee, W.-K.; Oh, E.; Lee, S.-M.; Oh, B.-T. Potential use of lactic acid bacteria *Leuconostoc mesenteroides* as a probiotic for the removal of pb (II) toxicity. *J. Microbiol.* **2017**, *55*, 296–303. [CrossRef] [PubMed]
22. Zhai, Q.; Wang, G.; Zhao, J.; Liu, X.; Tian, F.; Zhang, H.; Chen, W. Protective effects of *Lactobacillus plantarum* CCFM8610 against acute cadmium toxicity in mice. *Appl. Environ. Microbiol.* **2013**, *79*, 1508–1515. [CrossRef] [PubMed]
23. Zhai, Q.; Wang, G.; Zhao, J.; Liu, X.; Narbad, A.; Chen, Y.Q.; Zhang, H.; Tian, F.; Chen, W. Protective effects of *Lactobacillus plantarum* CCFM8610 against chronic cadmium toxicity in mice: Intestinal sequestration is not the only route of protection. *Appl. Environ. Microbiol.* **2014**, *14*, 00762.
24. Tian, F.; Zhai, Q.; Zhao, J.; Liu, X.; Wang, G.; Zhang, H.; Zhang, H.; Chen, W. *Lactobacillus plantarum* CCFM8661 alleviates lead toxicity in mice. *Biol. Trace Element Res.* **2012**, *150*, 264–271. [CrossRef] [PubMed]
25. Topcu, A.; Bulat, T. Removal of cadmium and lead from aqueous solution by *Enterococcus faecium* strains. *J. Food Sci.* **2010**, *75*, T13–T17. [CrossRef] [PubMed]
26. Abou-Shanab, R.; Van Berkum, P.; Angle, J. Heavy metal resistance and genotypic analysis of metal resistance genes in gram-positive and gram-negative bacteria present in Ni-rich serpentine soil and in the rhizosphere of alyssum murale. *Chemosphere* **2007**, *68*, 360–367. [CrossRef] [PubMed]
27. Chakravarty, R.; Banerjee, P.C. Mechanism of cadmium binding on the cell wall of an acidophilic bacterium. *Bioresour. Technol.* **2012**, *108*, 176–183. [CrossRef] [PubMed]
28. Vijayaraghavan, K.; Padmesh, T.; Palanivelu, K.; Velan, M. Biosorption of nickel (II) ions onto sargassum wightii: Application of two-parameter and three-parameter isotherm models. *J. Hazard. Mater.* **2006**, *133*, 304–308. [CrossRef] [PubMed]
29. Chatterjee, S.; Das, S.K.; Chakravarty, R.; Chakrabarti, A.; Ghosh, S.; Guha, A.K. Interaction of malathion, an organophosphorus pesticide with Rhizopus oryzae biomass. *J. Hazard. Mater.* **2010**, *174*, 47–53. [CrossRef] [PubMed]
30. Chakravarty, R.; Banerjee, P.C. Morphological changes in an acidophilic bacterium induced by heavy metals. *Extremophiles* **2008**, *12*, 279–284. [CrossRef] [PubMed]
31. Azar, A.; Trochimowicz, H.; Maxfield, M. Review of Lead Studies in Animals Carried Out at Haskell Laboratory: Two-Year Feeding Study and Response to Hemorrhage Study. In *Environmental Health Aspects of Lead: Proceedings of an International Symposium*; Commission of the European Communities: Luxembourg, 1972; pp. 199–210.
32. Flora, S.J.; Pande, M.; Mehta, A. Beneficial effect of combined administration of some naturally occurring antioxidants (vitamins) and thiol chelators in the treatment of chronic lead intoxication. *Chem. Biol. Interact.* **2003**, *145*, 267–280. [CrossRef]
33. Monachese, M.; Burton, J.P.; Reid, G. Bioremediation and tolerance of humans to heavy metals through microbial processes: A potential role for probiotics? *Appl. Environ. Microbiol.* **2012**, *78*, 6397–6404. [CrossRef] [PubMed]
34. Passot, S.; Gautier, J.; Jamme, F.; Cenard, S.; Dumas, P.; Fonseca, F. Understanding the cryotolerance of lactic acid bacteria using combined synchrotron infrared and fluorescence microscopies. *Analyst* **2015**, *140*, 5920–5928. [CrossRef] [PubMed]
35. Schär-Zammaretti, P.; Ubbink, J. The cell wall of lactic acid bacteria: Surface constituents and macromolecular conformations. *Biophys. J.* **2003**, *85*, 4076–4092. [CrossRef]
36. Mishra, V.; Balomajumder, C.; Agarwal, V.K. Dynamic, mechanistic, and thermodynamic modeling of Zn (II) ion biosorption onto zinc sequestering bacterium VMSDCM. *CLEAN Soil Air Water* **2013**, *41*, 883–889. [CrossRef]
37. Kazy, S.K.; D'souza, S.; Sar, P. Uranium and thorium sequestration by a *Pseudomonas* sp.: Mechanism and chemical characterization. *J. Hazard. Mater.* **2009** *163*, 65–72. [CrossRef] [PubMed]

38. Liu, M.; Dong, F.; Yan, X.; Zeng, W.; Hou, L.; Pang, X. Biosorption of uranium by saccharomyces cerevisiae and surface interactions under culture conditions. *Bioresour. Technol.* **2010**, *101*, 8573–8580. [CrossRef] [PubMed]
39. Ren, G.; Jin, Y.; Zhang, C.; Gu, H.; Qu, J. Characteristics of *Bacillus* sp. PZ-1 and its biosorption to pb (II). *Ecotoxicol. Environ. Saf.* **2015**, *117*, 141–148. [CrossRef] [PubMed]
40. Jin, Y.; Qu, J.; Li, Y.; Gu, H.; Yan, L.; Sun, X. Isolation, identification and pb (ii) biosorption characterization of a lead-resistant strain. *Acta Sci. Circumst.* **2013**, *33*, 2248–2255.
41. Tian, F.; Xiao, Y.; Li, X.; Zhai, Q.; Wang, G.; Zhang, Q.; Zhang, H.; Chen, W. Protective effects of *Lactobacillus plantarum* CCFM8246 against copper toxicity in mice. *PLoS ONE* **2015**, *10*, e0143318. [CrossRef] [PubMed]
42. Patra, R.; Swarup, D. Effect of lead on erythrocytic antioxidant defence, lipid peroxide level and thiol groups in calves. *Res. Vet. Sci.* **2000**, *68*, 71–74. [CrossRef] [PubMed]
43. Jomova, K.; Valko, M. Advances in metal-induced oxidative stress and human disease. *Toxicology* **2011**, *283*, 65–87. [CrossRef] [PubMed]
44. Valko, M.; Morris, H.; Cronin, M. Metals, toxicity and oxidative stress. *Curr. Med. Chem.* **2005**, *12*, 1161–1208. [CrossRef] [PubMed]
45. Odewabi, A.O.; Ekor, M. Levels of heavy and essential trace metals and their correlation with antioxidant and health status in individuals occupationally exposed to municipal solid wastes. *Toxicol. Ind. Health* **2016**. [CrossRef] [PubMed]
46. Vijayavel, K.; Balasubramanian, M.P. Fluctuations of biochemical constituents and marker enzymes as a consequence of naphthalene toxicity in the edible estuarine crab *Scylla serrata*. *Ecotoxicol. Environ. Saf.* **2006**, *63*, 141–147. [CrossRef] [PubMed]
47. Agrahari, S.; Gopal, K. Retracted: Fluctuations of certain biochemical constituents and markers enzymes as a consequence of monocrotophos toxicity in the edible freshwater fish, channa punctatus. *Pestic. Biochem. Physiol.* **2009**, *94*, 5–9. [CrossRef]
48. Klobukowski, J.; Modzelewska-Kapitula, M.; Kornacki, K. Calcium bioavailability from diets based on white cheese containing probiotics or synbiotics in short-time study in rats. *Pak. J. Nutr.* **2009**, *8*, 933–936. [CrossRef]
49. Kruger, M.C.; Fear, A.; Chua, W.-H.; Plimmer, G.G.; Schollum, L.M. The effect of *Lactobacillus rhamnosus* HN001 on mineral absorption and bone health in growing male and ovariectomised female rats. *Dairy Sci. Technol.* **2009**, *89*, 219–231. [CrossRef]

16

Mismatch between Probiotic Benefits in Trials versus Food Products

Mary J. Scourboutakos [1], Beatriz Franco-Arellano [1], Sarah A. Murphy [1], Sheida Norsen [1], Elena M. Comelli [1,2,*] and Mary R. L'Abbé [1,2,*]

1 Department of Nutritional Sciences, Faculty of Medicine, University of Toronto, Toronto, ON M1E 3S1, Canada; m.scourboutakos@mail.utoronto.ca (M.J.S.); beatriz.francoarellano@mail.utoronto.ca (B.F.-A.); sarah.murphy@mail.utoronto.ca (S.A.M.); sheida.norsen@alum.utoronto.ca (S.N.)

2 Center for Child Nutrition and Health, Faculty of Medicine, University of Toronto, Toronto, ON M1E 3S1, Canada

* Correspondence: elena.comelli@utoronto.ca (E.M.C.); mary.labbe@utoronto.ca (M.R.L.);

Abstract: Probiotic food products contain a variety of different bacterial strains and may offer different health effects. The objective was to document the prevalence and dosage of probiotic strains in the Canadian food supply and to review the literature investigating these strains in order to understand what health benefits these products may offer. The Food Label Information Program was used to identify probiotic-containing products in the food supply. PubMed, Web of Science, and Embase were searched for randomized controlled trials that tested the health effects of these strains in humans. There were six probiotic strains/strain combinations identified in the food supply. Thirty-one studies investigated these strains and found that they are associated with decreased diarrhea and constipation, improved digestive symptoms, glycemic control, antioxidant status, blood lipids, oral health, and infant breastfeeding outcomes, as well as enhanced immunity and support for *Helicobacter pylori* eradication. There were a limited number of studies investigating these strains. Many studies were funded by the food industry and tested dosages that were up to twenty-five times the dosage found in most food products. Probiotic food products could have health benefits not currently reported on their labels. However, many dosages are too low to provide the benefits demonstrated in clinical trials. Further research is needed to enable more effective use of these functional foods.

Keywords: probiotics; yogurt; functional foods; microbiome; dairy products; food supply; packaged foods; Canada; public health; preventive medicine

---

1. Introduction

Probiotics are "live microorganisms that when administered in adequate amounts confer a health benefit on the host" [1,2]. The benefits of consuming bacteria have been known since ancient times, when fermented milk was commonly prescribed to treat an upset stomach [3]. Today, the term "probiotic" has been defined and qualified by the World Health Organization, which put also forward guidelines to support their use. Accordingly, different probiotics have been shown to prevent or treat a wide range of health issues, including respiratory tract infections, infectious diarrhea, atopic eczema associated with cow's milk allergy, infant colic, necrotizing enterocolitis, pouchitis, bacterial vaginosis, *Clostridioides* (formerly *Clostridium*) *difficile*-associated diarrhea, and urinary tract infections [4–6].

Probiotic food products are one of the fastest growing product markets globally [7]. Currently, commercial probiotic food products contain a variety of different probiotic species and strains. Certain health benefits are common to most or all probiotic species. These effects are considered "core benefits" and include the regulation of intestinal transit, normalization of perturbed microbiota, turnover of enterocytes, competitive exclusion of pathogens, colonization resistance, and short-chain fatty acid production [2]. Meanwhile, some probiotic effects are found only among specific species of probiotics. Examples include vitamin synthesis, gut-barrier reinforcement, bile salt metabolism, enzymatic activity, and neutralization of carcinogens [2]. Lastly, certain benefits may only be found among specific strains of bacteria; this includes neurological effects, immunological effects, endocrinological effects, and the production of bioactives [2].

Therefore, probiotic food products currently in the marketplace may have the potential to offer a variety of different health benefits, depending on the specific species and strains of bacteria they contain. However, depending on in which country the products are being sold, consumers have varying degrees of information about the health benefit a probiotic product has been designed to provide.

The WHO has recommended that, where scientific evidence exists, strain specific probiotic health claims should be allowed to enable the linkage of a product to a specific health effect [8]. However, in the European Union, there are no approved probiotic health claims [9]. In fact, even the word "probiotic" is considered a health claim and is not permissible on food packages. In the US, products containing probiotics can state that they "support" the body or "maintain" general well-being (for instance, some products state; "help support your immune system" or "helps naturally regulate the digestive tract") [10]. Meanwhile, in Canada, products contain a general health claim (such as "promotes a healthy gut flora") but could provide more specific benefits depending on the species and strain(s) they contain [8,11,12].

To date, the majority of systematic reviews investigating probiotics have focused on the effects of different strains on a single health outcome or the effects of a single strain on different health outcomes. Furthermore, there have been no reviews focused exclusively on probiotics delivered in food formats.

This study had two objectives; first, to document the prevalence and dosage of probiotic species/strains in the Canadian food supply and, second, to review the literature investigating these species/strains in order to understand what health benefits consumers could potentially receive from the probiotic products in the marketplace.

2. Materials and Methods

2.1. *Investigation of Probiotic Strains in the Food Supply*

Data was derived from the Food Label Information Program (FLIP), a database of Canadian food package label information derived from major outlets of the three largest grocery chains in Canada (Loblaws, Metro, and Sobeys) and one major western retailer (Safeway) [13]. This database represents 75.4% of the grocery retail market share in Canada [14] and provides a detailed assessment of the nutrition information found on Canadian packaged food labels. Grocery store shelves were systematically scanned, and data for every food product with a Nutrition Facts table (NFt), including all available national and private label brands, were collected. Data for food products sold at multiple retailers were collected only once. When multiple sizes of a product were available, only one size was collected. However, all flavors and varieties of a product were collected. Information collected for each product included the Universal Product Code, company, brand, price, Nutrition Facts table information (serving size, calories etc.), ingredients, container size, nutrient content claims, disease risk reduction claims, function claims, front of pack symbols, children's marketing, and other claims (e.g., organic, natural, and gluten-free), in addition to the date and location of sampling. The FLIP database is updated every three years. Presently, two collections have been completed (in 2010 and 2013) and have been described in greater detail elsewhere [13,15]. The packages were visually inspected, and ingredient lists of the 15,341 unique products collected in 2013 were searched to identify probiotic-containing products. Fermented foods were not considered to be probiotic products unless they were labeled as being probiotic. The species, strain(s), and dosage found in the 92 probiotic-containing products were recorded and tabulated. In July 2016, Loblaws, Metro, and Sobeys were revisited to identify if any probiotic strain and dosage information had changed and to investigate if new probiotic products had entered the marketplace. Four new probiotic products were identified and included in this study. Companies that listed species names without strain information were contacted via e-mail to inquire whether strain data could be disclosed. One company provided strain information via e-mail.

2.2. *Review of Randomized Controlled Trials Testing the Probiotic Strains Found in the Canadian Food Supply*

A systematic search of the peer-reviewed literature investigating each strain/strain combination found in the food supply was conducted in 2016 in accordance with the preferred reporting items for systematic reviews and meta-analysis protocols (PRISMA) checklist (with the exception of items related to meta-analyses) [16]. The full detailed protocol for this is available at PROSPERO registry CRD42106042660 [17].

2.2.1. Eligibility Criteria

Study Design, Treatment, and Participants

Double-blind randomized-controlled trials that tested the effects of probiotic strains in the food supply were considered. The probiotic strains were required to be administered in a food format similar to the formats found in the food supply.

Studies that administered probiotics in supplement form, that tested synbiotics, or investigated the safety, tolerance, persistence, or viability of probiotics were not included.

Studies on humans of all ages were considered, with the exception of infants under six-months. Individuals with a chronic disease (like diabetes), infections (such as *Helicobacter pylori*), or conditions (like constipation or Irritable Bowel Syndrome) were included.

Outcome Measures

This was not a traditional systematic review. This was an exploratory review and descriptive synthesis that aimed to understand what health effects these food products may offer. Therefore, any and all health-related outcome measures in humans were recorded. This ranged from serum lipid and glycemic levels, to incidence/duration of infections and illness, to markers of inflammation. Effects detected in-vitro were not included. Effects on cellular immunomodulation (e.g., increased number of lymphocytes) were not included.

2.2.2. Literature Search

PubMed, Web of Science, and Embase were searched by two independent reviewers (Beatriz Franco-Arellano and Sarah Murphy) from the earliest record to July 2016. The following keywords were searched in the title/abstract: (multiple iterations of each strain name) and (yogurt OR yoghurt OR milk OR fermented milk OR dairy) with (randomized controlled trial) in any field. When the strain was not found in a dairy product, the dairy keywords were omitted. The search was limited to full-manuscripts in English. Only randomized controlled trials in humans were searched.

Study Selection

After the removal of duplicates, two independent reviewers (Beatriz Franco-Arellano and Sarah Murphy) screened the title and abstracts of retrieved studies against the a priori selection criteria. The selection criteria included any double-blind randomized controlled trial reported in a peer-reviewed journal that included strain/strain combinations found in the food supply, a control group, a quantified dose of the probiotic, a quantified measure of the food treatment, and oral administration of the probiotic via a food format. The study could test any clinical health endpoint on any human population (healthy or sick, including pregnant and breastfeeding mothers). Full-text screening was completed independently by two of the authors of this paper (Mary Scourboutakos and Sarah Murphy), with consensus required for inclusion or exclusion.

Data Extraction

The following information was extracted from each manuscript; information related to the article (complete citation plus author, country, and year of publication), the probiotic species and strain(s) tested, strain dosage, food format, population characteristics (e.g., adults, children, male, female, both), health status of the population (e.g., healthy, population with constipation, diabetic population), sample size, study duration, primary outcome measure, secondary outcome measure(s), significant outcomes, and source of funding. Data was independently extracted by one author (Mary Scourboutakos) and verified by a different author (Sarah Murphy). When articles reported insufficient information, attempts were made to contact their authors via-e-mail to retrieve further information.

Assessment of Methodological Quality

The study quality was independently assessed by one author (Mary Scourboutakos) using Health Canada's quality appraisal tool for intervention studies [18] and independently checked by another author (Sarah Murphy). This tool is used to evaluate the quality of studies that provide evidence to support health claim submissions. The risk of bias was assessed using the Cochrane risk-of-bias tool (Table A1) [19].

Data Synthesis

All studies were grouped according to the strain/strain combination they investigated, and health outcomes were recorded accordingly.

3. Results

The probiotic strains found in the Canadian food supply and a summary of their health effects are shown in Table 1. The initial search of the probiotic strains found in the food supply and their health benefits yielded 188 papers, with 95 remaining after the removal of duplicates (Figure 1). After reviewing the titles and abstracts, 59 remained for full-text review, 29 of which were eligible for inclusion (Table 2). All studies were deemed to be of a 'high quality' according to Health Canada's quality appraisal tool for intervention studies. The majority of studies were judged to have an overall low risk of bias (Table A1).

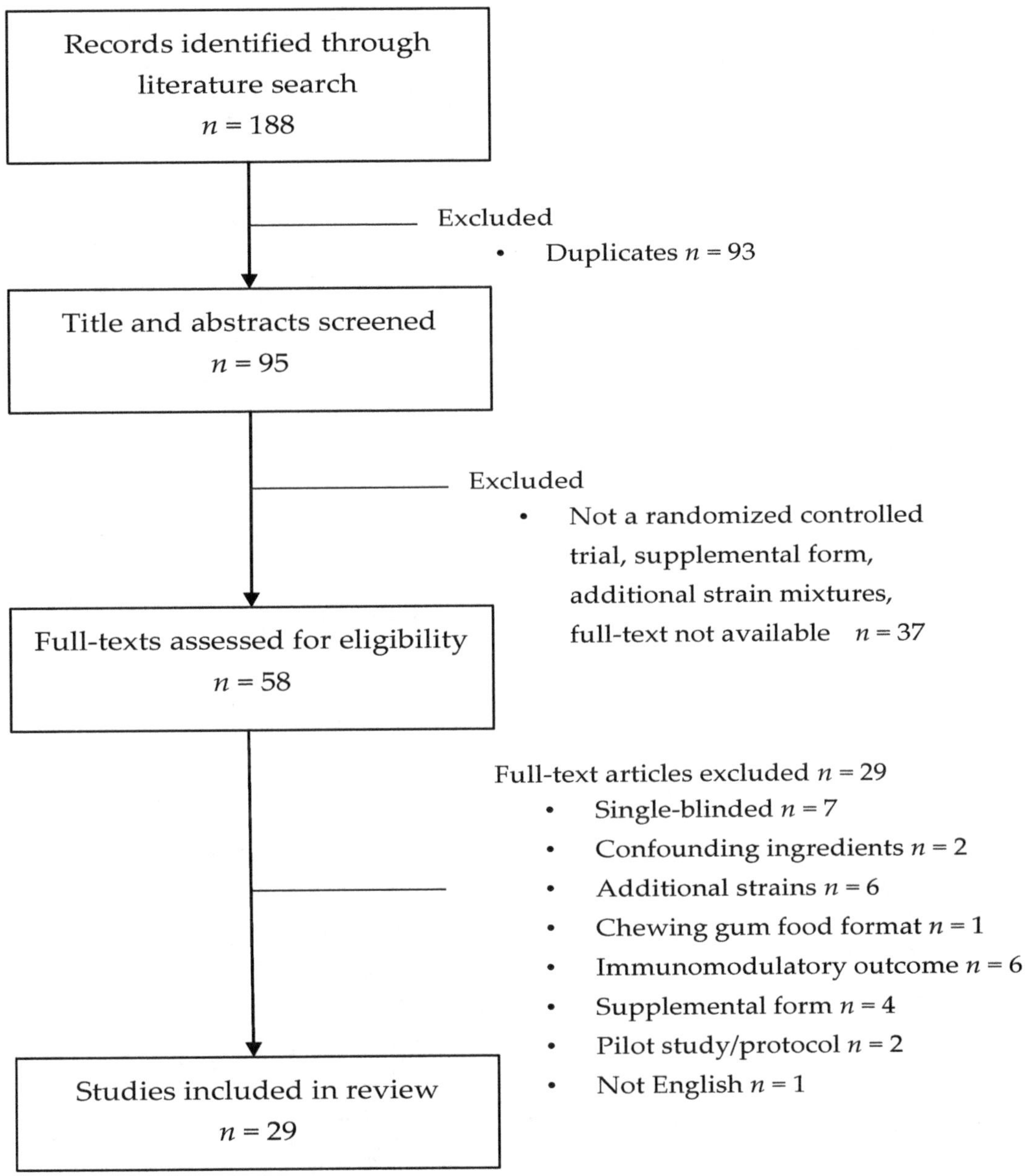

Figure 1. Identification of eligible studies.

Table 1. Strains in probiotic food products and reported health effects associated with these strains.

Strain(s)	Manufacturer and Product Brand	Food Type	Probiotic Dosage in Food (CFU */Serving)	Dosage Tested in Studies (CFU */Day)	Duration of Study	Health Effects Investigated in Healthy Populations										
						Acute Diarrhea	Antibiotic-Associated Diarrhea	Constipation	Digestive Symptoms	Glycemic Control	*Helicobacter pylori* Eradication	Immunity	Infant Breastfeeding Outcomes	Inflammation	Serum Lipids/Blood Pressure	Oral Health
Bifidobacterium lactis BB12 + *Lactobacillus acidophilus* LA-5	Yoplait's *Yoptimal*, Lucerne's *Organics* †	Yogurt	>1 × 10^9	2 × 10^6–3 × 10^9	7 days–6 weeks		X [20] $			O [21]	O [20] $				O [22,23]	x [24,25]
Bifidobacterium lactis BB12	Iogo's *Probio* **, Yoplait's *Minigo*	Yogurt	>1 × 10^9	1 × 10^{10}–3.5 × 10^{10}	10 days—3 months							o [26] $ [27]		O [28] $		X [29]
Lactobacillus casei DN 114-001	Danone's *DanActive*	Drinkable yogurt	1 × 10^{10}	1 × 10^{10}–3 × 10^{10}	2 weeks–6 months	x [30] $, [31] o [32] $	X [33] $				x [34] $	X [35,36] $ x [26,30] $	x [37] $			
Bifidobacterium lactis DN-173 010	Danone's *Activia*	Yogurt	>1 × 10^9	8 × 10^9–2.5 × 10^{10}	2–4 weeks			o [38] $	X [39,40] $ x [38] $							O [41] $
Lactobacillus acidophilus NCFM + *Bifidobacterium lactis* Bi-07	Astro's *BioBest*	Yogurt	1 × 10^9	1 × 10^{10}	6 months	o [42] $						x [42] $				
Lactobacillus acidophilus NCFM	President's Choice's *ProAdvantage* †	Yogurt	1 × 10^9	1 × 10^{10}	6 months	o [42] $						x [42] $				

X = beneficial effects observed in healthy adults; x = beneficial effects observed in healthy children, O = studies that have investigated this outcome and have found no significant effect in adults, o = studies that have investigated this outcome and found no significant effect in children, $ = indicates that the research was funded by the company that uses that particular strain in their products. A blank square indicates that no research investigating the effects of that strain/strain combination was identified during the systematic review of all literature published up to 21 July 2016, as described in the methods. All effects reported in this table were found in healthy populations that were not diagnosed with a chronic disease or condition. Definition of health effects: Constipation = improved stool frequency, consistency, or condition; Acute diarrhea = decreased incidence or severity of acute diarrhea; Antibiotic-associated diarrhea = decreased incidence of antibiotic-associated or *Clostridium difficile*-associated diarrhea; Digestive symptoms = decreased abdominal pain/discomfort, bloating, flatulence, or overall GI well-being; Glycemic control = improved fasting glucose, insulin, HbA1c (marker of long-term glycemic control), or HOMA-IR (measure of insulin sensitivity); *Helicobacter pylori* eradication = enhanced eradication of *Helicobacter pylori* infections; Immunity = decreased incidence and/or duration of common infectious diseases, including fever, cough, common respiratory infections (rhinitis, sore throat), common gastrointestinal infections (gastroenteritis, vomiting), asthma, or days missed from school; Infant breastfeeding outcomes = infants (2–6 months old) of mothers who consume this strain while breastfeeding had decreased incidence of gastrointestinal episodes and lower medication-use rates; Inflammation = decreased levels of inflammatory markers (ex. C-reactive protein); Lipids = decreased serum total cholesterol, low density lipoprotein (LDL), triglyceride levels, or increased high density lipoprotein (HDL); Oral health = decreased levels of cavity causing bacteria. * CFU = colony forming units. ** Iogo's *Probio* reported two strains on its label in 2013 (*Bifidobacterium lactis* BB12 + *Lactobacillus acidophilus* LA-5) and only one strain on its label in 2016. † These products were available in 2013 but may no longer be available in the Canadian market. Note: All cited references were deemed to be of high quality according to Health Canada's quality appraisal tool for intervention studies [18].

Table 2. Results of the review of randomized controlled trials investigating the health effects of probiotic strains found in the Canadian food supply [1].

Strain	Study, Country (Year)	Population (*n*)	Probiotic Dosage (CFU per Day)	Study Duration	Outcome Measures (Primary and Secondary)	Statistically Significant Effects (Relative to Placebo Group)	Funding Source
B. lactis BB12 + *L. acidophilus* LA-5	Ivey et al. [21] Australia (2014)	Overweight adults *n* = 156	3×10^9	6 weeks	**Primary:** Glycemic control (fasting blood glucose, insulin, HbA1c, and HOMA-IR)	Increased HOMA-IR (worsened insulin sensitivity)	Sir Charles Gairdner Hospital
	Sadrzadeh-Yeganeh et al. [23] Iran (2010)	Females *n* = 90	3.9×10^7	6 weeks	**Primary:** Serum total cholesterol, HDL, LDL, and triglycerides	No observed effects	Tehran University Grant
	Ivey et al. [22] Australia (2015)	Overweight adults *n* = 156	3×10^9	6 weeks	**Primary:** Blood pressure, total cholesterol, HDL, LDL, and triglycerides	No observed effects	Sir Charles Gairdner Hospital
	deVrese et al. [20] Germany (2011)	H pylori infected adults *n* = 88	5×10^6	5 weeks	**Primary:** *Helicobacter pylori* activity; **Secondary:** Frequency, intensity and duration of abdominal pain; stool frequency/consistency; duration of diarrhea episodes; IBS symptoms; orofecal transit time	Decreased duration of antibiotic-associated diarrhea episodes	Chr. Hansen GmbH J. & Co., KG, NOM AG [$]
	Ashwin et al. [24] India (2015)	Children *n* = 60	2×10^6	7 days	**Primary:** Salivary levels of streptococcus mutans (a cavity causing bacteria)	Reduced salivary *mutans streptococci*	Funded by study author
	Singh et al. [25] India (2011)	Children *n* = 40	5.4×10^7	10 days	**Primary:** Salivary levels of salivary *mutans streptococci* and *lactobacilli* (cavity causing bacteria)	Reduced salivary *mutans streptococci*	Not disclosed
	Ejtahed et al. [43] Iran (2011)	Type II Diabetics *n* = 64	$>1 \times 10^9$	6 weeks	**Primary:** Fasting blood glucose, HbA1c, insulin and antioxidant molecules (superoxide dismutase, glutathion peroxidase, catalase activity, malondialdehyde concentration, and total antioxidative status)	Decreased fasting blood glucose and HbA1c; increased activity of superoxide dismutase, glutathoine peroxidase, and total antioxidative status	Iran Dairy Industry [$]
	Mohamadshahi et al. [44] Iran (2014)	Type II Diabetics *n* = 44	$>1 \times 10^9$	8 weeks	**Primary:** Serum triglycerides, LDL, HDL, triglycerides, LDL:HDL	Decreased LDL:HDL, increased HDL	Nutrition Disease Research Center
	Ejtahed et al. [45] Iran (2012)	Type II Diabetics *n* = 60	6×10^8	6 weeks	**Primary:** total cholesterol, triglycerides, HDL, LDL, total cholesterol:HDL, LDL:HDL	Decreased total cholesterol, LDL, LDL:HDL and total cholesterol:HDL	Grant from Tabriz University
	Nabavi et al. [46] Iran (2014)	Non-alcoholic fatty liver disease patients *n* = 72	$>1 \times 10^9$	8 weeks	**Primary:** Blood levels of liver enzymes (alanine aminotransferase and aspartate aminotransferase); fasting blood glucose; total cholesterol, triglycerides, LDL, HDL.	Decreased blood levels of liver enzymes, total cholesterol, triglycerides, and LDL	Nutrition Research Center, Tabriz University
	Tonucci et al. [47] Brazil (2015)	Type II Diabetics *n* = 45	2×10^9	6 weeks	**Primary:** Glycemic control (fasting blood glucose, insulin, HOMA-IR, fructosamine, HbA1c); lipid profile (total cholesterol, LDL, VLDL, triglycerides, total cholesterol:HDL); total antioxidant status and cytokine concentrations (Il-6, Il-10, TNF-α, adiponectin, and resistin); fecal short-chain fatty acids	Decreased fructosamine, LDL, and total cholesterol; significant change in HbA1c	Brazilian Agri-Research; Foundation to Support the State of Miras Gerais
B. lactis BB12	Caglar et al. [29] Turkey (2008)	Healthy young adults *n* = 24	5×10^8	10 days	**Primary:** Salivary levels of *mutans streptococci* and *lactobacilli* (cavity causing bacteria)	Decreased salivary *mutans streptococi*	Funded by researchers
	Merenstein et al. [48] USA (2010)	Children *n* = 182	1×10^{10}	90 days	**Primary:** Missed days of school due to illness; **Secondary:** Diarrhea, stool consistency, respiratory infection, missed parental work, doctor visits, illnesses, and overall parental satisfaction	No observed effects	The Gerber Foundation [$]
	Merenstein et al. [27] USA (2011)	Healthy children *n* = 172	1×10^{10}	90 days	**Primary:** Missed days of school due to illness; **Secondary:** Diarrhea, stool consistency, respiratory infection, missed parental work, doctor visits, illnesses	No observed effects	USDA
	Kekkonen et al. [28] Finland (2008)	Healthy adults *n* = 62	3.5×10^{10}	3 weeks	**Primary:** Blood levels of inflammatory markers including C-reactive protein and cytokines (TNF-α, IL-6, IFN-γ, IL-10)	No observed effects	Resaerch Council Finland and Valio [$]
L. acidophilus NCFM + *B. lactis* Bi-07	Leyer et al. [42] China (2009)	Healthy children *n* = 326	1×10^{10}	6 months	**Primary:** Frequency and duration of fever, cough, rhinorrhea, vomiting, diarrhea, physicians' visits and antibiotic prescriptions; **Secondary:** School absences	Decreased incidence of fever, cough, rhinorrhea, antibiotic use, and days missed from school. Reduced symptom duration.	Danisco [$]

Table 2. *Cont.*

Strain	Study, Country (Year)	Population (n)	Probiotic Dosage (CFU per Day)	Study Duration	Outcome Measures (Primary and Secondary)	Statistically Significant Effects (Relative to Placebo Group)	Funding Source
B. lactis DN-173 010	Pinto et al. [41] Brazil (2013)	Healthy adults $n = 26$	not reported	2 weeks	**Primary:** Salivary levels of cavity-associated microorganisms (*mutans streptococci, lactobacilli* and total microorganisms) in saliva	No observed effects	Not Disclosed
	Tabbers et al. [38] Netherlands and Poland (2011)	Constipated children $n = 159$	$>8 \times 10^9$	3 weeks	**Primary:** Stool frequency; **Secondary:** Stool consistency, frequency of faecal incontinence, pain during defecation, abdominal pain, flatulence	Decreased flatulence	Danone $
	Guyonnet et al. [39] Germany (2009)	Healthy adult women $n = 192$	2.5×10^{10}	4 weeks	**Primary:** Overall GI well-being (intestinal transit, stool frequency and consistency, abdominal pain/discomfort, bloating, flatulence, stomach rumbling); **Secondary:** Frequency of digestive symptoms including abdominal pain/discomfort, bloating, flatulence, stomach rumbling; stool frequency and consistency; health-related quality of life	Improved overall GI well-being; decreased frequency of flatulence, stomach rumbling, improved stool consistency, and health-related quality of life.	Danone $
	Agrawal et al. [40] United Kingdom (2008)	Adult females with IBS $n = 34$	2.5×10^{10}	4 weeks	**Primary:** Abdominal distension and bloating; **Secondary:** Orocaecal and colonic transit times; incidence and severity of IBS symptoms (abdominal pain/discomfort, bloating, flatulence); overall IBS symptom severity; time and consistency of bowel movements; feelings of incomplete evacuation at time of stool passage	Decreased maximal abdominal distension, orocaecal and colonic transit times, overall IBS symptom severity, and abdominal pain/discomfort.	Danone $
L. casei DN 114-001	Guillemard et al. [35] Germany (2010)	Healthy adult shift workers $n = 1000$	$>2 \times 10^{10}$	3 months	**Primary:** Cumulative number of common infectious diseases (CID) (e.g., sore throat, sinusitus, nasal discharge, ear ache, influenza, pneumonia, cough, GI infection, diarrhea, nausea vomiting) **Secondary:** Occurrence of having at least one CID: time to first CID, severity, duration, cumulated duration; occurrence and duration of fever, sick days, medication use	Decreased occurrence and time to first CID; decreased duration of fever; decreased cumulative number of CIDs (post-hoc analysis)	Danone $
	Merenstein et al. [26] USA (2010)	Healthy children $n = 638$	$>2 \times 10^{10}$	3 months	**Primary:** Change in behaviour due to illness (e.g., missed school, missed sports activity); incidence of common infectious diseases (CIDs) **Secondary:** Absences from daycare or school, missed parental work, days with diarrhea, vomiting, stomach pain, constipation, runny nose, cough, decreasing appetite, fever, rash, medication use	Decreased incidence of CID	Danone $
	Guillemard et al. [36] France (2009)	Elderly adults $n = 1072$	$>2 \times 10^{10}$	3 months	**Primary:** Cumulative number of all common infectious diseases (CID) **Secondary:** The occurrence of CID (defined as the number of subjects experiencing at least one CID), duration of CID (cumulative and per episode), time to first CID, severity of CID, fever associated with CID, occurrence or duration of medication use	Decreased duration of CID episodes and cumulative duration of CID	Danone $
	Sykora et al. [34] Czech Republic (2005)	Children w/H Pylori $n = 86$	1×10^{10}	14 days	**Primary:** Eradication rate of *Helicobacter pylori* infection	Increased *Helicobacter pylori* eradication rates	Ministry of Health and Danone $
	Ortiz-Andrellucchi et al. [37] Spain (2008)	Breastfeeding infants $n = 104$	3×10^{10}	6 weeks	**Primary:** Immunomodulatory molecules in breast milk (not included in this review) **Secondary:** Infant growth and weight; incidence of gastrointestinal episodes, respiratory symptoms, medication use, allergies and dermatitis	Reduced incidence of gastrointestinal episodes and lower rate of medication use in infants	Danone $
	Agarwal et al. [31] India (2002)	Children $n = 150$	$2–3 \times 10^{10}$	9 months	**Primary:** Duration of acute diarrhea	Decreased duration of acute diarrhea	Not Disclosed
	Hickson et al. [33] United Kingdom (2007)	Elderly in-patients $n = 137$	2×10^{10}	2 weeks	**Primary:** Incidence of antibiotic-associated diarrhea and *Clostridium difficile* associated diarrhea	Decreased incidence of antibiotic- and *Clostridium*-associated diarrhea	Danone $
	Giovannini et al. [30] Italy (2007)	Children with asthma/rhinitis $n = 187$	1×10^{10}	12 months	**Primary:** Episodes and duration of asthma and rhinitis (runny/stuff nose) **Secondary:** Episodes and duration of abdominal symtoms, diarrhea and fever	Decreased asthma and rhinitis episodes, decreased duration of diarrhea in children with rhinitis	Danone $
	Giralt et al. [49] Spain (2008)	Gynecological cancer patients $n = 85$	2.8×10^{10}	6 months	**Primary:** Frequency and severity of radiation induced diarrhea **Secondary:** Time to the development of diarrhea, stool consistency	Improved stool consistency	Danone $

[1] All probiotic strains in the Canadian food supply were recorded and a systematic review of their health effects was conducted. All literature published up to 21 July 2016 was included, as described in the methods. All studies included in the review were deemed to be of a 'high quality' according to Health Canada's quality appraisal tool for intervention studies and thus are considered eligible to substantiate a health claim [18]. [$] Indicates that funding was provided by the food industry HbA1c = hemoglobin A1c, a long-term measure of glycemic control; HOMA-IR = a measure of insulin sensitivity; LDL = low-density lipoprotein; HDL = high-density lipoprotein; VLDL = very low-density lipoprotein; IBS = irritable bowel syndrome; CID = common infectious diseases.

Danone's *DanActive* contained one proprietary strain (*Lactobacillus casei* DN 114-001). This was one of the most well studied strains in the food supply with eleven studies, all funded by Danone, investigating its effects [35]. Three studies showed decreased incidence [26,35] and duration [36] of common infectious diseases (ranging from upper respiratory tract infections to sore throats and influenza) in adults, children, and seniors. Of these, one study showed decreased duration of acute diarrhea in children [31]. One study of hospitalized elderly adults showed decreased incidence of *Clostridium difficile* and antibiotic-associated diarrhea [33]. Other effects associated with this strain included decreased asthma and rhinitis episodes [30] and increased *Helicobacter pylori* eradication rates in children [34]. One study tested the effect of this strain when consumed by breastfeeding mothers and showed that their infants had a reduced incidence of gastrointestinal episodes and a lower rate of medication use [37]. The probiotic dosage administered in these studies was up to three times the dosage found in one serving of this product.

Danone's *Activia* contained a different proprietary strain, *Bifidobacterium lactis* DN-173 010. This strain was associated with improved overall GI well-being, including decreased flatulence [38], decreased stomach rumbling, and improved stool consistency [39]. In one study of women with irritable bowel syndrome (IBS), this strain was shown to decrease overall IBS symptom severity and to decrease maximal abdominal bloating [40].

President's Choice's *ProAdvantage* contained *Lactobacillus acidophilus* NCFM. One study tested this strain in children and found decreased incidence of fever, cough, rhinorrhea, antibiotic use, symptom duration, and days missed from school [42]. However, the dosage tested in the study (10 billion colony forming units (cfu) per day) was ten times the dosage found in the product (1 billion cfu per day). Astro's *BioBest* contained *Lactobacillus acidophilus* NCFM in combination with *Bifidobacterium lactis* Bi-07. This combination was tested in the same study reported above and was found to have the same effects and dosage discrepancy.

Bifidobacterium lactis BB-12 was found in two brands; Iogo's *Probio* and Yoplait's *Minigo* (a product intended for children). This strain was investigated in four studies. In one study, testing a dosage that was half of what is found in these products, this strain was associated with decreased levels of a cavity causing bacteria (*mutans streptococci*) in saliva [29]. Two studies tested the effect of this strain (at a dosage that was ten-times the dosage found in the product) on children's risk of illness and absences from school [27,48]. No effects were seen. One study tested a dosage that was thirty-five times the dosage found in the products containing this strain and showed no effect on inflammatory markers (C-reactive protein and cytokines) [28].

Bifidobacterium lactis BB-12 in combination with *Lactobacillus acidophilus* LA-5 was found in two brands (Yoplait's *Yoptimal* and Lucerne's *Organics*). Eleven studies investigated this strain combination. Three studies tested dosages that were substantially smaller than the dosage found in commercial products. Two of those studies showed reduced salivary levels of cavity causing bacteria (*Streptococcus mutans*) [24,25], while one showed decreased duration of antibiotic-associated diarrhea in patients infected with *Helicobacter pylori* [20]. Two studies investigated the impact of these strains on blood lipids and found no effects despite the fact that one study tested a dosage that was lower than found in commercial products and the other tested a dosage that was higher [22,23]. One study investigated the effect of these strains on glycemic control [21]. It tested a dosage that was three-times the dosage found in commercial products and found decreased insulin sensitivity. There were four studies that tested the effect of these strains on type-two diabetics and used dosages that were similar to those found in commercial products (Table 3). These studies showed improved glycemic control [43,47], improved blood lipid levels [44,45,47], and enhanced antioxidant status [43] in diabetics.

Nine brands labeled species names without identifying the strain (Table 4). Therefore, strain-specific health benefits could not be inferred for these products.

Table 3. Strains in probiotic food products and reported health effects in populations with a diagnosed non-communicable disease/condition.

Population	Strain/Strain Combination	Manufacturer and Product Brand	Probiotic Dosage in Food (CFU */Serving)	Dosage Tested in Studies (CFU */Day)	Health Effects Investigated in Populations with a Disease/Condition						
					Antioxidant Status	Digestive Symptoms	Glycemic Control	Inflammation	Liver Damage	Radiation Induced Diarrhea	Serum Lipids
Type II Diabetics	*Bifidobacterium lactis* BB12 + *Lactobacillus acidophilus* LA-5	Yoplait's *Yoptimal,* Lucerne's *Organics* †	>1 × 10^9	6 × 10^8–>1 × 10^9	X [43] $ O [47]		X [43] $, [47]	O [47]			X [44,45,47]
Patients with Non-Alcoholic Fatty Liver Disease				>1 × 10^9					X [46]		X [46]
Females with Irritable Bowel Syndrome	*Bifidobacterium lactis* DN-173 010	Danone's *Activia*	>1 × 10^9	2.5 × 10^9		X [40] $					
Gynecological Cancer patients undergoing radiation therapy	*Lactobacillus casei* DN 114-001	Danone's *DanActive*	1 × 10^{10}	2.8 × 10^{10}						X [49] $	

X = beneficial effects observed; O = studies have investigated this outcome and have found no significant effects; $ = indicates that the research was funded by the dairy industry. A blank square indicates that no research investigating the effects of that strain/strain combination was identified during the systematic review of all literature published up to 21 July 2016, as described in the methods. Effects reported in this table were observed in populations that were diagnosed with a disease or condition Definition of health effects: Antioxidant status = activity of superoxide dismutase, glutathoine peroxidase, and total antioxidant status; Digestive symptoms: decreased abdominal distension/pain/discomfort, decreased fecal transit time, reduced IBS symptom severity; Glycemic control = decreased fasting blood glucose, insulin, and/or HbA1c (long-term measure of blood glucose control); Inflammation = Increased levels of anti-inflammatory markers (cytokines: IL-6, IL-10, TNF-α, adiponectin, and resistin) Liver damage = decreased serum levels of liver enzymes (alanine aminotransferase and aspartate aminotransferase) [a marker of decreased liver damage]; Radiation Induced Diarrhea = incidence and severity; Serum Lipids = decreased serum total cholesterol, LDL, or triglyceride levels; increased HDL; improved lipid ratios. * CFU = colony forming units. † This product may no longer be available in the marketplace Note: All cited references were deemed to be of high quality according to Health Canada's quality appraisal tool for intervention studies [18].

Table 4. Additional probiotic products with undetermined health effects.

A: Products whose specific health effects are undetermined because there is no research on the strain/strain combination in their specific food format			
Bacterial strains identified in the food database *	Manufacturer and product brand	Food type	Probiotic dosage (CFU) per serving
Lactobacillus acidohpilus Bi-07	Irresistibles' *Life Smart*	Frozen fruit and yogurt blend	Not indicated
Lactobacillus acidophilus LA-5	Breuggens *Yog Active Cereal*	Cereal with yogurt flakes	1×10^9
Bacillus coagulans GBI-30 6086	ShaSha Co's *Spelt Ginger Snaps*	Cookies	Not indicated
Lactobacillus acidophilus ATCC 4356T *Lactobacillus helveticus* ATCC 10797 *Lactobacillus helveticus* ATCC 12046 *Lactobacillus helveticus* ATCC 15009T *Lactobacillus kefir* ATCC 35411T *Lactobacillus kefir* ATCC 8007 *Lactobacillus brevis* ATCC 14869T *Lactobacillus brevis* ATCC 13648 *Lactobacillus kefirgranum* LMG 15132T *Lactobacillus parakefir* LMG 15133T *Lactobacillus kefiranofaciens* ATCC 43761T *Leuconostoc mesenteroides* ATCC 8293T *Leuconostoc mesenteroides* LMG 14531 *Leuconostoc mesenteroides* LMG 6909T *Leuconostoc pseudomesenteroides* ATCC 12291T *Lactococcus lactis* subsp. *lactis* LMG 6890T *Lactococcus lactis* LMG 7931 *Lactococcus lactis* subsp. *cremoris* LMG 6897	† Liberte's *Kefir* (effervescent)	Fermented milk	4.5×10^{10}

Table 4. *Cont.*

B: Products whose specific health effects are undetermined because they only indicate the species and not the specific strain of the bacteria they contain			
Bifidobacterium	Lucerne's *Eating Right*	Yogurt	Not indicated
Lactobacillus casei	Liberte's *BioOrganic*	Yogurt	>1 × 10^9
Bifidobacterium lactis + *Lactobacillus acidophilus* + *Lactobacillus casei*	Liberte's *Classic*	Yogurt	>1 × 10^9
	Riviera's *Petit Pot Yogurt* **		1 × 10^9
Bifidobacterium lactis + *Lactobacillus acidophilus*	Liberte's *Goat Yogurt*	Yogurt	>1 × 10^9
	Skotidakis' *Greek Yogurt* **	Yogurt	not indicated
Lactobacillus casei *Lactobacillus acidophilus* *Bifidobacterium lactis* *Lactobacillus rhamnosus* *Lactococcus lactis* subsp. *cremoris* *Lactococcus lactis* subsp. *lactis biovar diacetylactis* *Lactobacillus delbrueckii* subsp. *lactis* *Lactobacillus delbruecki* subsp. *bulgaricus* *lauconostoc mesenteroides* subsp. *cremoris*	Liberte's *Kefir* (non-effervescent)	Fermented milk	>1 × 10^9
Bifidobacterium infantis *Bifidobacterium lactis* *Lactobacillus acidophillus* *Lactobacillus fermentum* *Lactobacillus lactis* *Lactobacillus paracasei* *Lactobacillus rhamonus* *Lactococcus lactis* subsp. *Cremoris* *Lactococcus lactis* subsp. *Lactis* *Lactococcus lactis* subsp. *lactis biovar diacetylactis* *Lactobacillus delbrueckii* subsp. *bulgaricus Leuconostoc mesenteroides* *Leuconostoc pseudomensenteroides*	Iogo's *Probio Kefir*	Fermented milk	2 × 10^9
Bifidobacterium bifidum + *Bifidobacterium longum* subsp *longum* + *Bifidobacterium animals* subsp. *lactis*	President's Choice's *Kefir* **	Fermented milk	2 × 10^9
Lactobacillus acidophilus + *Bifidobacterium lactis*	President's Choice's *Greek Probiotic* **	Yogurt	1 × 10^9

* Probiotic containing foods were identified in the Food Label Information Program (FLIP), a database of Canadian food package label information. FLIP data was collected in 2013 from major outlets of the four largest grocery retail chains in Canada. Probiotic species/strain information was obtained from the ingredients list and package of each probiotic product. Data was re-verified in 2016 to ensure that the species and dosage information had not changed. ** These products were not included in the 2013 database but were identified when grocery chains were revisited in 2016. † The strains associated with Liberte's effervescent Kefir are not listed on the product label. This data was obtained via an inquiry with the company. All companies that listed species names without strains were contacted to inquire whether strain data could be disclosed.

Most products contained one or two different strains. Kefir (here a fermented milk with added probiotics) products had the largest strain and species diversity, as well as the highest dosage (45 billion colony forming units per serving). However, not all kefir products contained this dosage and diversity.

4. Discussion

Probiotic food products in the Canadian marketplace contained bacterial strains that were associated with a wide variety of health benefits ranging from enhanced immunity to improved glycemic control in diabetics, suggesting that probiotic products could potentially offer health benefits that are not advertised on their labels. However, many of the current probiotic dosages in products were lower than the dosages tested in randomized controlled trials.

4.1. Dosage

In order to obtain many of the health benefits reported in the randomized controlled trials that were reviewed in this study, consumers would need to eat anywhere from two to twenty-five servings of these products each day. The WHO has recommended that "the suggested serving size (on the product label) must deliver the effective dose of probiotics related to the health claim" [8]. Currently most products contain one billion colony forming units (CFU) of probiotics because that is the minimum required in order to provide core benefits and thus be eligible to display the probiotic health claim "promotes a healthy gut flora" in Canada [12]. Therefore, if strain-specific health claims were implemented (in addition to the existing general probiotic health claim), companies would have greater incentive to provide the higher dosages needed to convey some of the health benefits reported in this review.

4.2. Strain Diversity

Most products contained one or two strains. However, research has shown that, in some cases, strain mixtures can be more effective than single strains [50–54], as "different strains (that are) targeted toward different ailments can be blended into one preparation", enabling cultures to complement each other's health effects and produce synergistic benefits [55]. For instance, *Bifidobacterium lactis* BB-12 (found in the food supply) has been shown to have greater gut-adherence when accompanied by *Lactobacillus rhamnosus* GG (one of the most well-studied probiotic strains [4], which is mainly available in supplement form) [56]. Furthermore, evidence from Leyer et al.'s investigation of *Lactobacillus acidophilus* NCFM alone and in combination with *Bifidobacterium lactis* Bi-07 showed that the combination of strains resulted in a lower risk of fever, coughing, and rhinorrhea when compared to the single strain [42]. It is understandable that our results found that fewer products contained strain mixtures, as, presently, food companies have no incentive to utilize strain synergies. Not to mention that single strain probiotics are more easily patentable than multi-strain probiotics [52]. Therefore, current health claims that are based on a single strain encourage the addition of single strains and could therefore be partially responsible for promoting a potentially suboptimal pharmaceutical-like approach to probiotic foods. That being said, it should be noted that not all strain mixtures are beneficial, as strains can antagonize one another. Therefore, research is needed to verify if mixtures are synergistic or antagonistic [50]. It has been previously noted that there is a lack of research on multi-strain probiotics because such research is more difficult to conduct and thus more expensive [57].

4.3. Strengths and Limitations

A strength of this study is the use of FLIP to derive information on all marketed products, which is why we chose to focus on the Canadian market as a model. Obviously, different markets will have different probiotic-containing products, which may come with benefits that overlap or differ from those discussed here. It is important that future research focuses on these other markets to the benefit of both the consumers and the industry. Furthermore, many probiotic benefits could vary depending on an individual's lifestyle and baseline microbiome. Therefore, it is expected that the health effects noted in this review may not benefit all consumers equivalently.

Limitations include the fact that studies in this review tested various strains, dosages, and health outcomes. Therefore, at this point in time, there is no consensus on what strain, dose, or product is best. For example, while our review showed that one strain (*Bifidobacterium lactis* DN-173 010) was associated with decreased digestive symptoms, this was the only strain for which this outcome was assessed. Hence, we cannot conclude that other strains/products would not also have these benefits. Therefore, these results show what is known according to the limited amount of literature that currently exists. Additionally, since much of the current research was funded by the companies that sell probiotic products and therefore dictated which strains were studied, there is a need for further research on a broader range of species/strains that is supported by alternate funding bodies.

Despite the WHO's recommendation that genus, species, and strain should be designated on a product's label [8], nearly half of the brands in this study did not disclose strain information. Thus, the potential health benefits for these products could not be deduced.

Previous research has shown that industry funded nutrition-related research may bias conclusions in favor of the sponsors' products [58]. Most of the studies included in this review were funded by the companies making the products [26,30,32–37,40,59] or were published in journals that are funded by the food industry (Table 1) [45,46]. Many of these studies investigated a large number of outcome measures but did not make statistical adjustments to control for testing multiple hypotheses. Furthermore, in many of these studies, the primary outcome measure was not significant, and, instead, significance was detected in secondary outcomes or through post-hoc analyses. Therefore, while these studies were deemed to be of high quality and were published in peer-reviewed journals, elements of their analysis suggest that their results should be interpreted with caution.

5. Conclusions

Probiotic food products sold in Canada could offer a variety of health benefits depending on the strain(s) and dosage they contain. That being said, the probiotic dosages contained in most food products are currently too low to provide the benefits shown in clinical trials. Therefore, with higher dosages, or with trails substantiating the current dosage, there is potential for the strains that are already in food products to provide more benefits to the consumer.

Currently there is only a small volume of literature investigating the health benefits of the probiotic strains used in the Canadian food supply. Thus, additional clinical trials, particularly ones that are not sponsored by the food industry, are needed. Hopefully this work will encourage funding and regulatory agencies to fund more research investigating probiotics. A larger number of well conducted studies and clear evidence-based labeling regulations will ultimately help the consumers to make informed choices and derive substantiated benefits form the products they choose to consume.

Overall, considering the wide range of diseases and health conditions for which probiotics have been shown to have benefits, further research to promote the optimal design of probiotic food products is needed to enable more effective use of these functional foods.

Acknowledgments: The project was supported by the Canadian Institutes of Health Research Vanier Scholarship (MS), the McHenry Endowed Chair Award (ML), the Lawson Family Chair in Microbiome Nutrition Research (EC), the Department of Nutritional Sciences Graduate Student Fellowship (BFA), the Canadian Institutes of Health Research Master's Award (SN), and finally, in part, by the Center for Child Nutrition and Health, Faculty of Medicine, University of Toronto (EC, ML). Thank you to the L'Abbé lab FLIP data collection team who assembled the 2013 FLIP database. Elena M. Comelli has received funds from a probiotic company to support research; however, the company was not involved in this study.

Author Contributions: Scourboutakos and L'Abbe had full access to all of the data in the study and take responsibility for the integrity of the data and the accuracy of the data analysis. Scourboutakos and Comelli conceived and designed the study; Scourboutakos, Norsen, Franco-Arellano, Murphy, and L'Abbé acquired the data; Scourboutakos, Comelli, and L'Abbé analyzed and interpreted the data; Scourboutakos wrote the manuscript; Scourboutakos, Norsen, Franco-Arellano, Murphy, and L'Abbé reviewed the manuscript for important intellectual content; L'Abbé and Comelli obtained funding; L'Abbé and Comelli supervised the study.

Appendix A

Table A1. Appraisal of the risk of bias of the included studies using the Cochrane risk-of-bias tool.

Strain Studied	Study	Sequence Generation	Allocation Concealment	Blinding	Incomplete Outcome Data	Selective Reporting	Overall
Bifidobacterium lactis BB12	Caglar et al. [29]	L	L	L	L	L	L
	Merenstein et al. [48]	L	L	L	U	L	L
	Merentstein et al. [27]	L	L	L	U	L	L
	Kekkonen et al. [28]	U	U	L	L	L	U
Bifidobacterium lactis DN-173 010	Pinto et al. [41]	L	L	L	L	L	L
	Tabbers et al. [38]	L	L	L	L	L	L
	Guyonnet et al. [39]	U	U	L	L	L	U
	Agrawal et al. [40]	U	U	L	L	L	U
Lactobacillus acidophilus NCFM + *Bifidobacterium lactis* Bi-07	Leyer et al. [42]	L	U	L	L	L	L
Bifidobacterium lactis BB12 + *Lactobacillus acidophilus* LA-5	Ivey et al. [21]	L	L	L	L	L	L
	Ivey et al. [22]	L	L	L	L	L	L
	Sadrzadeh-Yeganeh et al. [23]	U	U	L	U	L	U
	de Vrese et al. [20]	U	U	L	L	L	U
	Ashwin et al. [24]	U	U	L	U	L	U
	Singh et al. [25]	L	L	L	U	L	L
	Ejtahed et al. [45]	L	L	L	L	H	L
	Mohamadshahi et al. [44]	L	L	L	U	L	L
	Ejtahed et al. [43]	L	L	L	L	H	L
	Nabavi et al. [46]	L	L	L	L	U	L
	Tonucci et al. [47]	L	U	L	L	L	L
Lactobacillus casei DN 114-001	Guillemard et al. [36]	L	U	L	L	L	L
	Merenstein et al. [26]	L	L	L	L	U	L
	Guillemard et al. [35]	L	U	L	L	L	L
	Sykora et al. [34]	L	H	L	L	L	L
	Ortiz-Andrellucchi et al. [37]	U	L	L	L	U	U
	Agarwal et al. [31]	L	U	L	L	L	L
	Hickson et al. [33]	L	L	L	U	L	L
	Giovannini et al. [30]	L	H	L	L	L	L
	Giralt et al. [49]	L	L	L	L	L	L

Note: H = high risk of bias, L = low risk of bias, and U = unclear risk of bias.

References

1. Joint FAO/WHO Expert Consultation on Evaluation of Health and Nutritional Properties of Probiotics in Food Including Powder Milk with Live Lactic Acid Bacteria Probiotcs in Food—Health and Nutritional Properties and Guidelines for Evaluation. Available online: http://www.fao.org/3/a-a0512e.pdf (accessed on 8 September 2016).
2. Hill, C.; Guarner, F.; Reid, G.; Gibson, G.R.; Merenstein, D.J.; Pot, B.; Morelli, L.; Canani, R.B.; Flint, H.J.; Salminen, S.; et al. Expert consensus document. The international scientific association for probiotics and prebiotics consensus statement on the scope and appropriate use of the term probiotic. *Nat. Rev. Gastroenterol. Hepatol.* **2014**, *11*, 506–514. [CrossRef] [PubMed]
3. Butel, M.J. Probiotics, gut microbiota and health. *Med. Mal. Infect.* **2014**, *44*, 1–8. [CrossRef] [PubMed]
4. Goldin, B.R.; Gorbach, S.L. Clinical indications for probiotics: An overview. *Clin. Infect. Dis.* **2008**, *46*, S96–S100. [CrossRef] [PubMed]
5. Kaur, I.P.; Kuhad, A.; Garg, A.; Chopra, K. Probiotics: Delineation of prophylactic and therapeutic benefits. *J. Med. Food* **2009**, *12*, 219–235. [CrossRef] [PubMed]
6. Taibi, A.; Comelli, E.M. Practical approaches to probiotics use. *Appl. Physiol. Nutr. Metab.* **2014**, *39*, 980–986. [CrossRef] [PubMed]
7. Grand View Research Probiotics Market Analysis by Application (Probiotic Functional Foods & Beverages, Probiotic Dietary Supplements, Animal Feed Probiotics), by End-Use (Human Probiotics, Animal Probiotics) and Segment Forecasts to 2020. Available online: http://www.grandviewresearch.com/industry-analysis/probiotics-market (accessed on 11 August 2016).

8. World Health Organization. Guidelines for the Evaluation of Probiotics in Food. Available online: http://www.who.int/foodsafety/fs_management/en/probiotic_guidelines.pdf (accessed on 25 January 2016).
9. Glanville, J.; King, S.; Guarner, F.; Hill, C.; Sanders, M.E. A review of the systematic review process and its applicability for use in evaluating evidence for health claims on probiotic foods in the european union. *Nutr. J.* **2015**, *14*, 16. [CrossRef] [PubMed]
10. Saldanha, L.G. Us food and drug administration regulations governing label claims for food products, including probiotics. *Clin. Infect. Dis.* **2008**, *46*, S119–S121; discussion: S144–S151. [CrossRef] [PubMed]
11. Canadian Food Inspection Agency Health Claims—Probiotic Claims. Available online: http://www.inspection.gc.ca/food/labelling/food-labelling-for-industry/health-claims/eng/1392834838383/1392834887794?chap=9 (accessed on 25 January 2016).
12. Health Canada Guidance Document—The Use of Probiotic Microorganisms in Food. Available online: http://www.hc-sc.gc.ca/fn-an/alt_formats/hpfb-dgpsa/pdf/legislation/probiotics_guidance-orientation_probiotiques-eng.pdf (accessed on 25 January 2016).
13. Bernstein, J.; Schermel, A.; Mills, C.; L'Abbe, M. Total and free sugar content of canadian prepackaged foods and beverages. *Nutrients* **2016**, *8*, 582. [CrossRef] [PubMed]
14. Canadian Grocer. *Executive Report, Canadian Grocery Industry 2012–2013*; Rogers Publishing Limited: Toronto, ON, Canada, 2012.
15. Schermel, A.; Emrich, T.E.; Arcand, J.; Wong, C.L.; L'Abbe, M.R. Nutrition marketing on processed food packages in canada: 2010 food label information program. *Appl. Physiol. Nutr. Metab.* **2013**, *38*, 666–672. [CrossRef] [PubMed]
16. Shamseer, L.; Moher, D.; Clarke, M.; Ghersi, D.; Liberati, A.; Petticrew, M.; Shekelle, P.; Stewart, L.A. Preferred reporting items for systematic review and meta-analysis protocols (prisma-p) 2015: Elaboration and explanation. *Br. Med. J.* **2015**, *349*, g7647. [CrossRef] [PubMed]
17. PROSPERO International Prospective Register of Systematic Reviews. Available online: http://www.crd.york.ac.uk/PROSPERO/display_record.asp?ID=CRD42016042660 (accessed on 28 June 2016).
18. Health Canada Guidance Document for Preparing a Submission for Food Health Claims. Available online: http://www.hc-sc.gc.ca/fn-an/legislation/guide-ld/health-claims_guidance-orientation_allegations-sante-eng.php (accessed on 10 July 2016).
19. Higgins, J.P.; Altman, D.G.; Gotzsche, P.C.; Juni, P.; Moher, D.; Oxman, A.D.; Savovic, J.; Schulz, K.F.; Weeks, L.; Sterne, J.A. The cochrane collaboration's tool for assessing risk of bias in randomised trials. *Br. Med. J.* **2011**, *343*, d5928. [CrossRef] [PubMed]
20. De Vrese, M.; Kristen, H.; Rautenberg, P.; Laue, C.; Schrezenmeir, J. Probiotic lactobacilli and bifidobacteria in a fermented milk product with added fruit preparation reduce antibiotic associated diarrhea and helicobacter pylori activity. *J. Dairy Res.* **2011**, *78*, 396–403. [CrossRef] [PubMed]
21. Ivey, K.L.; Hodgson, J.M.; Kerr, D.A.; Lewis, J.R.; Thompson, P.L.; Prince, R.L. The effects of probiotic bacteria on glycaemic control in overweight men and women: A randomised controlled trial. *Eur. J. Clin. Nutr.* **2014**, *68*, 447–452. [CrossRef] [PubMed]
22. Ivey, K.L.; Hodgson, J.M.; Kerr, D.A.; Thompson, P.L.; Stojceski, B.; Prince, R.L. The effect of yoghurt and its probiotics on blood pressure and serum lipid profile; a randomised controlled trial. *Nutr. Metab. Cardiovasc. Dis. NMCD* **2015**, *25*, 46–51. [CrossRef] [PubMed]
23. Sadrzadeh-Yeganeh, H.; Elmadfa, I.; Djazayery, A.; Jalali, M.; Heshmat, R.; Chamary, M. The effects of probiotic and conventional yoghurt on lipid profile in women. *Br. J. Nutr.* **2010**, *103*, 1778–1783. [CrossRef] [PubMed]
24. Ashwin, D.; Ke, V.; Taranath, M.; Ramagoni, N.K.; Nara, A.; Sarpangala, M. Effect of probiotic containing ice-cream on salivary mutans streptococci (sms) levels in children of 6–12 years of age: A randomized controlled double blind study with six-months follow up. *J. Clin. Diagn. Res. JCDR* **2015**, *9*, ZC06–ZC09. [CrossRef] [PubMed]
25. Singh, R.P.; Damle, S.G.; Chawla, A. Salivary mutans streptococci and lactobacilli modulations in young children on consumption of probiotic ice-cream containing bifidobacterium lactis bb12 and lactobacillus acidophilus la5. *Acta Odontol. Scand.* **2011**, *69*, 389–394. [CrossRef] [PubMed]
26. Merenstein, D.; Murphy, M.; Fokar, A.; Hernandez, R.K.; Park, H.; Nsouli, H.; Sanders, M.E.; Davis, B.A.; Niborski, V.; Tondu, F.; et al. Use of a fermented dairy probiotic drink containing lactobacillus casei

(DN-114-001) to decrease the rate of illness in kids: The drink study. A patient-oriented, double-blind, cluster-randomized, placebo-controlled, clinical trial. *Eur. J. Clin. Nutr.* **2010**, *64*, 669–677. [CrossRef] [PubMed]

27. Merenstein, D.; Gonzalez, J.; Young, A.G.; Roberts, R.F.; Sanders, M.E.; Petterson, S. Study to investigate the potential of probiotics in children attending school. *Eur. J. Clin. Nutr.* **2011**, *65*, 447–453. [CrossRef] [PubMed]
28. Kekkonen, R.A.; Lummela, N.; Karjalainen, H.; Latvala, S.; Tynkkynen, S.; Jarvenpaa, S.; Kautiainen, H.; Julkunen, I.; Vapaatalo, H.; Korpela, R. Probiotic intervention has strain-specific anti-inflammatory effects in healthy adults. *World J. Gastroenterol.* **2008**, *14*, 2029–2036. [CrossRef] [PubMed]
29. Caglar, E.; Kuscu, O.O.; Selvi Kuvvetli, S.; Kavaloglu Cildir, S.; Sandalli, N.; Twetman, S. Short-term effect of ice-cream containing bifidobacterium lactis bb-12 on the number of salivary mutans streptococci and lactobacilli. *Acta Odontol. Scand.* **2008**, *66*, 154–158. [CrossRef] [PubMed]
30. Giovannini, M.; Agostoni, C.; Riva, E.; Salvini, F.; Ruscitto, A.; Zuccotti, G.V.; Radaelli, G. A randomized prospective double blind controlled trial on effects of long-term consumption of fermented milk containing lactobacillus casei in pre-school children with allergic asthma and/or rhinitis. *Pediatr. Res.* **2007**, *62*, 215–220. [CrossRef] [PubMed]
31. Agarwal, K.N.; Bhasin, S.K. Feasibility studies to control acute diarrhoea in children by feeding fermented milk preparations actimel and indian dahi. *Eur. J. Clin. Nutr.* **2002**, *56*, S56–S59. [CrossRef] [PubMed]
32. Pedone, C.A.; Bernabeu, A.O.; Postaire, E.R.; Bouley, C.F.; Reinert, P. The effect of supplementation with milk fermented by lactobacillus casei (strain DN-114-001) on acute diarrhoea in children attending day care centres. *Int. J. Clin. Pract.* **1999**, *53*, 179–184. [PubMed]
33. Hickson, M.; D'Souza, A.L.; Muthu, N.; Rogers, T.R.; Want, S.; Rajkumar, C.; Bulpitt, C.J. Use of probiotic lactobacillus preparation to prevent diarrhoea associated with antibiotics: Randomised double blind placebo controlled trial. *Br. Med. J.* **2007**, *335*, 80. [CrossRef] [PubMed]
34. Sykora, J.; Valeckova, K.; Amlerova, J.; Siala, K.; Dedek, P.; Watkins, S.; Varvarovska, J.; Stozicky, F.; Pazdiora, P.; Schwarz, J. Effects of a specially designed fermented milk product containing probiotic lactobacillus casei DN-114-001 and the eradication of h. Pylori in children: A prospective randomized double-blind study. *J. Clin. Gastroenterol.* **2005**, *39*, 692–698. [CrossRef] [PubMed]
35. Guillemard, E.; Tanguy, J.; Flavigny, A.; de la Motte, S.; Schrezenmeir, J. Effects of consumption of a fermented dairy product containing the probiotic lactobacillus casei DN-114-001 on common respiratory and gastrointestinal infections in shift workers in a randomized controlled trial. *J. Am. Coll. Nutr.* **2010**, *29*, 455–468. [CrossRef] [PubMed]
36. Guillemard, E.; Tondu, F.; Lacoin, F.; Schrezenmeir, J. Consumption of a fermented dairy product containing the probiotic lactobacillus casei DN-114001 reduces the duration of respiratory infections in the elderly in a randomised controlled trial. *Br. J. Nutr.* **2010**, *103*, 58–68. [CrossRef] [PubMed]
37. Ortiz-Andrellucchi, A.; Sanchez-Villegas, A.; Rodriguez-Gallego, C.; Lemes, A.; Molero, T.; Soria, A.; Pena-Quintana, L.; Santana, M.; Ramirez, O.; Garcia, J.; et al. Immunomodulatory effects of the intake of fermented milk with lactobacillus casei DN-114-001 in lactating mothers and their children. *Br. J. Nutr.* **2008**, *100*, 834–845. [CrossRef] [PubMed]
38. Tabbers, M.M.; Chmielewska, A.; Roseboom, M.G.; Crastes, N.; Perrin, C.; Reitsma, J.B.; Norbruis, O.; Szajewska, H.; Benninga, M.A. Fermented milk containing bifidobacterium lactis DN-173 010 in childhood constipation: A randomized, double-blind, controlled trial. *Pediatrics* **2011**, *127*, e1392–e1399. [CrossRef] [PubMed]
39. Guyonnet, D.; Schlumberger, A.; Mhamdi, L.; Jakob, S.; Chassany, O. Fermented milk containing bifidobacterium lactis DN-173 010 improves gastrointestinal well-being and digestive symptoms in women reporting minor digestive symptoms: A randomised, double-blind, parallel, controlled study. *Br. J. Nutr.* **2009**, *102*, 1654–1662. [CrossRef] [PubMed]
40. Agrawal, A.; Houghton, L.A.; Morris, J.; Reilly, B.; Guyonnet, D.; Goupil Feuillerat, N.; Schlumberger, A.; Jakob, S.; Whorwell, P.J. Clinical trial: The effects of a fermented milk product containing bifidobacterium lactis DN-173 010 on abdominal distension and gastrointestinal transit in irritable bowel syndrome with constipation. *Aliment. Pharmacol. Ther.* **2009**, *29*, 104–114. [CrossRef] [PubMed]
41. Pinto, G.S.; Cenci, M.S.; Azevedo, M.S.; Epifanio, M.; Jones, M.H. Effect of yogurt containing bifidobacterium animalis subsp. Lactis DN-173 010 probiotic on dental plaque and saliva in orthodontic patients. *Caries Res.* **2014**, *48*, 63–68. [CrossRef] [PubMed]

42. Leyer, G.J.; Li, S.; Mubasher, M.E.; Reifer, C.; Ouwehand, A.C. Probiotic effects on cold and influenza-like symptom incidence and duration in children. *Pediatrics* **2009**, *124*, e172–e179. [CrossRef] [PubMed]
43. Ejtahed, H.S.; Mohtadi-Nia, J.; Homayouni-Rad, A.; Niafar, M.; Asghari-Jafarabadi, M.; Mofid, V. Probiotic yogurt improves antioxidant status in type 2 diabetic patients. *Nutrition* **2012**, *28*, 539–543. [CrossRef] [PubMed]
44. Mohamadshahi, M.; Veissi, M.; Haidari, F.; Javid, A.Z.; Mohammadi, F.; Shirbeigi, E. Effects of probiotic yogurt consumption on lipid profile in type 2 diabetic patients: A randomized controlled clinical trial. *J. Res. Med. Sci.* **2014**, *19*, 531–536. [PubMed]
45. Ejtahed, H.S.; Mohtadi-Nia, J.; Homayouni-Rad, A.; Niafar, M.; Asghari-Jafarabadi, M.; Mofid, V.; Akbarian-Moghari, A. Effect of probiotic yogurt containing lactobacillus acidophilus and bifidobacterium lactis on lipid profile in individuals with type 2 diabetes mellitus. *J. Dairy Sci.* **2011**, *94*, 3288–3294. [CrossRef] [PubMed]
46. Nabavi, S.; Rafraf, M.; Somi, M.H.; Homayouni-Rad, A.; Asghari-Jafarabadi, M. Effects of probiotic yogurt consumption on metabolic factors in individuals with nonalcoholic fatty liver disease. *J. Dairy Sci.* **2014**, *97*, 7386–7393. [CrossRef] [PubMed]
47. Tonucci, L.B.; Olbrich Dos Santos, K.M.; Licursi de Oliveira, L.; Rocha Ribeiro, S.M.; Duarte Martino, H.S. Clinical application of probiotics in type 2 diabetes mellitus: A randomized, double-blind, placebo-controlled study. *Clin. Nutr.* **2017**, *36*, 85–92. [CrossRef] [PubMed]
48. Merenstein, D.J.; Smith, K.H.; Scriven, M.; Roberts, R.F.; Sanders, M.E.; Petterson, S. The study to investigate the potential benefits of probiotics in yogurt, a patient-oriented, double-blind, cluster-randomised, placebo-controlled, clinical trial. *Eur. J. Clin. Nutr.* **2010**, *64*, 685–691. [CrossRef] [PubMed]
49. Giralt, J.; Regadera, J.P.; Verges, R.; Romero, J.; de la Fuente, I.; Biete, A.; Villoria, J.; Cobo, J.M.; Guarner, F. Effects of probiotic lactobacillus casei DN-114-001 in prevention of radiation-induced diarrhea: Results from multicenter, randomized, placebo-controlled nutritional trial. *Int. J. Radiat. Oncol. Biol. Phys.* **2008**, *71*, 1213–1219. [CrossRef] [PubMed]
50. Chapman, C.M.; Gibson, G.R.; Rowland, I. Health benefits of probiotics: Are mixtures more effective than single strains? *Eur. J. Nutr.* **2011**, *50*, 1–17. [CrossRef] [PubMed]
51. Juntunen, M.; Kirjavainen, P.V.; Ouwehand, A.C.; Salminen, S.J.; Isolauri, E. Adherence of probiotic bacteria to human intestinal mucus in healthy infants and during rotavirus infection. *Clin. Diagn. Lab. Immunol.* **2001**, *8*, 293–296. [CrossRef] [PubMed]
52. Timmerman, H.M.; Koning, C.J.; Mulder, L.; Rombouts, F.M.; Beynen, A.C. Monostrain, multistrain and multispecies probiotics—A comparison of functionality and efficacy. *Int. J. Food Microbiol.* **2004**, *96*, 219–233. [CrossRef] [PubMed]
53. Zoppi, G.; Cinquetti, M.; Benini, A.; Bonamini, E.; Minelli, E.B. Modulation of the intestinal ecosystem by probiotics and lactulose in children during treatment with ceftriaxone. *Curr. Ther. Res.* **2001**, *62*, 418–435. [CrossRef]
54. Perdigon, G.; Nader de Macias, M.E.; Alvarez, S.; Oliver, G.; Pesce de Ruiz Holgado, A.A. Prevention of gastrointestinal infection using immunobiological methods with milk fermented with lactobacillus casei and lactobacillus acidophilus. *J. Dairy Res.* **1990**, *57*, 255–264. [CrossRef] [PubMed]
55. Sanders, M.E. Summary of conclusions from a consensus panel of experts on health attributes of lactic cultures: Significance to fluid milk products containing cultures. *J. Dairy Sci.* **1993**, *76*, 1819–1828. [CrossRef]
56. Ouwehand, A.C.; Isolauri, E.; Kirjavainen, P.V.; Tolkko, S.; Salminen, S.J. The mucus binding of bifidobacterium lactis bb12 is enhanced in the presence of lactobacillus gg and lact. Delbrueckii subsp. Bulgaricus. *Lett. Appl. Microbiol.* **2000**, *30*, 10–13. [CrossRef] [PubMed]
57. Klaenhammer, T.R.; Kullen, M.J. Selection and design of probiotics. *Int. J. Food Microbiol.* **1999**, *50*, 45–57. [CrossRef]
58. Lesser, L.I.; Ebbeling, C.B.; Goozner, M.; Wypij, D.; Ludwig, D.S. Relationship between funding source and conclusion among nutrition-related scientific articles. *PLoS Med.* **2007**, *4*, e5. [CrossRef] [PubMed]
59. Pedone, C.A.; Arnaud, C.C.; Postaire, E.R.; Bouley, C.F.; Reinert, P. Multicentric study of the effect of milk fermented by lactobacillus casei on the incidence of diarrhoea. *Int. J. Clin. Pract.* **2000**, *54*, 568–571. [PubMed]

Permissions

All chapters in this book were first published by MDPI; hereby published with permission under the Creative Commons Attribution License or equivalent. Every chapter published in this book has been scrutinized by our experts. Their significance has been extensively debated. The topics covered herein carry significant findings which will fuel the growth of the discipline. They may even be implemented as practical applications or may be referred to as a beginning point for another development.

The contributors of this book come from diverse backgrounds, making this book a truly international effort. This book will bring forth new frontiers with its revolutionizing research information and detailed analysis of the nascent developments around the world.

We would like to thank all the contributing authors for lending their expertise to make the book truly unique. They have played a crucial role in the development of this book. Without their invaluable contributions this book wouldn't have been possible. They have made vital efforts to compile up to date information on the varied aspects of this subject to make this book a valuable addition to the collection of many professionals and students.

This book was conceptualized with the vision of imparting up-to-date information and advanced data in this field. To ensure the same, a matchless editorial board was set up. Every individual on the board went through rigorous rounds of assessment to prove their worth. After which they invested a large part of their time researching and compiling the most relevant data for our readers.

The editorial board has been involved in producing this book since its inception. They have spent rigorous hours researching and exploring the diverse topics which have resulted in the successful publishing of this book. They have passed on their knowledge of decades through this book. To expedite this challenging task, the publisher supported the team at every step. A small team of assistant editors was also appointed to further simplify the editing procedure and attain best results for the readers.

Apart from the editorial board, the designing team has also invested a significant amount of their time in understanding the subject and creating the most relevant covers. They scrutinized every image to scout for the most suitable representation of the subject and create an appropriate cover for the book.

The publishing team has been an ardent support to the editorial, designing and production team. Their endless efforts to recruit the best for this project, has resulted in the accomplishment of this book. They are a veteran in the field of academics and their pool of knowledge is as vast as their experience in printing. Their expertise and guidance has proved useful at every step. Their uncompromising quality standards have made this book an exceptional effort. Their encouragement from time to time has been an inspiration for everyone.

The publisher and the editorial board hope that this book will prove to be a valuable piece of knowledge for researchers, students, practitioners and scholars across the globe.

List of Contributors

Jacek Piatek, Hanna Krauss, Paulina Wojtyla-Buciora and Henning Sommermeyer
Department of Medicine, The President Stanisław Wojciechowski State University of Applied Sciences in Kalisz, Nowy Świat 4, 62-800 Kalisz, Poland

Arleta Ciechelska-Rybarczyk
District Sanitary-Epidemiological Station in Jarocin, Waska 2, 63-200 Jarocin, Poland

Malgorzata Bernatek
State Hospital Jarocin, Szpitalna 1, 63-200 Jarocin, Poland

Miranda Green and Satya Prakash
Biomedical Technology and Cell Therapy Research Laboratory, Department of Biomedical Engineering, Faculty of Medicine, McGill University, 3775 University Street, Montreal, QC H3A 2B4, Canada

Karan Arora
Biomedical Technology and Cell Therapy Research Laboratory, Department of Biomedical Engineering, Faculty of Medicine, McGill University, 3775 University Street, Montreal, QC H3A 2B4, Canada
Department of Bioengineering, Faculty of Engineering, McGill University, 3775 University Street, Montreal, QC H3A 2B4, Canada
Biena Inc., 2955 Rue Cartier, Saint-Hyacinthe, QC J2S 1L4, Canada

Beata Olas
Department of General Biochemistry, Faculty of Biology and Environmental Protection, University of Lodz, Pomorska 141/3, 90-236 Lodz, Poland

Girish Deshpande
Department of Neonatology, Nepean Hospital, Kingswood, NSW 2747, Australia
Sydney Medical School Nepean, University of Sydney, Kingswood, NSW 2747, Australia

Gayatri Athalye-Jape and Sanjay Patole
Department of Neonatology, King Edward Memorial Hospital for Women, Perth, WA 6008, Australia

Pamela Vernocchi, Federica Del Chierico and Andrea Quagliariello
Unit of Human Microbiome, Bambino Gesù Children's Hospital, IRCCS, Viale San Paolo 15, 00146 Rome, Italy

Danilo Ercolini
Department of Agricultural Sciences, Division of Microbiology, University of Naples Federico II, Via Università 100, Portici, 80055 Napoli, Italy

Vincenzina Lucidi
Cystic Fibrosis Unit, Bambino Gesù Children's Hospital, IRCCS, Piazza Sant' Onofrio 4, Rome 00165, Italy

Lorenza Putignani
Unit of Human Microbiome, Bambino Gesù Children's Hospital, IRCCS, Viale San Paolo 15, 00146 Rome, Italy
Unit of Parasitology Bambino Gesù Children's Hospital, IRCCS, Piazza Sant' Onofrio 4, Rome 00165, Italy

Valentina Leccioli, Mara Oliveri and Paola Rossi
Department of Biology and Biotechnology "L. Spallanzani", University of Pavia, via Ferrata 1, 27100 Pavia, Italy

Marcello Romeo
C.E.R.H.M. Center for Experimental Research for Human Microbiome Ludes H.E.I., Pietro Stiges Palace, Strait Street, 1436 Valletta, Malta

Massimiliano Berretta
Department of Medical Oncology, CRO-Aviano, National Cancer Institute, Via Franco Gallini 2, 33081 Aviano, Italy

Bonnie L. Taylor, Georgia E. Woodfall, Katherine E. Sheedy, Meggan L. O'Riley, Kelsie A. Rainbow, Elsa L. Bramwell and Nicole J. Kellow
Be Active Sleep & Eat (BASE) Facility, Department of Nutrition, Dietetics & Food, Monash University, Notting Hill, VIC 3168, Australia

Hideaki Shima, Shizuka Masuda, Mizuho Kajikawa and Taisei Kanamoto
The Laboratory of Microbiology, Showa Pharmaceutical University, Machida, Tokyo 194-8543, Japan

Amiu Shino and Yuuri Tsuboi
RIKEN Center for Sustainable Resource Science, 1-7-22 Suehiro-cho, Tsurumi-ku, Yokohama, Kanagawa 230-0045, Japan

Ivano Mezzaroma
Department of Clinical Medicine, University of Rome "Sapienza", 00185 Rome, Italy

Yasuhiro Date
RIKEN Center for Sustainable Resource Science, 1-7-22 Suehiro-cho, Tsurumi-ku, Yokohama, Kanagawa 230-0045, Japan
Graduate School of Medical Life Science, Yokohama City University, 1-7-29 Suehiro-cho, Tsurumi-ku, Yokohama, Kanagawa 230-0045, Japan

Yoshihiro Inoue
Laboratory of Pharmaceutical Sciences and Education, Showa Pharmaceutical University, Machida, Tokyo 194-8543, Japan

Jun Kikuchi
RIKEN Center for Sustainable Resource Science, 1-7-22 Suehiro-cho, Tsurumi-ku, Yokohama, Kanagawa 230-0045, Japan
Graduate School of Medical Life Science, Yokohama City University, 1-7-29 Suehiro-cho, Tsurumi-ku, Yokohama, Kanagawa 230-0045, Japan
Graduate School of Bioagricultural Sciences, Nagoya University, 1 Furo-cho, Chikusa-ku, Nagoya, Aichi 464-0810, Japan

Giancarlo Ceccarelli, Eugenio Nelson Cavallari, Giuseppe Corano Scheri, Claudia Pinacchio, Ivan Schietroma, Saeid Najafi Fard, Vincenzo Vullo and Gabriella d'Ettorre
Department of Public Health and Infectious Diseases, University of Rome "Sapienza", Rome (Italy) and Azienda Policlinico Umberto I, 00161 Rome, Italy

Jason M. Brenchley
Laboratory of Parasitic Diseases, National Institute of Allergy and Infectious Diseases, NIH, Bethesda, MD 20892, USA

Mariangela Fratino
Department of Neurology, University of Rome "Sapienza", 00185 Rome, Italy

Carolina Scagnolari
Department of Molecular Medicine, Laboratory of Virology, University of Rome "Sapienza", 00185 Rome, Italy

Bin Kwon
Research Center, BIFIDO Co. Ltd., Hongcheon 250-804, Korea

Tomás Cerdó
Department of Paediatrics, School of Medicine, University of Granada, 18016 Granada, Spain
EURISTIKOS Excellence Centre for Paediatric Research, Biomedical Research Centre, University of Granada, 18016 Granada, Spain

Alicia Ruíz
EURISTIKOS Excellence Centre for Paediatric Research, Biomedical Research Centre, University of Granada, 18016 Granada, Spain
Department of Biochemistry and Molecular Biology 2, Biomedical Research Centre, University of Granada, 18016 Granada, Spain

Antonio Suárez
Department of Biochemistry and Molecular Biology 2, Biomedical Research Centre, University of Granada, 18016 Granada, Spain

Cristina Campoy
Department of Paediatrics, School of Medicine, University of Granada, 18016 Granada, Spain
EURISTIKOS Excellence Centre for Paediatric Research, Biomedical Research Centre, University of Granada, 18016 Granada, Spain
Spanish Network of Biomedical Research in Epidemiology and Public Health (CIBERESP), Carlos III Institute, 18016 Granada, Spain
Department of Paediatrics, Faculty of Medicine, University of Granada, Av. de la Investigación, 11, 18016 Granada, Spain

Flavia Indrio, Maria Ficarella and Ruggiero Francavilla
Department of Pediatric, Aldo Moro University of Bari, Ospedale Pediatrico Giovanni XXIII via Amendola 276, 70125 Bari, Italy

Giuseppe Riezzo
Laboratory of Nutritional Physiopathology, National Institute for Digestive Diseases, Istituto di Ricerca e Cura a Carattere Scientifico (I.R.C.C.S.), Saverio de Bellis, 70013 Castellana Grotte (BA), Italy

Silvio Tafuri
Department of Biomedical Sciences and Human Oncology, Section of Hygiene, Aldo Moro University of Bari, 70125 Bari, Italy

Barbara Carlucci
Division of Neonatology, Ospedale Perrino, 72100 Brindisi, Italy

Massimo Bisceglia
Department of Pediatrics, Neonatology Division San Giovanni di Dio Hospital, 88900 Crotone, Italy

Lorenzo Polimeno
Department of Organ Transplantation, Gastroenterology Section, University Aldo Moro Bari, 70125 Bari, Italy

Alicia Huazano-García and Mercedes G. López
Departamento de Biotecnología y Bioquímica, Centro de Investigación y de Estudios Avanzados del IPN, Unidad Irapuato 36821, México

Hakdong Shin
Faculty of Food Science and Biotechnology, College of Life Science, Sejong University, Seoul 05006, Korea

Myeong Soo Park
Department of Hotel Culinary Arts, Yeonsung University, Anyang 430-749, Korea

Seockmo Ku
Fermentation Science Program, School of Agribusiness and Agriscience, College of Basic and Applied Sciences, Middle Tennessee State University, Murfreesboro, TN 37132, USA

Geun Eog Ji
Research Center, BIFIDO Co. Ltd., Hongcheon 250-804, Korea
Department of Food and Nutrition, Research Institute of Human Ecology, Seoul National University, Seoul 151-742, Korea

Eva Maier and Rachel C. Anderson
Food Nutrition & Health Team, Food & Bio-Based Products Group, AgResearch Grasslands, Palmerston North 4442, New Zealand
Riddet Institute, Massey University, Palmerston North 4442, New Zealand

Nicole C. Roy
Food Nutrition & Health Team, Food & Bio-Based Products Group, AgResearch Grasslands, Palmerston North 4442, New Zealand
Riddet Institute, Massey University, Palmerston North 4442, New Zealand
High-Value Nutrition National Science Challenge, Auckland 1142, New Zealand

Bailiang Li, Da Jin, Shangfu Yu, Zafarullah Muhammad and Fei Liu
Key Laboratory of Dairy Science, Ministry of Education, Northeast Agricultural University, Harbin 150030, China

Smith Etareri Evivie
Key Laboratory of Dairy Science, Ministry of Education, Northeast Agricultural University, Harbin 150030, China
Food Science and Nutrition Unit, Department of Animal Science, Faculty of Agriculture, University of Benin, PMB 1154 Benin City, Nigeria

Guicheng Huo
Key Laboratory of Dairy Science, Ministry of Education, Northeast Agricultural University, Harbin 150030, China
Food College, Northeast Agricultural University, Harbin 150030, China

Elena M. Comelli and Mary R. L'Abbé
Department of Nutritional Sciences, Faculty of Medicine, University of Toronto, Toronto, ON M1E 3S1, Canada
Center for Child Nutrition and Health, Faculty of Medicine, University of Toronto, Toronto, ON M1E 3S1, Canada

Mary J. Scourboutakos, Beatriz Franco-Arellano, Sarah A. Murphy and Sheida Norsen
Department of Nutritional Sciences, Faculty of Medicine, University of Toronto, Toronto, ON M1E 3S1, Canada

Index

N

O

P

R

S

T

U

www.ingramcontent.com/pod-product-compliance
Lightning Source LLC
LaVergne TN
LVHW060549210926
848485LV00005B/1287